Go online to watch in-depth technique videos at MediaCenter.Thieme.com!

Simply visit MediaCenter.Thieme.com and, when prompted during the registration process, enter the code below to get started today.

TY74-CD65-2D95-M92T

	WINDOWS & MAC	TABLET
Recommended Browser(s)	Recent browser versions on all major platforms and any mobile operating system that supports HTML5 video playback. *All browsers should have JavaScript enabled.*	
Flash Player Plug-in	Flash Player 9 or higher. *For Mac users, ATI Rage 128 GPU doesn't support full-screen mode with hardware scaling.*	Tablet PCs with Android OS support Flash 10.1.
Recommended for optimal usage experience	Monitor resolutions: • Normal (4:3) 1024×768 or higher • Widescreen (16:9) 1280×720 or higher • Widescreen (16:10) 1440×900 or higher A high-speed internet connection (minimum 384 Kps) is suggested.	WiFi or cellular data connection is required.

Connect with us on social media

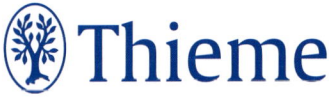

The Art of Combining Surgical and Nonsurgical Techniques in Aesthetic Medicine

Julius W. Few Jr., MD
Director
The Few Institute for Aesthetic Plastic Surgery
Clinical Professor
Department of Surgery
Division of Plastic Surgery
University of Chicago Pritzker School of Medicine
Health Science Clinician
Division of Plastic Surgery
Northwestern University Feinberg School of Medicine
Chicago, Illinois

205 illustrations

Thieme
New York • Stuttgart • Delhi • Rio de Janeiro

Managing Editor: Haley Paskalides
Director, Editorial Services: Mary Jo Casey
Developmental Editor: Kathleen Sartori
Production Editor: Naamah Schwartz
International Production Director: Andreas Schabert
Editorial Director: Sue Hodgson
International Marketing Director: Fiona Henderson
International Sales Director: Louisa Turrell
Director of Institutional Sales: Adam Bernacki
Senior Vice President and Chief Operating Officer: Sarah Vanderbilt
President: Brian D. Scanlan

Library of Congress Cataloging-in-Publication Data

Names: Few, Julius, author.
Title: The art of blending surgical and nonsurgical techniques in aesthetic medicine / Julius Few, MD.
Description: New York : Thieme, [2017] | Includes bibliographical references and index.
Identifiers: LCCN 2017054011 (print) | LCCN 2017055891 (ebook) | ISBN 9781626237698 (ebook) | ISBN 9781626236820 (print : alk. paper) | ISBN 9781626237698 (ebook : alk. paper)
Subjects: LCSH: Surgery, Plastic–Methodology.
Classification: LCC RD119 (ebook) | LCC RD119 .F49 2017 (print) | DDC 617.9/5–dc23
LC record available at https://lccn.loc.gov/2017054011

© 2018 Thieme Medical Publishers, Inc.
Thieme Publishers New York
333 Seventh Avenue, New York, NY 10001 USA
+1 800 782 3488, customerservice@thieme.com

Thieme Publishers Stuttgart
Rüdigerstrasse 14, 70469 Stuttgart, Germany
+49 [0]711 8931 421, customerservice@thieme.de

Thieme Publishers Delhi
A-12, Second Floor, Sector-2, Noida-201301
Uttar Pradesh, India
+91 120 45 566 00, customerservice@thieme.in

Thieme Publishers Rio de Janeiro
Thieme Publicações Ltda.
Edifício Rodolpho de Paoli, 25º andar
Av. Nilo Peçanha, 50 – Sala 2508
Rio de Janeiro 20020-906 Brasil
+55 21 3172-2297 / +55 21 3172-1896

Cover design: Thieme Publishing Group
Typesetting by Thomson Digital, India

Printed in India by Replika Press Pvt Ltd   5 4 3 2 1

ISBN 978-1-62623-682-0

Also available as an e-book:
eISBN 978-1-62623-769-8

Important note: Medicine is an ever-changing science undergoing continual development. Research and clinical experience are continually expanding our knowledge, in particular our knowledge of proper treatment and drug therapy. Insofar as this book mentions any dosage or application, readers may rest assured that the authors, editors, and publishers have made every effort to ensure that such references are in accordance with **the state of knowledge at the time of production of the book.**

Nevertheless, this does not involve, imply, or express any guarantee or responsibility on the part of the publishers in respect to any dosage instructions and forms of applications stated in the book. **Every user is requested to examine carefully** the manufacturers' leaflets accompanying each drug and to check, if necessary in consultation with a physician or specialist, whether the dosage schedules mentioned therein or the contraindications stated by the manufacturers differ from the statements made in the present book. Such examination is particularly important with drugs that are either rarely used or have been newly released on the market. Every dosage schedule or every form of application used is entirely at the user's own risk and responsibility. The authors and publishers request every user to report to the publishers any discrepancies or inaccuracies noticed. If errors in this work are found after publication, errata will be posted at www.thieme.com on the product description page.

Some of the product names, patents, and registered designs referred to in this book are in fact registered trademarks or proprietary names even though specific reference to this fact is not always made in the text. Therefore, the appearance of a name without designation as proprietary is not to be construed as a representation by the publisher that it is in the public domain.

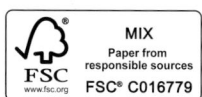

This book, including all parts thereof, is legally protected by copyright. Any use, exploitation, or commercialization outside the narrow limits set by copyright legislation, without the publisher's consent, is illegal and liable to prosecution. This applies in particular to photostat reproduction, copying, mimeographing, preparation of microfilms, and electronic data processing and storage.

I would like to dedicate this book to my family—Miles, Maxwell, Julius Sr., Gladys, Mark, and Kris; Team TFI—Shay, Charisse, Elizabeth, and Carly; my past and present fellows—LaNesha, Denis, Sheri, Diane, Diana, Marie K.; Megan (my first employee); and all the patients who believed in our vision.

4-23-18.

To ~~my~~ parents —
T~~hank~~ you for all you are & have been!

Love always,
J.

Contents

    Video Contents ix

    Preface xi

    Acknowledgments xiii

    Contributors xv

1   **Concepts of Beauty** 1
      Julius W. Few Jr. and Michael P. Ogilvie

2   **Nonsurgical Cervicofacial Rejuvenation of a Traditional Surgical Candidate** 6
      Sahar Nadimi and Corey S. Maas

      Commentary by *Julius W. Few Jr.* 26

3   **Background of Noninvasive Technology: Evolving Patient Selection** 30
      Julius W. Few Jr.

4   **Blending and Sequencing Considerations** 36
      Daniel R. Butz and Julius W. Few Jr.

5   **Diverse Skin Type Considerations and Applications for Nonsurgical Combinations** 42
      Valerie D. Callender, Moneé Thomas, and Susan C. Taylor

      Commentary by *Julius W. Few Jr.* 52

6   **Noninvasive Devices Used in Combination with Volumizing** 60
      Rachel N. Pritzker, Shraddha Desai, and Brian S. Biesman

      Commentary by *Julius W. Few Jr.* 67

7   **Microneedling and Platelet-Rich Plasma** 69
      Johnson C. Lee and Z. Paul Lorenc

      Commentary by *Julius W. Few Jr. and Alec Semersky* 72

8   **Use of Light- and Energy-Based Therapies with Cosmetic Surgery** 74
      Michael I. Kulick and Natasha Kulick

      Commentary by *Julius W. Few Jr.* 93

9   **Blending Nonsurgical Treatments with Surgery for Facial Rejuvenation** 95
      Lawrence S. Bass, Jason N. Pozner, and Barry E. DiBernardo

      Commentary by *Julius W. Few Jr.* 102

10 **Blending Nonsurgical Treatments with Surgery for Skin Lifting on the Body** 104
      Lawrence S. Bass, Barry E. DiBernardo, and Jason N. Pozner

      Commentary by *Julius W. Few Jr.* 109

Contents

11 **Nonsurgical Salvage and Enhancement of a Surgical Result** 111
David A. Sieber, John E. Hoopman, and Jeffrey M. Kenkel

Commentary by *Julius W. Few Jr.* 124

12 **Integrating Technology in Facial Plastic Surgery** 126
Jonathan M. Sykes and Amir Allak

Commentary by *Julius W. Few Jr.* 130

13 **Cryolipolysis** 132
W. Grant Stevens, Michelle Manning Eagan, Cory Felber, Deniz Sarhaddi, and Marc Vincent Orlando

Commentary by *Julius W. Few Jr.* 148

14 **Minimally Invasive Techniques: Preventing and Managing Adverse Events** 150
Mark S. Nestor, Paige Paparone, and Mitchell Manway

Commentary by *Julius W. Few Jr.* 157

15 **Future Considerations** 159
Michael P. Ogilvie and Julius W. Few Jr.

16 **Product Index: Fillers** 167

17 **Product Index: Lasers** 176

Index 199

Video Contents

1.1 Where are We? My Perspective on Facial Rejuvenation with Soft Tissue Fillers and Neuromodulators
     Julius W. Few Jr.

2.1 Aesthetic Evaluation and Facial Treatment Midface (Restylane Lyft, Restylane Silk)
     Julius W. Few Jr.

2.2 Aesthetic Evaluation and Facial Rejuvenation Midface (Voluma)
     Julius W. Few Jr.

2.3 Aesthetic Evaluation and Facial Rejuvenation Lower Face (Voluma)
     Julius W. Few Jr.

2.4 Choosing a Botulinumtoxin A Product
     Julius W. Few Jr.

2.5 Aesthetic Evaluation and Injections of Botulinumtoxin A in The Face and Neck (Botox Cosmetic)
     Julius W. Few Jr.

2.6 Demonstration of Silhouette InstaLift in the Midface: Evaluation
     Julius W. Few Jr.

2.7 Demonstration of Silhouette InstaLift in the Midface: Placing the Sutures
     Julius W. Few Jr.

2.8 Demonstration of Silhouette InstaLift in the Midface: Setting the Sutures
     Julius W. Few Jr.

2.9 Demonstration of Silhouette InstaLift in the Lower Face and Neck, Part 1
     Julius W. Few Jr.

2.10 Demonstration of Silhouette InstaLift in the Lower Face and Neck, Part 2
     Julius W. Few Jr.

2.11 Corset Platysmaplasty With Facial Ulthera
     Julius W. Few Jr.

2.12 Nonsurgical Division of Platysma Bands
     Julius W. Few Jr.

2.13 Halo 1080 Fractional Laser Animation (*Courtesy Sciton, Inc.*)

2.14 Halo Fractional Laser (*Courtesy Sciton, Inc.*)

4.1 Submental Skin Flap Elevation (In preparation for corset submental platysmaplasty prior to full face and neck Ulthera in the same clinical setting)
     Julius W. Few Jr.

4.2 Submental Corset Platysmaplasty
     Julius W. Few Jr.

Video Contents

4.3 Nonsurgical Chin Augmention with Juvederm Voluma (*Courtesy Allergan, Inc.*)

5.1 African American Rhinoplasty
Julius W. Few Jr.

11.1 Nonsurgical Salvage
Julius W. Few Jr.

15.1 Morph showing the average of 116 female faces from 20 to 30 years of age animated with 100 female faces from 68 years of age and up (average age: 76).
Val Lambros

I.1 Cellfina: Clinical Demonstration (*Cellfina is a registered trademark of Ulthera, Inc.*)

Preface

The quote "We all stand on the shoulder of giants" was first told to me by some of my early surgical idols, Bob Bartlett, Norm Thompson, and Lazar Greenfield, more than 2 decades ago while I was completing general surgery training at the University of Michigan. Although this was taken from the famous quote by Sir Isaac Newton in 1676, it hit me as one of the most profound statements and left a desire to make a difference in the world of medicine that still burns today.

A desire to make a difference in the world of medicine and to give back to a specialty that has been so good to me has come very naturally as a result of very early impressions on me. This book discusses the idea of combining nonsurgical techniques in a surgical way—much like a text would describe the techniques for a patient having a facelift. The surgeon outlines the combination of blepharoplasty, fat grafting, laser resurfacing, and of course SMAS repositioning with skin removal. So why would there be initial resistance to the concept? There have been so many innovations in the world of cosmetic medicine, and not all of them have delivered as promised, leaving many surgeons skeptical and believing that only surgery can deliver for the cosmetic patient. Much of the skepticism is valid if one looks at single modalities in a less-than-ideal candidate, but I challenge the reader to consider this no different than thinking a facelift alone will address the older face with end-stage sun damage. Another issue has been the overuse of a single nonsurgical modality to achieve a "good correction," which, in many cases, only creates unnatural results.

What do you do for the patient who wants more results but absolutely refuses surgery? This question brings about the birth of "The Stackable Treatment," an attempt to address the nonsurgical patient by using surgical reasoning to formulate a treatment strategy. *The Art of Combining Surgical and Nonsurgical Techniques in Aesthetic Medicine* is for all aesthetic specialists, novice and expert alike, wanting to deliver more for their patients in a thoughtful, scientifically supported manner.

This book presents the techniques and is the result of the work of some of the brightest minds in the world of cosmetic plastic surgery, dermatology, and oculofacial and facial plastic surgery. These are authors who are not afraid to look at disruptors in their world of expertise and cosmetic medicine. My colleagues who have contributed to this book are true visionaries who have looked at a very challenging, dynamic subject and developed approaches that will revolutionize the field—I am forever grateful!

The Art of Combining Surgical and Nonsurgical Techniques in Aesthetic Medicine presents practical, real-life case studies, and is supported by science and practical strategy. There are more than 200 vivid photos and colorful illustrations, technical video, and a comprehensive product index with full-color product images and case studies.

Although there are many books that look at cosmetic medicine, this is the first book to look specifically at techniques and to strategically combine them with or without surgery. We hope our readers find it beneficial.

Julius W. Few Jr., MD

Acknowledgments

As I continue to be a part of educating future plastic surgeons, I realize how much these amazing men and women are educating me. Their inquisitive nature and spirit is infectious. And while this textbook is cosmetic in nature, I must pay respect to my reconstructive and restorative roots.

First, "do no harm" and the pursuit of a clinical solution originate in the art of reconstruction and restorative medicine. I have been blessed to be surrounded by truly incredible minds, starting with the faculty and staff at the University of Chicago Department of Surgery, led by the late George Block, and then at the University of Michigan under the leadership of Lazar Greenfield. The past and current faculty of Northwestern University and the University of Chicago plastic surgery divisions continue to be a source of pride for me as a faculty member today.

I appreciate Thomas Mustoe for giving me my first job, as both Plastic Surgery Resident and then Assistant Professor. Laurie Casas, Neil Fine, and Gregory Dumanian were major sources of inspiration and guidance during the early years of my career in plastic surgery—Thank You.

David Song, one of the most powerful minds in our specialty, brought me back to the University of Chicago and supported me during very challenging times, for which I will always be grateful; I could not ask for a better friend or colleague. I thank Dan Baker and Sherrell Aston for allowing me to see their magic at work.

Shay Moinuddin, my senior aesthetic nurse and clinical manager in Chicago, has been a respected voice of reason for my clinical pursuits, and I am most appreciative for her valuable contribution to the practices' innovation. Thank you, Carly Bruno, for helping to secure valuable material for this text.

I am forever grateful to Robert Flowers, Glenn and Elizabeth Jelks, Clinton McCord, Mark Codner, and Foad Nahai, who showed me the true art of ophthalmic plastic surgery. They are like family to me now.

Finally, I must acknowledge some of my dearest friends and confidants who have been there for me: Morris Velilla, DDS; Sanjay Gupta, MD; Thomas Sarakatsannis, JD; Jeff Marcus, MD; Michael Lee, MD; Al Lin, DDS; Matt Murphy; David Greenwald, JD; James Chandler, MD; Robert Gramins, DDS; James Platis, Lainchen Friese, and Sean O'Connor, the senior authors of this textbook, and Emilio Salvi. Thank you, Genevieve Bulev, for being the best administrative assistant that anyone could hope to have. This book would have not come together without your support.

Contributors

Amir Allak, MD, MBA
Fellow Surgeon
Facial Plastic and Reconstructive Surgery
University of California Davis Medical Center
Sacramento, California

Lawrence S. Bass, MD, FACS
Clinical Assistant Professor of Plastic Surgery
Hofstra Northwell School of Medicine
Department of Plastic Surgery
Lenox Hill/Manhattan Eye, Ear and Throat Hospital
New York, New York

Brian S. Biesman, MD, FACS
Assistant Clinical Professor of Ophthalmology,
  Dermatology, Otolaryngology
Vanderbilt University Medical Center
Past President
American Society for Laser Medicine and Surgery
Nashville, Tennessee

Daniel R. Butz, MD
Plastic and Reconstructive Surgeon
Private Practice
Milwaukee, Wisconsin

Valerie D. Callender, MD
Professor of Dermatology
Howard University College of Medicine
Washington, DC
Medical Director
Callender Dermatology and Cosmetic Center
Glenn Dale, Maryland

Shraddha Desai, MD
Physician
Private Practice
The Dermatology Institute
Naperville, Illinois

Barry E. DiBernardo, MD, FACS
Director
New Jersey Plastic Surgery
Montclair, New Jersey USA
Clinical Associate Professor
Division of Plastic Surgery
Rutgers New Jersey Medical School
Newark, New Jersey

Cory Felber, PA-C
Clinical Research Coordinator
Marina Plastic Surgery Associates
Marina del Rey, California

Julius W. Few Jr., MD
Director
The Few Institute for Aesthetic Plastic Surgery
Clinical Professor
Department of Surgery
Division of Plastic Surgery
University of Chicago Pritzker School of Medicine
Health Science Clinician
Division of Plastic Surgery
Northwestern University Feinberg School of Medicine
Chicago, Illinois

John E. Hoopman, CLMSO
Laser Safety Officer
University of Texas Southwestern Medical Center
Dallas, Texas

Jeffrey M. Kenkel, MD
Professor and Chairman
Department of Plastic Surgery
University of Texas Southwestern Medical Center
Dallas, Texas

Michael I. Kulick, MD
Director
Bay Area Plastic Surgery Medical Center
San Francisco, California

Natasha Kulick, EMT
Student
Department of Neuroscience
Research Assistant
Center for Catalysis and Surface Science
President
Northwestern Emergency Medicine Organization
Northwestern University
Evanston, Illinois

Val Lambros, MD, FACS
Plastic Surgeon
Private Practice
Cosmetic and Reconstructive Surgery
Corona Del Mar, California

Johnson C. Lee, MD
Private Practice
Johnson C. Lee, MD Plastic Surgery
Beverly Hills, California

Contributors

Z. Paul Lorenc, MD, FACS
Director
Lorenc Aesthetic Plastic Surgery Center
New York, New York

Corey S. Maas, MD, FACS
Associate Clinical Professor
Facial Plastic and Reconstructive Surgery
University of California, San Francisco
Aesthetic and Facial Plastic Surgery
The Maas Clinic
San Francisco, California

Michelle Manning Eagan, MD
Aesthetic Plastic Surgery Fellowship
University of Southern California
Los Angeles, California

Mitchell Manway, DO
Fellow
Center for Cosmetic Enhancement
Center for Clinical and Cosmetic Research
Aventura, Florida

Sahar Nadimi, MD
Assistant Clinical Professor
Facial Plastic and Reconstructive Surgery
Loyola University Medical Center
Aesthetic and Facial Plastic Surgery
Oakbrook Aesthetic, PC
Oakbrook Terrace, Illinois

Mark S. Nestor, MD, PhD
Center for Cosmetic Enhancement
Center for Clinical and Cosmetic Research
Aventura, Florida USA
Department of Dermatology and Cutaneous Surgery
Department of Surgery
Division of Plastic and Reconstructive Surgery
University of Miami Miller School of Medicine
Miami, Florida

Michael P. Ogilvie, MD, MBA
Aesthetic Surgery Fellow
The Few Institute for Aesthetic Plastic Surgery
Chicago, Illinois

Marc Vincent Orlando, MD
Marina Plastic Surgery Associates
Marina del Rey, California

Paige Paparone, DO, MSBS
Center for Cosmetic Enhancement
Center for Clinical and Cosmetic Research
Aventura, Florida

Jason N. Pozner, MD, FACS
Director
Sanctuary Plastic Surgery
Boca Raton, Florida
Adjunct Clinical Faculty
Department of Plastic Surgery
Cleveland Clinic Florida
Weston, Florida

Rachel N. Pritzker, MD
Dermatologist
Chicago Cosmetic Surgery and Dermatology
Chicago, Illinois

Deniz Sarhaddi, MD
Resident Physician
Department of Plastic and Reconstructive Surgery
Saint Louis University Hospital
Saint Louis, Missouri

Alec Semersky
Undergraduate Student
University of North Carolina at Chapel Hill
Chapel Hill, North Carolina

David A. Sieber, MD
Plastic Surgeon
Sieber Plastic Surgery
San Francisco, California

W. Grant Stevens, MD, FACS
Clinical Professor of Surgery
University of Southern California
Keck School of Medicine
Division of Plastic Surgery
Director USC Aesthetic Surgery Fellowship
Chairman, Marina Plastic Surgery
Marina del Rey, California

Jonathan M. Sykes, MD
Professor
University of California Davis Medical Center
Sacramento, California

Susan C. Taylor, MD
Associate Professor of Medicine
Department of Dermatology
Perelman School of Medicine
University of Pennsylvania
Philadelphia, Pennsylvania

Moneé Thomas, MD
Dermatology Resident
Howard University Hospital
Washington, DC

1 Concepts of Beauty

Julius W. Few Jr. and Michael P. Ogilvie

Summary

This chapter provides the understanding that beauty is the central concept behind aesthetic surgery, but that beauty is very difficult to define. With today's modern technology and medical advancements, creating greater beauty can be achieved. Today, aesthetic surgeons possess the same passion to redefine beauty by improving a patient's aesthetic qualities with a finesse few others can produce. Ultimately, natural beauty is best (**Video I.1**).

Keywords: beauty, history of aesthetic surgery, symmetry, proportion, harmony, Golden Ratio, Divine Proportion

> **Key Points**
>
> **Concepts of Beauty**
> - Understanding beauty is a central concept behind aesthetic surgery.
> - Attempted explanations that describe beauty include creating symmetrical images, proportions (Golden Ratio), harmony, and an individual's own intrinsic beliefs.
> - There are significant social effects that surround beauty.
> - Aesthetic surgery has transformed into the new generation of art that combines a scientific approach and a keen eye to create beauty.

1.1 Introduction

Elena Dmitrievna Diakonova met Salvador Dalí in 1929 in Paris, France.[1] Known as "Gala" by her close friends, Diakonova was a prominent figure in the Paris art scene and known to be a muse for many artists. However, Dalí saw more in her (▶ Fig. 1.1). In his autobiography,[1] Dalí writes, "'It is mostly with your blood, Gala, that I paint my pictures,' I said to her one day, and since then I have always used her name with mine in signing my work." Gala helped Dalí refine his artistic skills and push boundaries that others were incapable of reaching. Specifically, Dalí was fascinated by the idea of depicting any image, idea, or concept in his imagination and illustrating it as unaltered and realistically as possible. Dalí took this to heart when painting his wife.

Gala makes numerous appearances in Dalí's art. From Gala Contemplating the Mediterranean Sea to Dalí from the Back Painting Gala (▶ Fig. 1.1), Salvador Dalí transcribes Gala's beauty as natural and raw.[1] Dalí did not have to imagine Gala's beauty—he saw it. Concluding his memoire, Dalí[1] profoundly declares, "Gala, you are reality." With that simple line, one finally comprehends the main pursuit of Dalí's life. For Dalí, like many other artists, the obsession to translate an idea or image to an artistic representation dominates who they are as a person. Artists are never satisfied until the image they see with their eyes matches the image found in their innermost self. Dalí

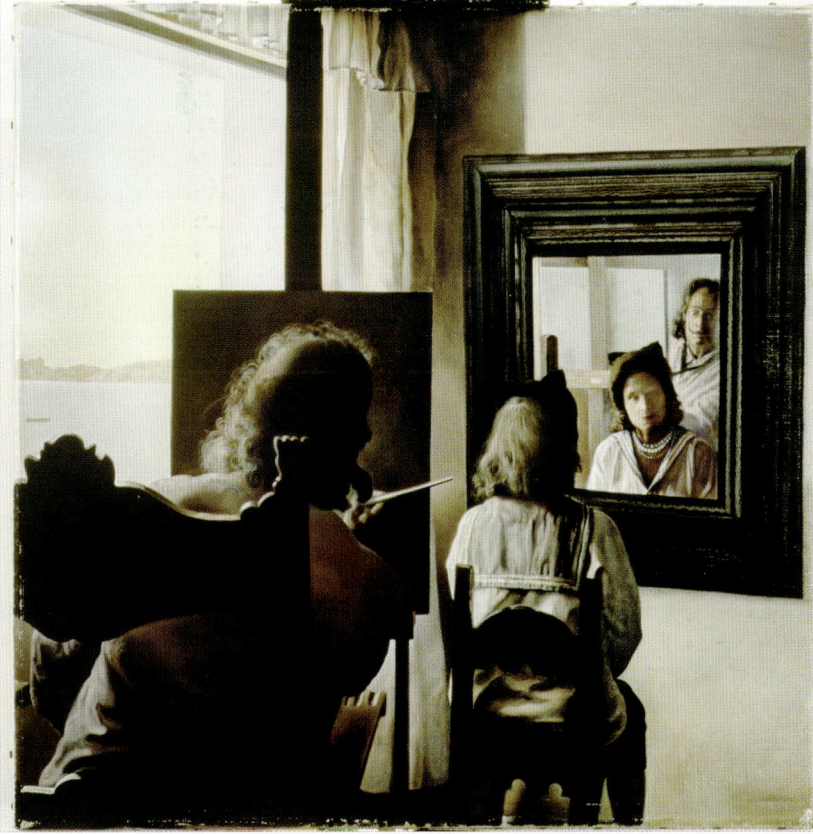

Fig. 1.1 Dalí Seen from the Back Painting Gala from the Back Eternalized by Six Virtual Corneas Provisionally Reflected by Six Real Mirrors. (Reproduced with permission from Dali de espaldas pintando a Gala–Dali paints Gala in front of a mirror, 1972-1973. Museo Dali, Figueras, Spain. Erich Lessing / Art Resource, NY. Salvador Dalí, Fundació Gala-Salvador Dalí, Artists Rights Society [ARS], New York 2017.)

was consumed by this ideology, especially when drawing Gala—the artist's true embodiment of beauty.

Dalí was of course a product of his time period and its respective technology. Imagine what vivid cinematography Dalí could have generated with computer-generated imagery at his fingertips. Could Dalí have created a divine, unearthly representation of beauty?

With today's modern technology and medical advancements, creating greater beauty can be achieved. Today, aesthetic surgeons possess the same passion to redefine beauty by improving a patient's aesthetic qualities with a finesse few others can produce. Perceived as a new generation of art, aesthetic surgery carries the fire that Dalí and his fellow innovative artists ignited.

Today's new aesthetic of art utilizes a needle laser, and energy-firming technology to substitute for a brush, oil pastels, and palate. With a calm, careful demeanor, aesthetic surgeons create an artistic work located one layer beneath the skin's epidermis. Rather than creating a single dimension that remains lifeless on a painting, aesthetic surgeons create masterpieces with blood flowing through the individual's veins. This cannot be accomplished, however, without many unusual yet effective methods. For instance, skilled professionals carefully inject micro-doses of Clostridium botulinum toxin (Botox) around the orbicularis oculi (muscles surrounding the eye).

The toxin, the same neuromodulator that causes flaccid paralysis in other situations, relaxes the muscles, thus diminishing wrinkling and accentuating the eye's beauty. Similarly, hyaluronic acid, a substance that is found naturally outside a cell, can be applied under the skin to smoothen almost any aging signs. A frequent concern for patients includes nasolabial lines or smile lines. Strategically inserted at an angle, the blunted cannula tip spreads out hyaluronic acid while causing little to no side effects. Any of these nonsurgical procedures reveal the modern era of aesthetic tools that have limited downsides.

The beginning days of plastic surgery were coarse. Aesthetic surgeons would primarily focus on surgically altering and not enhancing an individual's natural beauty. A common procedure, the traditional facelift alone, resulted in a homogeneous population. In some cases, incorrectly, a physician would pull the skin removing not only wrinkles but also the patient's basic individuality. A doctor certified in aesthetics must be in tune to rapidly changing trends and be able to cater to patient's desires. Also, a true professional understands that not every patient is a candidate for a specific procedure or surgery, even if a patient is adamant about it. A genuine physician will be honest with the patient and advocate for procedures that follow his or her best interests. In order to avoid the stigma negatively associated with aesthetic medicine, one has to understand the goal of natural-appearing alteration and enhancement. The primary reason for this divide between the aesthetic physician and the public is rooted in the perplexing question: what is beauty?

1.2 "Beauty Is in the Eye of the Beholder"

This simple yet effective statement demonstrates how one's perception of beauty is a personal choice. A man may find a woman appealing, although his friend does not feel the same way. What factors determine this? Is it the appeal of Hollywood actresses in extravagant wedding dresses shown on tabloid magazines? Or is it the athletic build of a football player that makes him handsome? Whether it is from the simplicity apparent in the DNA's helical structure to the complexity apparent in a rosebud, beauty's presence permeates every corner of the universe. One cannot argue that Michelangelo's grandiose, dramatic representation shown in La Pietà or his sculpture David outdoes the elegant timelessness that Alexandros of Antioch captures in the Venus de Milo. Clearly, it is impossible to define beauty in an absolute manner. However, there are a number of algorithms that have been developed to attempt to define an answer.

An infinite number of examples illustrate beauty, so there must be at least one unifying aspect that helps produce it. In actuality, some have theorized that there is a reproducible element that attempts to define beauty's presence—symmetry. *Symmetry* refers to exact mirror image between two parts separated by an axis or line. The linkage between symmetry and beauty is quite logical. Since its creation, humanity has an intrinsic predisposition toward symmetrical images. People are inclined to favor equality, because it has less dichotomy and disorder. As visualized in nature, countless examples of symmetry are seen in various animals, insects, or even the sun's shape. Consequently, it appears rational to make human features similar when comparing contralateral sides. By understanding that a genetic code for perceived attractiveness may exist, could one unlock the map for creating natural, humanistic masterpieces?

However, symmetrical proportions are not the main foundation for achieving beauty. A study conducted in Italy explored the three-dimensional (3D) facial asymmetry in subjects deemed "attractive" and "normal."[2] With digital computer technology, researchers demonstrated how asymmetrical features undermine an individual's beauty. Most importantly, though, they saw a general trend showing no exact correlation with higher symmetry with "attractive" people (▶ Fig. 1.2). Although this is convoluted, their data[2] expressed that "asymmetric faces deviate from attractiveness because they deviate from averageness [defined as similarity to the basic appearance of respective genders]...In synthesis, humans' symmetry may be a good sign of health, but not necessarily for attractiveness, also considering intrinsic asymmetry of our brain, and, therefore, of our perception."

Furthermore, symmetry, although significant, unfortunately does not equate to real-life applications of beauty. Theoretically, even if a patient were a 100% symmetrical, they may not be identified as beautiful by a lay observer. Artist Alex John Beck[3] reveals this in his photographic series entitled "Both Sides Of," a photography project that juxtaposes side-by-side portraits of models whose faces have been Photoshopped to be mirror images of the left and right sides of their faces. Beck[3] perfectly describes his finding by stating, "I think they [mirror image] lack character— beauty is more based on character than an arbitrary data point." "Humanity is messy and should remain as such. I, for one, am not a fan of center-parting, for example. And even the greatest tennis players favor one arm."[3]

Alternatively, beauty's foundations might lay more in proportion and harmony. A powerful idea that has dominated art of all aspects has been the Golden Ratio and Phi.[4,5] Conceptualized by the ancient Greek sculptor Phidias, Phi is the irrational number 1.618 and its respective Golden Ratio is 1.618:1. The ratio is

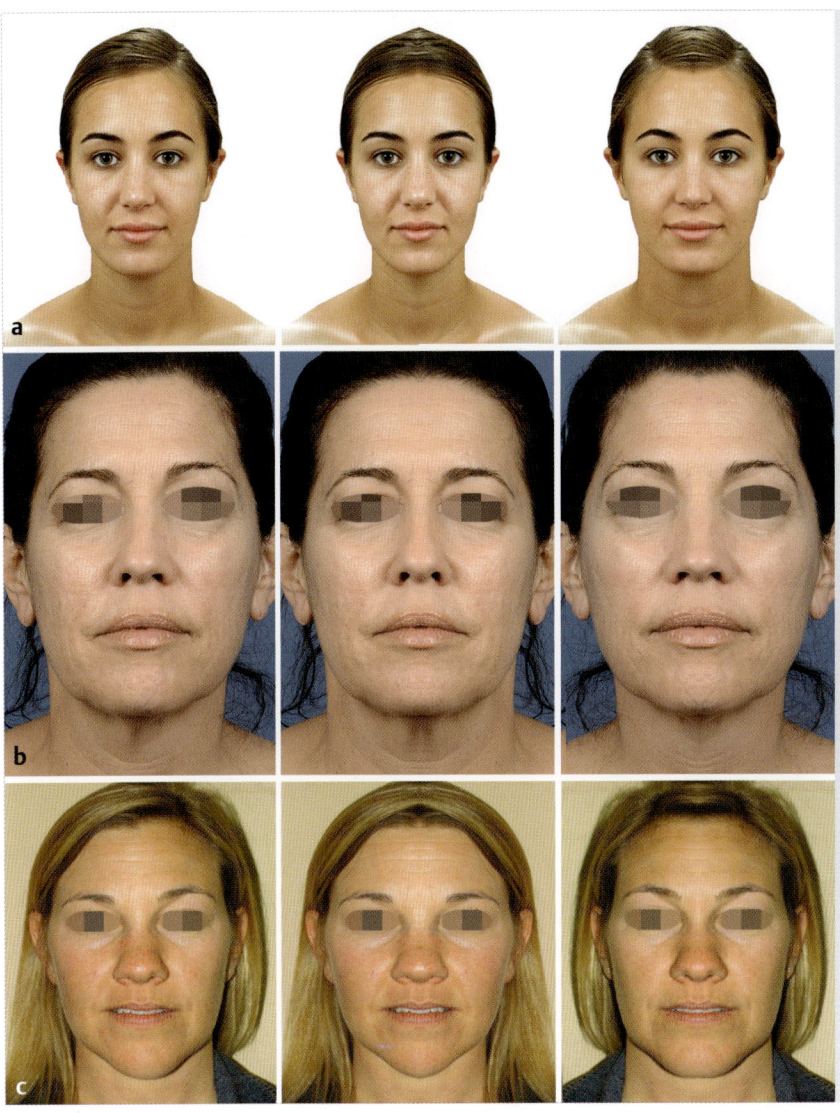

Fig. 1.2 (a-c) Each photo shows a mirror image of the individual's left and right sides, respectively. ((a) Reproduced with permission from Nahai F. The Art of Aesthetic Surgery: Principles and Techniques, ed 2. St. Louis, MO: Thieme Publishing Group, 2011.)

strictly based on numerous mathematical relationships and in concert with other ratios can generate "Divine Proportions." Nonetheless, it seems that its applications for creating beauty are endless. The Divine Proportion's presence resonates in everything from the faces of models to the spiral structure of a sunflower. Aesthetic surgeons utilize the ratio while approaching the patients' desires. Dr. Arthur Swift[4] has dedicated a significant portion of his practice to addressing the power of phi, including the famed calipers that measure the ratio patterns of the face. He describes, "In general, ideal facial width for most ethnicities falls approximately Phi (1.618) times the intercanthal distance [distance between the inner corners of eyes] from the medial canthus [inner corner of eye] to the ipsilateral cheek [same sided cheek]."[4] At his actual practice, Dr. Swift commonly uses golden calipers when utilizing fillers to achieve the most aesthetically pleasing results for his patients. When proportion works in conjugation with harmony, the ambiguity of beauty is cleared (▶ Fig. 1.3).

Harmony is the instrumental facet that allows diverse features to flow together. Harmony adds life to the beauty created by symmetry and proportion. With a multitude of different factors affecting the overall image, it is necessary to have a common theme that unifies them. Sexual dimorphism, "the degree to which a particular face resembles the prototype to his or her sex," plays a key role in harmony.[5] When painting a female figure, an artist relies on accentuating feminine qualities: higher cheekbones, larger lips, and a smaller nose. Conversely, a prominent jaw, smaller lips, and a dominant nose will define a male's figure. Despite a true explanation that describes how these qualities work synchronously with one another, any human has the innate ability to appreciate harmony.

The questions one has to ask is how does the clarity of the skin affect one's perception of beauty, given that phi does not answer surface findings. In addition, for a long time in the history of humankind, one was considered unattractive if his or her skin was anything more than very fair and free of any signs of sun-induced pigmentation. One must acknowledge their given bias regarding beauty, whether it is related to pigment, alteration to skin caused by body art, or other findings in modern society. If one goes back far enough in the time of medical textbooks, it is easy to find "experts" who felt that there were ways to "correct a black nose" to achieve ideal beauty. Clearly, bias affected the given aesthetic physicians' perception of ideal beauty and in turn their goals for aesthetic enhancement. With

Concepts of Beauty

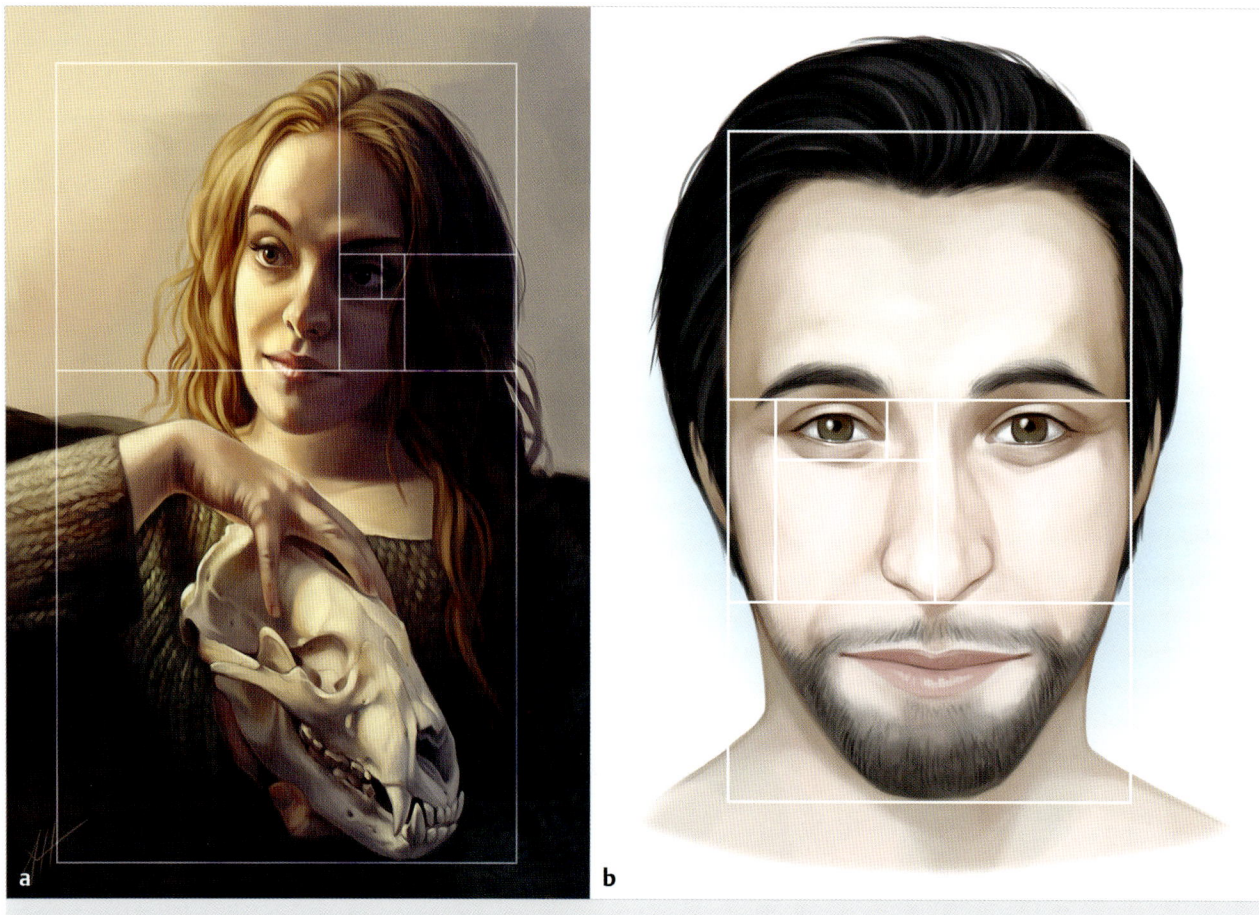

Fig. 1.3 (a,b) Depict applications of the Golden Ratio.

the above being said, one must realize that any given scale of beauty is simply a crude reference point that has been developed centuries ago. Ultimately, technology will continue to evolve and computer technology, such as IBM's Watson computer, may hold the key to these questions and more, but like art, we are dealing with the definition of subjectivity.

As discussed, the beautification process can appear daunting. Humankind's attempt to define beauty with irrational numbers, ratios, and geometric shapes displays our fascination and misconceptions about this amorphous concept. Because "beauty is in the eye of the beholder," humanity may never fully define what beauty exactly is from a mathematical relationship or sentence of words, but nevertheless it is something that humans can visualize and acknowledge (**Video 1.1**). In his article, Dr. Swift[4] explains, "regardless of nationality, age, or ethnic background, for the most part people universally share a sense of what is attractive."

Regardless of the methodology behind beauty's creation, the ends may justify the means. Appearance plays a strong role in today's culture. "It apparently takes only 150 milliseconds and no eye movement for a person to decide whether a face is attractive," says Constantian.[5] With a first impression made almost immediately, one's aesthetic qualities may be a substantial proponent to how others react to him or her. Moreover, not only do aesthetically pleasing people acquire higher economic positions but also more importantly they exude a more self-confident attitude toward life. Undeniably, patients pleased or even ecstatic about their results look at themselves in a brighter light.

There is substantial evidence that discusses how perceived "attractiveness" effectively benefits a patient. A group of psychologists from the University of Minnesota[6] wrote in their journal article What is Beautiful is Good, "A person's physical appearance, along with his sexual identity, is the personal characteristic most obvious and accessible to others in social interaction." Interestingly, they find statistical data pointing toward social attractiveness and the perceived ability to have "more prestigious jobs...as well as experiencing happier marriages...and enjoying more fulfilling social and occupational lives."[6] Although a human being should never be simplified to his or her external features, it is difficult to dispute the importance of appearance in social interactions.

Ultimately, natural beauty is best. Aesthetic surgeons irrevocably need to have this "eye" for beauty that permits them to transcribe beauty. The most efficient surgeons use their high attention to detail to shape out intended outcomes. Top physicians state that it is better to err on the side of gradual improvements rather than overshoot the "fine line" that exists. Wrinkles are part of the human face as imperfections are part of beauty. There has to be balance. While perfection is an unrealistic expectation, slight modifications will lead to a significant improvement toward balanced features.

Patients do not want to lose their self-identity when undergoing a procedure.[5] "It thus appears that any patient's desired aesthetic goals may derive, more than anything else, from their own DNA," writes Constantian.[5] An effective aesthetic surgeon does not intend to erase every fine line, but instead meshes every facial aspect to create a more holistic image. An idea surrounding rhinoplasty is that it extends to any area within aesthetic surgery and states, "Not all noses were meant to be identical," Constantian continues.[5] With 99% of a person's genetic makeup similar to any other being, it is the duty of a capable aesthetic surgeon to retain the patient's unique 1%.

Although the actual field is known as "plastic" surgery, there is nothing artificial about this profession (The word plastic originally was derived from the Greek term *plastikos*, which means "to sculpt or give form."). Unlike the past with obvious pulled facial skin, the current age of aesthetic surgery creates beauty more discretely. No longer do family and friends question the patient if they had a facelift but rather wonder if the patient slept more, lost weight, and perhaps changed their hairstyle. Additionally, beautification methods are no longer restricted for A-list celebrities or prominent musicians but rather everyday mothers, firefighters, or small business owners. Most significantly, it is noteworthy to emphasize the hallmark goal of this profession. An aesthetic surgeon never intends to prey on a patient's insecurities. They seek to resolve the patient's frustrations, therefore helping the patient feel more in touch with their outer and inner beauty.

The future of aesthetic surgery is remarkably nonsurgical and/or minimally invasive (**Video 2.11**). This field transforms as quickly as its patients transform. A new laser technology for resurfacing can be outdated in a matter of a year or even a few months. Today, an absorbable suture material that mimics a facelift's effectiveness at a third of the cost is replacing the facelift. Combining focused ultrasound, laser resurfacing and necessary volume to the face can produce an incredible makeover in one sitting. Furthermore, aesthetic surgeons hint upon the horizons of aesthetic surgery to include the use of stimulating nature cells by using stem cells. There will be less emphasis on fixing the problem, but instead greater emphasis on hyper-focusing on preventative measures.

Salvador Dalí's presence reveals how "rich the world can be when you dare to embrace pure, boundless creativity."[7] The concept of beauty may always be one of the world's greatest mysteries. It changes with time and will always be dynamic. Aesthetic medicine should not strive to reverse time; good aesthetic medicine strives to make a patient age with grace and beauty. Undeniably, aesthetic surgeons will be at the forefront of humanity's attempt to understand the concept of beauty.

References

[1] Dalí S. The Secret Life of Salvador Dalí. Reprint edn. New York: Dover Publications; March 3, 1993
[2] Sforza C, Laino A, Grandi G, et al. Three-dimensional facial asymmetry in attractive and normal people from childhood to young adulthood. Symmetry (Basel). 2010; 2:1925–1944
[3] Stampler L. Here's what faces would actually look like if they were perfectly symmetrical. Time. 2014. Accessed 06 Feb, 2016
[4] Swift A, Remington K. BeautiPHIcation™: a global approach to facial beauty. Clin Plast Surg. 2011; 38(3):347–377, v. Web. 7 Feb. 2016
[5] Constantian MB. Rhinoplasty: Craft & Magic. St. Louis, MO: Thieme Publishing Group; 2009:289–290
[6] Dion K, Berscheid E, Walster E. What is beautiful is good. J Pers Soc Psychol. 1972; 24(3):285–290
[7] Unparalleled Collection of Salvador Dali Art Works - The Dali Museum. St., Petersburg, FL. www.thedali.org. Accessed 08 Feb, 2016

2 Nonsurgical Cervicofacial Rejuvenation of a Traditional Surgical Candidate

Sahar Nadimi and Corey S. Maas

Summary

This chapter will discuss how the blending of various technologies, such as injective bioactive agents, lipolytic therapies, lasers and laserlike devices for laser skin resurfacing, radiofrequency (RF) technology, and hyaluronic acid (HA), and synthetic fillers, offer an excellent means of facial rejuvenation, may significantly enhance surgical results, and/or delay the need for surgery in the proper patient.

Keywords: neuromodulators, soft tissue fillers, lypolytic therapies, kybella, cytolytic, facial rejuvenation, ablative lasers, nonablative lasers, hyaluronic acid fillers, synthetic fillers, nonsurgical

Key Points

- One of the most significant changes in the recent history for facial plastic surgery is the greater demand from patients for aesthetic improvement without surgery.
- The use of injectable bioactive agents (such as neuromodulators and soft tissue fillers), along with numerous lasers and "laserlike devices," has continued to increase in cosmetic surgery practices.
- It is important to select patients carefully and discuss expected benefits and limitations prior to treatment to avoid patient disappointment, because many aspects of facial rejuvenation still require surgical intervention.
- A thorough review of the patient's history is the first step in this process. In addition, it is important to know that the patient has realistic expectations.
- The blending of the technologies discussed in the chapter offers an excellent means of facial rejuvenation, may significantly enhance surgical results, and/or may delay the need for surgery in some patients.

2.1 Introduction

Minimally invasive procedures have revolutionized the treatment paradigm for facial rejuvenation and may be one of the most significant changes in the recent history for facial plastic surgery.

The use of injectable bioactive agents including neuromodulators and soft tissue fillers has continued to increase in cosmetic surgery practices as a result of the greater demands from patients for aesthetic improvement without surgery.[1,2,3,4,5,6,7] This is due to the growing indications and availability of neuromodulators and soft tissue fillers, along with the desire for rejuvenation from a wider patient population among varying ages and ethnicities.[1] The last decade has seen a dramatic increase in the number of facial fillers approved by the U.S. Food and Drug Administration (FDA) in response to the growing popularity of minimally invasive procedures.[8] According to The American Society of Plastic Surgeons (ASPS), 15.6 million cosmetic procedures, including both minimally invasive and surgical procedures, were performed in the United States in 2014. Of those 15.6 million cosmetic procedures, injectable treatments comprise 9 million, which is a 4% increase from 2013.[8]

A new category of injectable agents is lipolytic therapies. Currently this category is limited to one product, Kybella (deoxycholic acid, Allergan, Inc.). Kybella is a cytolytic drug indicated for improvement in the appearance of moderate to severe fullness associated with submental fat in adults (see Product Index (p.170)). In 2015, deoxycholic acid subcutaneous injections received approval from the FDA for the treatment of submental liposis.

Other noninvasive devices for facial rejuvenation that merit mention include Ulthera (Ulthera, Inc.) and numerous lasers and "laserlike devices" (ablative and nonablative lasers in both fractionated and unfractionated forms as well as RF technologies).

These products and devices are an attractive office procedure for providers because of their ease, cost, and minimal discomfort involved in treatment. With all the various products and devices now available, it can be anticipated that both demand and use will continue to increase, because the variety of options affords clinicians and patients greater versatility in tailoring therapy to individual needs and goals.

It is important to select patients carefully and to discuss expected benefits and limitations prior to treatment to avoid patient disappointment, because many aspects of facial rejuvenation still require surgical intervention.

This chapter will discuss how the blending of the previously mentioned technologies offers an excellent means of facial rejuvenation, may significantly enhance surgical results, and/or may delay the need for surgery in the proper patient.

2.2 Technologies for Rejuvenation: A Review

2.2.1 Neuromodulators

Botulinum neuromodulator (BoNT), first used for the management of strabismus in the 1980s by Dr. Allen Scott in San Francisco, is the workhorse of injectable agents for facial rejuvenation.[9] The neuromodulator's biologic action occurs at the neurosynaptic cleft responsible for muscle contraction by cleaving proteins involved in the active transport of acetylcholine.[10,11] Originally these proteins were described as toxins due to the illness botulism, which was associated with consuming large amounts of *Clostridium botulinum*–contaminated food. Their desired action is selective weakening, relaxation, or paralysis of treated muscles. As a result, unwanted lines and socially undesirable facial expressions can be suppressed or eliminated.

There are seven serotypes of BoNT (A-G), and only A and B have been developed for routine clinical use. The B serotype neuromodulator Myobloc (rimabotulinumtoxinB, Solstice Neurosciences) is less suitable for cosmetic use because of its shorter duration of effect and injection discomfort associated with its acidity (pH of 5.6).[12,13] The A serotype of botulinum neurotoxin (BoNTA) has demonstrated the longest duration of effect (90–120 days) and least discomfort with injection. Three formulations of BoNTA have been studied and used extensively for cosmetic and therapeutic indications (see Product Index (p. 167)): Botox Cosmetic, Dysport, and Xeomin. Botox (botulinum toxin type A) Cosmetic (Allergan, Inc.), approved for the reduction of hyperfunctional glabellar lines in 2002, set the standard for neuromodulators by demonstrating a proven safety and efficacy record. Dysport (abobotulinumtoxinA, Galderma Laboratories, L.P.) became FDA approved in 2009, followed by Xeomin (incobotulinumtoxinA, Merz, Inc.) in July 2011 (see Product Index (p. 169)). Although these three formulations are not interchangeable, and reportedly cannot be substituted by one another by any fixed-dose conversion ratio, most agree that the ratio is 2.5 to 3 units of Dysport to 1 unit of Botox and 1 to 1.3 units of Xeomin to 1 unit of Botox.[14,15]

Patient Selection

Proper patient selection is important to having satisfied patients and reducing undesired outcomes. A thorough review of the patient's history is the first step in this process, and it is important to know that the patient has realistic expectations. Allergies or hypersensitivities to any of the formulation ingredients (BoNTA, sodium chloride, human albumin) are contraindications for BoNT treatment. Neurodegenerative and neuromuscular disorders are typically absolute contraindications to therapy. Patients and providers should be made aware of any preexisting lid or brow ptosis if they are present and educated on the risk of exacerbation.[15]

2.2.2 Soft Tissue Fillers

Initially utilized for the treatment of fine lines and wrinkles, manufactured or commercially available fillers have expanded to include the correction of volume loss and augmentation of the aging face.[16] Since bovine collagen (Zyderm, Inamed Corp.) was introduced as an injectable filler in the early 1970s, several other products have been developed for soft tissue augmentation, particularly in the last decade. The ideal soft tissue filler is[17]

- Effective.
- Nonimmunogenic.
- Nontoxic.
- Noncarcinogenic.
- Nonmigratory.
- Easily applied.
- Nonpalpable.
- Painless.
- Long-lasting.

Currently available fillers can be broadly classified into the following three different categories: hyaluronic acid (HA) derivatives, synthetic fillers, and autologous fat (▶ Table 2.1).

Hyaluronic Acid Fillers

The currently available HA fillers in the United States are Restylane, Restylane Lyft, Juvéderm XC, Juvéderm Voluma, Belotero Balance, and Restylane Silk (see Product Index (p. 167)). HA is a naturally occurring substance in the human body and serves as the ground substance of dermis, fascia, and other tissues. There

Table 2.1 Comparison of Soft Tissue Fillers

	Filler	Manufacturer	Composition	Needle Size	Depth
Hyaluronic Acid	Restylane	Galderma Laboratories, L.P.	20 mg/mL hyaluronic acid; 330–430 um particle size	29–30 gauge	Mid-to-deep dermis
	Perlane (Restylane Lyft)	Galderma Laboratories, L.P.	20 mg/mL hyaluronic acid; 750–1,000 um particle size	27–29 gauge	Deep dermis, superficial subcutis
	Restylane Silk	Galderma Laboratories, L.P.	20 mg/mL hyaluronic acid; 50–220 um particle size	30 gauge	Mid-to-deep dermis
	Juvéderm XC	Allergan, Inc.	24 mg/mL with 0.3% lidocaine	27 gauge	Mid-to-deep dermis
	Juvéderm Voluma	Allergan, Inc.	20 mg/mL with 0.3% lidocaine	27–29 gauge	Deep (subcutaneous, supraperiosteal)
	Belotero	Merz North America	22.5 mg/mL	30 gauge	Mid-to-deep dermis
Synthetic Fillers	Radiesse	Merz, Inc.	30% calcium hydroxylapatite microspheres / 70% carrier gel	25–27 gauge	Subdermal
	Sculptra	Galderma Laboratories, L.P.	367.5 mg powder of poly-L-lactic acid microspheres	26 gauge	Deep dermis
	Bellafill (ArteFill)	Suneva Medical	20% polymethyl-methacrylate suspended in 80% solution with 3.5% bovine collagen and 0.3% lidocaine	26 gauge	Dermal-subdermal junction
Autologous Fat	Autologous Fat	Autologous	Liposuctioned fat	18–gauge needle with blunt cannula	Subcutaneous

are several advantages in using the HA fillers, including the immediate reversibility with hyaluronidase and the lack of antigenic specificity, decreasing the risk of allergic response. Another property that makes these products useful clinically is the hydrophilic nature, allowing 1 g HA to bind up to 6 L water (**Video 2.1**).[16,18]

Properties of HAs that are important in determining their clinical performance include the concentration of HA and the degree of cross-linking, which affect longevity and stability; gel hardness (G'), which helps determine flow properties, the extrusion force required, and the structure and stiffness of the finished product; and the degree of gel swelling, or the ability to resist dilution, which also influences longevity.[19] The stiffer the material then the higher the G'. This is determined by the degree and strength of interaction in the cross-linking HA as well as the HA concentration.[16]

HA typically must be cross-linked to avoid rapid degradation by hyaluronidase, temperature, or free radicals, and different HA fillers vary by the cross-linking density and resultant stiffness. HA fillers with a higher cross-linking density can be used for deep wrinkles, whereas HA fillers with a lower cross-linking density are preferable for fine lines.[16]

The Restylane family (Galderma Laboratories, L.P.) maintains an HA concentration of 20 mg/mL and includes Restylane, Restylane Lyft, and Restylane Silk (▶ Table 2.1, **Video 2.1**). Restylane was introduced in 1996 as the first non–animal-stabilized HA. Derived from the fermentation of *Streptococcus* species, the molecules are cross-linked by the addition of 1, 4-butanediol diglycidyl ether to increase surface area and slow down the natural breakdown of the product.[18]

Restylane Lyft is similar to Restylane but has a larger particle size. Because of the larger particle size, Restylane Lyft is better suited for deeper levels of injection such as treatment for deep cutaneous depressions, whereas Restylane can be used for these applications and more superficially. Overall, both Restylane and Restylane Lyft have a higher G', and therefore more firmness with less spreading of the product, making it better suited for placement in the subdermal level. Restylane Lyft needs to be injected through a 27-gauge needle compared with a 30-gauge needle used for Restylane.[11] Restylane Silk, FDA approved in June 2014, can be differentiated from other products in the Restylane family by its smaller particle size. It is intended for lip augmentation and correction of perioral rhytids. Restylane Silk is injected intradermally with a 31-gauge needle due to the small particle size for the correction of fine lines.[6,16,18]

Juvéderm (Allergan, Inc.) is currently available in two types: Juvéderm XC and Juvéderm Voluma, with an HA concentration of 24 and 20 mg/mL, respectively (▶ Table 2.1, **Video 2.2**). Both of the Juvéderm products have an intermediate G' and viscosity, which leads to a higher likelihood of spreading after implantation and a softer feel.[16,20] Because Juvéderm XC has a lower G' and viscosity than Juvéderm Voluma, it is ideal for areas where palpability is less desirable, such as medium-depth wrinkles (forehead and glabellar lines, nasolabial folds, and moderate nasal furrows).[16,20,21] Juvéderm Voluma, FDA approved in October 2013, consists of a low- and high-molecular-weight HA, which allows for efficient cross-linking, resulting in a highly cohesive gel with greater hardness (G') than other Juvéderm products, greater lift capability, and long in vivo duration optimized for midface volumizing.[22,23]

Two other HA fillers currently available in Europe that will likely be on the market in the Unites States include Juvéderm Volbella and Volift (Allergan, Inc.). Juvéderm Volbella has a much lower concentration at 15 mg/mL, and a lower G' and cohesivity, allowing it to be used in a more superficial spreading fashion for the lips, rhytids, and more subtle depressions. Volift at 17.5 mg/mL HA allows more subtle lift capacity but retains an element of spread, making it a useful agent for the perioral region and in the treatment of fine lines.

Belotero (Merz North America) is a HA gel filler that was FDA approved in 2011 for treatment of moderate-to-severe nasolabial folds and wrinkles.[24] Belotero has a higher concentration of non–cross-linked HA, and is considered poly-densified because the cross-linking is not uniform throughout.[25] This results in a low viscosity and the lowest G' (gel hardness) of the currently available HA fillers.[24] With these properties, Belotero is utilized mainly in areas for superficial intradermal or subdermal injection, because it is a softer product (due to the low G') that allows it to spread more evenly because of its low viscosity. Clinically, Belotero is useful for very fine lines such as the forehead, vermilion border, and tear trough.[16,24,25]

Synthetic Fillers

In addition to HA fillers, two other classes of fillers merit mention. Calcium hydroxylapatite (Radiesse, Merz, Inc.) and poly-L-lactic acid (Sculptra, Galderma Laboratories, L.P.) are larger molecule fillers, ranging from 25 to 63 um in particle size (see Product Index (p.173)).[18] These products work primarily by causing foreign body reaction and an increase in fibroblasts and collagen deposition. Radiesse is composed of calcium hydroxylapatite (CaHA) particles suspended in a carboxymethylcellulose gel, and should be injected subdermally near or well below the dermal-subcutaneous junction.[18] Injection too superficially can lead to visibility of the white material and nodularity.[26] After injection, the carrier gel that fills the interstitial space eventually dissipates and is replaced with soft tissue ingrowth, with the CaHA acting as a scaffold.[27,28] Sculptra (Galderma Laboratories, L.P.) is an injectable form of poly-L-lactic acid, a compound that has been used in absorbable suture material for over 40 years.[16] The microspheres eventually gets dissolved into carbon dioxide (CO_2) and water. Sculptra was approved in the treatment of shallow to deep nasolabial folds, facial wrinkles and lines, and improvement of the contour deficiencies with placement recommended subcutaneously.[16,29]

Injection techniques include serial puncture, linear threading, fanning, and cross-hatching, with fanning and cross-hatching being used primarily for facial contouring (▶ Fig. 2.1). All four techniques can be used to create a layered approach, with relatively thin product being used superficially and thicker, larger particle filler being used deeper.

Patient Selection

As with any procedure, it is important to ensure that the patient has realistic expectations. A history of excessive bleeding, bruising, or abnormal scar formation should be documented, and the patient should be aware that this may occur as a result of dermal filler injection. History of anaphylactoid reactions and lidocaine hypersensitivity should be elicited from the patient.

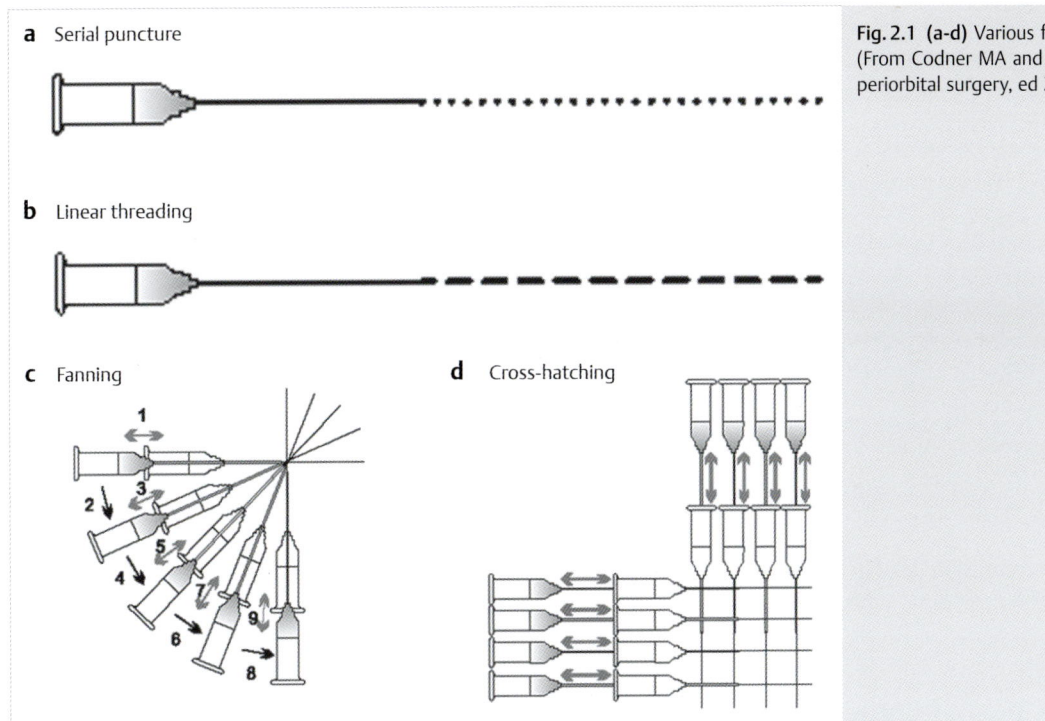

Fig. 2.1 (a-d) Various filler injection techniques. (From Codner MA and McCord CD. Eyelid & periorbital surgery, ed 2, 2016. Thieme, St. Louis)

2.2.3 Kybella

Although injectable lipolytic therapies such as deoxycholate with or without phosphatidylcholine have been performed for many years for the reduction of small areas of fat, none of the formulations used have been subject to appropriate pharmaceutical development and detailed clinical evaluation. Kybella is the first adipocytolitic drug for injection that was FDA approved for the treatment of submental liposis in 2015.

Kybella contains sodium deoxycholate, a naturally occurring bile acid that solubilizes dietary fat in humans and other animals, thereby aiding in its digestion. Deoxycholate induces pores in cellular membranes, producing leakage of cytoplasmic contents, membrane destabilization, and subsequent lysis. These lytic effects occur within minutes and account for the brisk, localized inflammatory response after injection. Replacement of grossly injured adipose tissue with fibrosis may account for subsequent fat reduction and skin retraction observed after treatment.[30,31,32]

Four large multicenter, randomized, double-blind Phase III trials confirmed the efficacy of Kybella subcutaneous injections to reduce submental fat and improve submental profile and skin laxity.[30,31,32,33,34,35,36,37] Kybella is a promising, less invasive alternative to liposuction for the reduction of submental fat.

Patient Selection

Kybella is indicated for improvement in the appearance of moderate to severe convexity or fullness associated with submental fat in adults. Careful consideration must be given for the use of Kybella in patients with excessive skin laxity or prominent platysmal bands for which the reduction of submental fat may result in an aesthetically undesirable outcome. Kybella is contraindicated in the presence of infection at the injection sites.

2.2.4 Ulthera

Ultrasound use as a therapeutic modality has evolved from its early neurologic applications in the 1950s.[38,39] The application for facial rejuvenation utilizes thermal injury through intense focused ultrasound. This is accomplished through a shorter pulse duration of 50 to 200 ms, a higher frequency of 4 to 7 MHz, and a decreased energy quantity of 0.5 to 10 J.[40] This technology was commercialized as the Ulthera System in 2004, and several clinical studies refined the device and supported its ability to create thermal coagulation points (TCPs) at specific tissue depths (see Product Index (p. 185)).[41,42,43,44] Intense focused ultrasound energy is delivered through the skin's surface with the selective creation of thermal injury zones in the superficial musculoaponeurotic system (SMAS), heating the fascia in a pinpoint way, resulting in contraction of the fascia. This results in lifting and tightening of the skin on the neck, under the chin, along the jawline, and on the brow.[45]

In 2009, a study by Alam et al[46] resulted in FDA approval for a brow lift indication. Kenkel[47] demonstrated improvement in the neck, giving the device an FDA-approved neck lift indication.

Patient Selection

An ideal patient is usually younger with a robust wound healing response, mild lipoptosis, and good skin elasticity. Ulthera is also a nice option for patients who have already had a facelift and need a "touch-up" procedure. An older patient with

Table 2.2 Ablative Nonfractionated Lasers

Wavelength & Type	Manufacturer & Product	Key Features	Clinical Indications
10,600 nm CO_2 laser	Sandstone Medical Technologies Matrix LS-40	Up to 100-ms pulses; 40 W; UltraFine-FS fractional scanner available	Facial photodamage (dyschromia / lentigines / rhytides)
	Lumenis UltraPulse & AcuPulse	Nonfractionated or fractionated modes	Facial atrophic scars
2,940 nm Er:YAG laser	Focus Medical NaturaLase ER	3J; includes fractional handpiece	Epidermal lesions (seborrheic keratoses / verrucae)
	Quantel Derma GmbH BURAINE	350-µs pulses; up to 2 J; fractional handpiece available	
	Sandstone Medical Technologies Whisper 3-G	300-µs pulses; 600 J/cm2; 1-/3-/6-/9-mm spot sizes	
	Sciton Contour TRL	Up to 50-ms pulses; up to 40 W; tunable resurfacing laser (TRL); computerized scanner	
	Syneron Candela SmoothPeel	2-/4-/6-Hz pulses; up to 750 mJ energy; 5- and 9-mm spot sizes	

extensive photoaging, severe skin laxity, marked platysmal banding, and a very heavy neck is generally not an ideal candidate.[45]

2.2.5 Laser Skin Resurfacing (Ablative and Nonablative)

The primary goal of skin rejuvenation is to combat aging and photodamaged skin, which manifest as facial lines, irregular pigmentation, telangiectasias, and textural changes. Five major classes of lasers are in common use: ablative and nonablative lasers in both fractionated and unfractionated forms as well as RF technologies.

The introduction of ablative laser skin resurfacing techniques with high-energy, pulsed CO_2 and erbium-doped yttrium aluminum garnet (Er:YAG) devices was met with great enthusiasm because of their excellent clinical outcomes in the treatment of scars and photodamaged facial skin, but the prolonged recovery and the risk of potential side effects made them less attractive treatment alternatives. The subsequent development of nonablative laser devices improved recovery and tolerability, although limited clinical efficacy was associated with these less invasive treatments.[48,49]

The concept of fractional photothermolysis, coined by Manstein and colleagues,[50] has revolutionized the field of laser skin resurfacing by providing the ability to obtain significant clinical results with minimal posttreatment recovery. Advantages of fractional over fully ablative lasers include faster re-epithelialization after treatment, shorter posttreatment skin care, less frequent acneiform eruptions, and quicker resolving postoperative erythema.[51,52]

In fractional technology, the laser beam creates microscopic treatment zones (MTZs) of controlled width, depth, and densities in the skin.[50] Only fractions of skin are treated by inducing small zones of thermal damage, resulting in an improved safety profile and shortened recovery times. Collateral damage is controlled and healing is rapid, because the tissue surrounding each tiny wound is undamaged and the keratinocytes have only short distances to migrate during re-epithelialization. Collagen contracts and neocollagenesis is initiated.[50,53]

Fractionated technology has led to the development of a number of nonablative and ablative devices (▶ Table 2.2). For patients with severely photodamaged skin, ablative resurfacing is the best treatment. Texture, tone, dyschromias, and mild to moderate wrinkles can all be improved after a single treatment.

CO_2 lasers emit light at 10,600 nm in the far infrared electromagnetic spectrum. The emitted energy is preferentially absorbed by intracellular water, which leads to rapid heating and vaporization of tissue. CO_2 lasers were introduced in the 1960s and were initially used in the continuous wave (CW) mode for cutting tissue. These CW systems produced significant thermal damage to the surrounding tissue and led to the development of high-energy pulsed and scanned systems in the early 1990s. The pulsed CO_2 lasers caused discrete areas of tissue vaporization while minimizing collateral thermal injury that was associated with fewer unwanted side effects such as scarring and hypopigmentation.[54,55]

The Er:YAG laser was approved for skin resurfacing by the FDA in 1996. Its 2940-nm wavelength is absorbed 12 to 18 times more efficiently than is the CO_2 laser, allowing more superficial absorption with less penetration. This allows even less collateral damage. At typical Er:YAG treatment parameters, dermal healing is limited with subsequent reduced effect on tissue tightening, but postoperative healing times are shortened compared with CO_2 lasers.[54]

Numerous studies using CO_2 and Er:YAG lasers have been performed to evaluate the efficacy and safety of ablative resurfacing. Most studies demonstrated marked (80% or greater) improvement in treated areas, with the periorbital and perioral regions showing the best results and areas of dynamic wrinkling, such as the glabella, showing the least[55,56,57,58,59,60,61] (▶ Table 2.3).

Nonablative laser technology was subsequently developed in an attempt to limit the prolonged postoperative recovery period associated with ablative laser skin resurfacing. Nonablative remodeling rejuvenates skin without superficial epidermolysis by targeting tissue beneath the surface. A direct dermal wound with new collagen formation effacing wrinkles and acne scarring is the goal. Some nonablative lasers also target irregular pigmentation, abnormal blood vessels, and telangiectasias.[55] Because nonablative lasers have limited thermal tissue effect,

Table 2.3 Nonablative Nonfractionated Lasers

Wavelength & Type	Manufacturer & Product	Key Features	Clinical Indications
1319-nm Pulsed energy	Sciton ThermaScan	5–200-ms pulses; 30 J/cm2; 6-mm spot; nonsequential scanning to reduce heat buildup between laser pulses	Mild facial photodamage
1320-nm Nd:YAG	CoolTouch Brand - Syneron Candela CT3Plus	450-µs pulses; 3 to 10 mm adjustable spot; burst and continuous modes	Mild facial atrophic scars
	Alma Lasers Harmony XL	Long-pulse; 5 to 40 J/cm2; 6-mm spot	
1450-nm diode	Syneron Candela SmoothBeam	210-ms pulses; 8 to 25 J/cm2; 4- or 6-mm spot	

Table 2.4 Nonablative Fractionated Lasers

Wavelength & Type	Manufacturer & Product	Key Features	Clinical Indications
1410 nm	Solta Medical Fraxel re:fine	700 µm depth; 20 mJ / MTZ	Facial photodamage
1440 nm Nd:YAG	Cynosure Affirm Laser	1,000 micro-pulses / 10-mm spot	Facial scars (atrophic / traumatic / burns)
	Palomar (Cynosure) StarLux	Includes both 1440 nm and 1540 nm handsets	Melasma
1540 nm	Palomar (Cynosure) StarLux	Includes both 1540 nm and 1440 nm handsets	
	Palomar Icon	Includes 2940 nm fractional ablative handset	
1550 nm Erbium glass and 1927 nm thulium fiber	Solta Medical Fraxel re:store and DUAL	1550 nm:1.4 mm depth; 70 mJ / MTZ 1927 nm:0.23 mm depth; 20 mJ / MTZ	
1440 nm and 1927 nm diode	Solta Medical Clear + Brilliant	2 handpieces available: Original: 200 to 300 µm depth Perméa: 170 µm depth	

treatments are commonly delivered in a series of three or more monthly sessions to produce mild clinical results. Most studies reported clinical improvement averaging 30% to 50% after a series of treatments.[55,62,63,64,65,66,67,68] Severely photodamaged patients with advanced wrinkles are better candidates for ablative resurfacing.

Most of the nonablative systems emit light in the infrared portion of the electromagnetic spectrum, including the intense pulsed light (500 to 1200 nm), Nd:YAG (1064 and 1320 nm), diode (980 and 1450 nm), and Er:glass (1540 nm) lasers. Intense pulsed light (IPL) is a noncoherent (thus not categorized as a laser), high-energy broadband-pulsed flashlamp that emits light in the range of 500 to 1200 nm. Absorption filters are selected to block wavelengths of light below the selected number. Spot size and energy also effect depth of penetration. The primary chromophores are hemoglobin with peak absorption between 577 to 585 nm and melanin with a range of 500 to 850 nm. Appropriate filters can be selected to target superficial vessels and melanin. The 1064 nm Nd:YAG laser affects larger blood vessels and deeper collagen, and may improve wrinkles. The 1320 nm Nd:YAG laser functions by avoiding damage to the epidermis and instead targeting the dermal layers to stimulate new collagen growth. The water in the skin absorbs the 1320 nm wavelength in particular, creating an even distribution of energy without damaging melanin or hemoglobin. The 1450 nm diode laser focuses on the water in the skin and is effective for the treatment of facial acne as well as for improving the appearance of scarring.

There is minimal to no downtime with nonablative lasers. Some edema and erythema may last for a few days, but it can usually be covered with makeup. Each system has specific parameters for the number and duration of treatments (▶ Table 2.4).

Fractionated technology has led to the development of a number of nonablative and ablative devices, and it has virtually replaced pulsed and scanned systems due to their excellent clinical effects and low risk profiles.

Significant improvement of facial rhytids, scars, and dyspigmentation has been demonstrated in several published studies of nonablative fractionated lasers. By increasing the energy delivered, greater depth of dermal penetration (and tissue effect) is achieved. Increasing the density (or area of coverage) also serves to increase the clinical effect without significantly altering postoperative recovery. Clinical assessment scores corresponding to 50% to 75% improvement or more are typically reported after a series of three or more treatments on facial rhytids.[55,69] Atrophic acne scars have shown improvement (50% and higher) after a treatment series using either a 1550-nm erbium-doped fiber laser or a number of other fractionated diode and Nd:YAG lasers (1410–1540 nm).[70,71,72]

The Clear + Brilliant (Solta Medical, Inc.) fractionated diode laser comes in two different handpieces: Original and Perméa. The Original handpiece utilizes a 1440 nm wavelength that is absorbed by the water in the skin. The stratum corneum remains functionally intact, which translates into a safe, low-risk treatment that heals quickly. Because the handpiece depth

Table 2.5 Ablative Fractionated Lasers

Wavelength & Type	Manufacturer & Product	Key Features	Clinical Indications
10,600 nm fractional CO_2	Alma Lasers Harmony Platform Pixel CO_2	Short/medium/long pulses; 300 to 2,500 mJ/p	Facial photodamage (dyschromia / lentigines / rhytides)
	Cynosure. SmartSkin +	150 to 20,000-μs pulses; up to 30 W power; multiple scanning patterns	Facial atrophic scars
	DEKA Medical Inc. SmartXide DOT 30 W/50 W	0.2-μs to 80-μs pulse; 150 W; multiple scanning modes	Epidermal lesions (seborrheic keratoses / verrucae)
	Ellman International, Inc.(Cynosure) Ellumine Fractional CO_2 laser system	2 to 7-ms pulse; up to 105 mJ	
	Focus Medical NaturaLase CO_2	Up to 10-ms pulse; 50 W	
	Hironic Co., Ltd. MIXEL	Up to 5000-μs pulse; 60 mJ	
	ILOODA CO., Ltd. FRAXIS	0.1 to 5-ms pulse; up to 30 W	
	Lasering USA MiXto Pro Slim Evolution II	2.5 to 16-ms CW pulse; 0.5 to 30 W; 180-μm or 300-μm spot size	
	Lumenis UltraPulse Encore (ActiveFX/ DeepFX/ TotalFX)	<1-ms pulse; 240 W; ActiveFX mode with 1.3-mm spot size; DeepFX with 0.12-mm spot size; TotalFX combines ActiveFX and DeepFX	
	Lumenis AcuPulse MultiMode	CW scanning robot-assisted laser; 0.01 to 1.00-s pulse; 30 W and 40 W models available; 1.3-mm and 0.12-mm spot sizes handpiece	
	Lutronic eCO2	2 to 240 mJ	
	Solta Medical Fraxel re:pair	Up to 70 mJ/MTZ	
	Syneron Candela CO2RE	60 W; 7 different treatment modes	
2940 nm Fractional Er: YAG	Alma Lasers Harmony Platform Pixel 2940	Short/medium/long pulses; 300 to 2,500 mJ/p; 11 mm2 pixel tips	
	INDUSTRA Technologies 2940 DualMode	300 μs to 5 milliseconds pulses; up to 60 mJ/ mtz; ablative and coagulative effects	
	Palomar (Cynosure) Icon Aesthetic System 2940 Fractional laser handpiece	0.25 to 5-ms pulses; 2 to 5.5 mJ / 0.1 mm	
	Sciton ProFractional (XC)	Variable pulse; up to 400 J/cm^2	

is 200 to 300 μm, it effectively targets the layers of the skin most compromised by early signs of aging such as uneven pigmentation, fine lines, and textural changes. On the other hand, the Clear + Brilliant Perméa handpiece utilizes a 1927 nm wavelength that has a significantly higher absorption coefficient than the Original. Although the stratum corneum remains intact, the Perméa handpiece creates wider and shallower lesions, causing greater superficial disruption, which increases skin permeability. The Perméa handpiece depth is fixed at 170 μm. Clear + Brilliant is safe on all skin types, because its longer wavelength penetrates to the dermis and avoids epidermal melanin absorption[55] (▶ Table 2.5). The stackable treatment approach is a combination of botulinum toxin injections and dermal fillers to smooth out wrinkles, along with energy-based tools such as laser skin resurfacing (**Video 2.3**). Stackable treatments and HA fillers can be used to restore volume to the cheeks, with nonsurgical lifting of the face and neck, and then simultaneously combine laser skin resurfacing.

The popularity of this approach was reflected in the 2015 cosmetic surgery data from the American Society for Aesthetic Plastic Surgery (ASAPS), which showed that the use of injectables (dermal fillers and botulinum toxin) increased by 21% from the previous year while laser skin resurfacing remained 1 of the top 10 nonsurgical treatments.[8]

Even more impressive improvement of photoaged skin has been demonstrated with ablative CO_2 and Er:YAG fractionated laser technology compared with the nonablative fractionated devices.[55,73,74,75] Previous studies have shown good long-term clinical results 5 years after fractional CO_2 laser skin resurfacing in the treatment of facial photoaging.[49]

The UltraPulse Encore (Lumenis) is an advanced fractional CO_2 laser system with three modes of delivering the laser's energy.[76] The first, ActiveFX, uses a 1.3-mm spot size that ablates the superficial tissue and is useful for treating fine lines and actinic keratosis. The second, DeepFX, focuses the lasers energy into a 0.12-mm spot size and allows for deep ablation

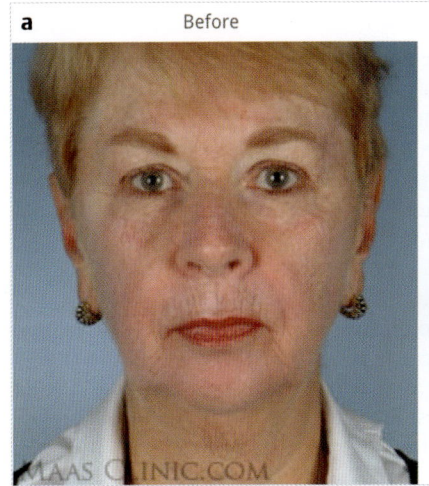
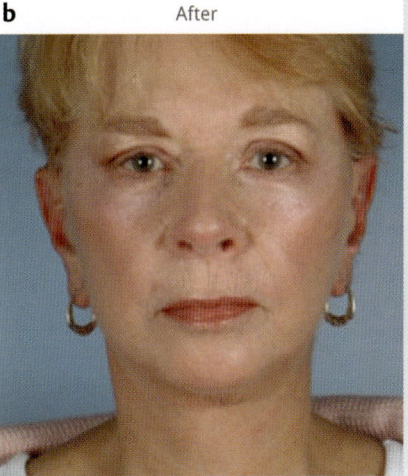

Fig. 2.2 (a) Before and (b) after photographs of upper blepharoplasty, facelift, and fractional CO_2 laser skin resurfacing of the face and neck.

that is useful for treating deep rhytides. DeepFX is particularly useful for treating perioral and periocular fine lines, and scars. This mode can ablate up to 2 mm into the tissue. The TotalFX mode uses both the ActiveFX and DeepFX modes simultaneously and is useful for treating scars and rhytides.[76] Modest power settings are important when treating around the eyelids and the neck. For superficial areas on the face and neck, the ActiveFX component of the UltraPulse is most commonly used with the following parameters: 90 to 125 mJ, 100 Hz, scan size 4 to 8, density 3 to 4. For deeper areas, the DeepFX component is most commonly used with the following parameters: 17.5 to 20 mJ, 300 Hz, scan size 4 to 8, density 15 to 20% (▶ Fig. 2.2).

The Fraxel re:pair fractional CO_2 laser system (Solta Medical, Inc.) works much like the UltraPulse Encore's DeepFX mode. The pulse duration on this laser can range from 0.15 to 3 ms. By using a short pulse duration, the laser system can deliver more energy quicker and ablate deeper. By combining its small 0.14-mm spot sizes and a short 0.15-ms duration, this laser ablates to depths of 1.6 mm. Fractional technology can be applied to Er:YAG lasers in much the same way that it was developed for CO_2 lasers[76] (▶ Table 2.6).

RF systems are unique in that they are thermal heating systems, working more like microwaves rather than lasers. They have the advantage of having a higher penetration depth, while aiming for collagen shrinkage and skin tightening. The RF largely passes through the skin surface, sparing it from heating.[76] Much like the laser systems, the RF systems achieve results by denaturing existing collagen and stimulating the production of newer and shorter collagen, leading to lasting tissue tightening.[76,77] This modality is often combined with other modalities to achieve a synergistic effect. For example, RF has been combined with diode systems (Polaris WR, Syneron Candela). A major limitation of this modality is that currently there is not enough published data regarding the optimal temperature and duration of treatment at that temperature to obtain ideal results. In fact, most data is currently anecdotal, and further research is necessary to determine the optimal parameters for this treatment modality.

Patient Selection

Patients should be educated about the course and importance of their postoperative care and potential complications. Indications for laser skin resurfacing include improvement in sun-damaged skin, facial rhytids, dyschromias, and scar revision. The senior author routinely performs ablative fractional laser skin resurfacing on patients of all skin types (Fitzpatrick I-VI).

Table 2.6 Radiofrequency Systems

Wavelength & Type	Manufacturer & Product	Key Features
10,600-nm CO_2 laser, RF excited tube	Eclipse Aesthetics Equinox CO_2	0.05 to 10-ms pulse; 350-μm spot fractional scanner
Multiphase RF fractional sublative	Eclipse Aesthetics EndyMed Pro	70 ms per pulse, 6 W RF output
4.0 MHz high-frequency monopolar RF	Ellman International (Cynosure) Pellevé Wrinkle Reduction System	Four handpiece sizes ranging from 7.5 mm to 20 mm
Radiofrequency	EndyMed EndyMed PRO / GLOW	65 W
Monopolar / Bipolar RF	ILOODA CO., Ltd. Lunar-N	0 to 150 ms pulses; 75 W
Radiofrequency	Invasix Fractora	62 mJ/pin
Bipolar RF	Lumenis Aluma	1 to 5-s pulse; 2 to 20 W
Bipolar RF	Syneron Candela ePrime	460 nm, 5 kHz
580 to 980-nm Optical/RF	Syneron Candela eMax/eLight SR(A)	Up to 46 J/cm2 / up to 25 J/cm2
900-nm Diode/RF	Syneron Candela eMax/eLaser WRA	Up to 50 J/cm2 / up to 100 J/cm2
1 MHz Fractional RF	Viora V-touch	50 to 200-ms pulses; up to 25 J

Patients with darker skin phototypes (Fitzpatrick III-VI) have a higher likelihood of developing postinflammatory hyperpigmentation (PIH), although this has never been permanent in the senior author's experience, and is easily treated with topical creams. PIH is much less frequent with fractional laser skin resurfacing than with other ablative procedures.[78] These patients should be informed about PIH, with treatment initiated when indicated. Any factors that may affect the pilosebaceous glands, such as previous facial radiation or the use of oral retinoids for 1 year in advance, can increase the risk for poor healing after treatment. Other contraindications include active skin infections, vitiligo, and a history of keloids or hypertrophic scars. Antivirals should be started 1 day prior to the procedure and continued for 1 week.[79]

2.2.6 Nonsurgical Blepharoplasty and Browplasty

The periorbital region is one of the early and more dramatic regions demonstrating signs of facial aging. Surgical and nonsurgical options such as blepharoplasty, browplasty, and skin resurfacing remain mainstays for the primary management of age-related changes in the eyelids and adjacent areas. However, we strongly feel that such interventions can be significantly enhanced or even delayed by using noninvasive products and devices.

2.3 Treatment Plans and Results

2.3.1 Neuromodulators

Lateral Orbital Rhytids (Crow's-Feet)

The orbicularis oculi muscle is a flat, wide muscle that encircles each orbit, and has been arbitrarily divided into two parts: orbital and palpebral. The part of the orbicularis oculi that is located along the lateral orbit is responsible for creating the lateral radial lines, known as *crow's-feet*. In addition, the orbital segment of the orbicularis oculi is a depressor of the lateral brow.

The most common treatment for lateral orbital rhytids is BoNTA. Two goals should be kept in mind regarding the use of BoNTA:
1. Relaxing the radial crow's-feet lines by targeting the lateral, vertically oriented portion of the orbicularis oculi.
2. Providing brow elevation by neuromodulation of the brow depressor function by treating the entire length of the lateral orbicularis oculi.

Studies have demonstrated the effect of BoNTA treatment of the lateral orbicularis oculi on brow position (also known as a *chemical browlift*).[80,81] Because the lateral orbicularis oculi muscle acts as a sphincter, careful attention must be paid to the vectors of force during contraction. The contraction vectors at 12 and 6 o'clock are predominantly horizontal, whereas the vectors at 3 and 9 o'clock are primarily vertical. With BoNTA treatment, the lateral frontalis muscle is now unopposed and will create a brow elevation. The medial brow position can be manipulated as well through treatment of the corrugator supercilii muscle. The crow's-feet wrinkles are treated by injecting the lateral orbicularis oculi at several sites lateral to the orbital rim. A typical dose is 10 units of Botox/Xeomin or Dysport equivalent per side, divided into 4 or 5 aliquots (▶ Fig. 2.3).

Glabellar Complex

The vertical glabellar lines are primarily formed by the actions of the paired corrugator supercilii muscles. The corrugator supercilii originates from the procerus medially and inserts laterally into the orbicularis oculi muscle and the soft tissue at and slightly above the medial eyebrow. This muscle is nearly horizontal in most individuals; thus, contraction of the corrugator supercilii produces a vertical wrinkle. It is crucial that BoNTA be injected properly into the corrugator supercilii muscle. A common mistake is to inject the corrugator supercilii too far superiorly and thus actually treat the frontalis. The frontalis relaxation may cause a mephisto, or "Spock-like," unattractive appearance (▶ Fig. 2.4). The correct placement of BoNTA into the corrugator supercilii muscle is just at or slightly above the medial clubhead of the eyebrow. A second small dose is given 3 to 5 mm lateral to the first injection to treat the entire length of the corrugator muscle. Typically, 10 units of Botox/Xeomin or Dysport equivalent is injected per side.

Furrows created at the base of the nose are created by the procerus muscle. If a patient has transverse furrows, 3 to 5 units of Botox/Xeomin or Dysport equivalent is injected into the belly of this muscle in 1 or 2 aliquots.

Frontalis Muscle

The frontalis is a thin, quadrangular muscle originating from the galea aponeurotica superiorly and inserting into the brow inferiorly. It is contiguous with the procerus muscle centrally and interdigitates with the corrugator and orbicularis oculi muscles at the brow. Its fibers are vertical in orientation, and contraction causes elevation of the brow. Hyperfunctional lines in this area cause classic horizontal forehead furrows.

Ten units of Botox/Xeomin or Dysport equivalent, divided into 4 aliquots, are used to treat the frontalis. The location of the injections is critical to achieving optimal results. The patient should raise the brow to better define the forehead lines, and injections immediately above the most inferior horizontal line is recommended. Laterally, the point at which the forehead curves temporally is the lateral injection point. Medially, the medial canthus is the medial injection point. Three additional injection points (2 units of Botox/Xeomin or Dysport equivalent) can be added as extension therapy in patients with numerous forehead lines or greater forehead height. One extension therapy injection is added in the midline, whereas the other is added between the medial and lateral injection points bilaterally. It is important to explain to the patient that BoNTA treatment of the frontalis can result in brow ptosis. Therefore, treatment of the frontalis involves walking a fine line between undertreatment of the forehead and persistent lines versus ptosis of the brow (▶ Fig. 2.3).

2.3.2 Soft Tissue Fillers

Glabellar Complex, Crow's-Feet, Forehead Lines

With the advent of BoNTA, soft tissue fillers have taken on a more limited role in the treatment of horizontal forehead lines, lateral orbital rhytids, and glabellar lines. It is important to distinguish between dynamic and nondynamic lines. Although dynamic lines are better treated with BoNTA, the superficial

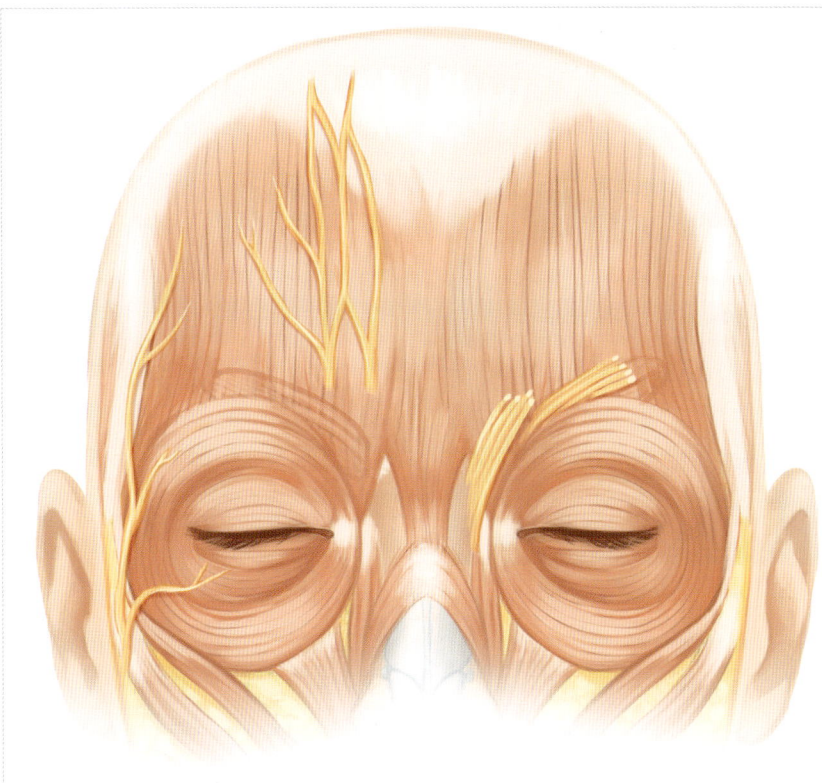

Fig. 2.3 Anatomy of the upper face demonstrating recommended neuromodulator injection sites and dosages.

lines caused by actinic damage may qualify for treatment with soft tissue fillers. Fine-line treatment using serial point intradermal injections with Belotero or Restylane Silk offers the best results for these superficial lines. The serial puncture technique, whereby small aliquots of filler are given to achieve even distribution, is particularly effective in accurate filler placement. When combining BoNTA and filler, it is advisable to stage the treatment. Most experienced injectors will use BoNTA first, and after it has taken effect, a better determination of filler application can be made.

Nasojugal Groove/Tear Trough

As one ages, the midface structures become ptotic and expose the nasojugal groove and orbital rim. Often pseudoherniation of orbital fat is present, accentuating the lower eyelid–cheek complex. Volume replacement can be an excellent option or supplement to surgery for patients with mild to moderate deformities.[82]

HA products such as Restylane are commonly used to fill the tear trough (▶ Fig. 2.5). Juvéderm has a smoother consistency, but in the senior author's experience, it is more hydrophilic than Restylane. Hyaluronic acid products will hold more water and result in more edema. This can complicate the correction and lead to undercorrection and a shorter duration than anticipated.

Filling the nasojugal groove is a delicate procedure requiring precision and artistry, and one must possess a clear understanding of the anatomy. Topical anesthetic creams and ice offer the best anesthesia. Anesthetic injections can distort the anatomy and interfere with proper filler injection. The patient should be seated upright, and his or her gaze should be fixed on the horizon, because fat pads can be reoriented by upward and downward gaze and by gravity. The product is injected along

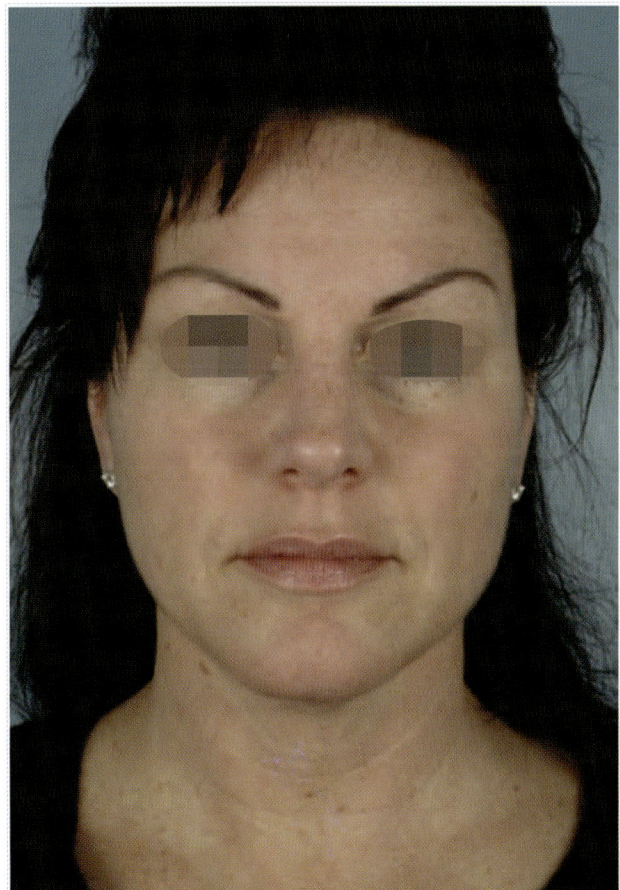

Fig. 2.4 Botox brow deformity demonstrating medial brow ptosis and medial eyelid hooding.

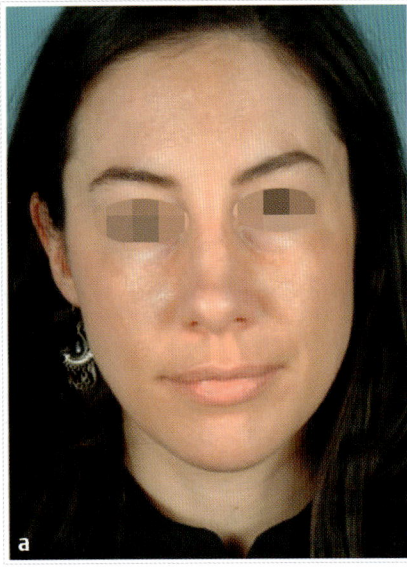
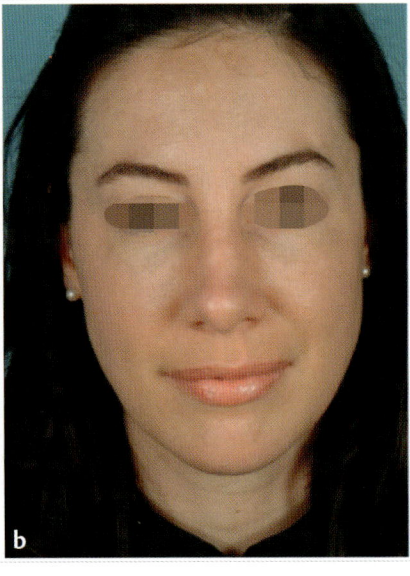

Fig. 2.5 (a) Before and (b) after Restylane injection into the nasojugal groove area.

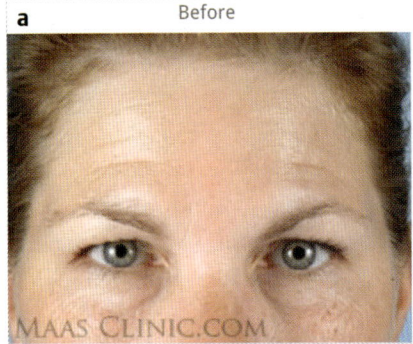
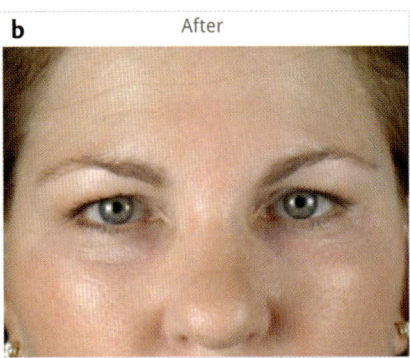

Fig. 2.6 (a) Before and (b) after fractional CO_2 laser skin resurfacing of the face.

the orbital rim, staying preseptal to avoid exacerbating the pseudoherniation of orbital fat that causes the deformity. The lower eyelid skin must be avoided. Ecchymosis may occur in this area because of the thin skin and the needle passing through the orbicularis muscle. If bruising becomes evident, the injection should be halted, and pressure should be applied to the area for several minutes. After the injection is complete, the area should be massaged to ensure even product distribution.

The senior author prefers to use serial puncture and linear threading techniques. It is important to inject slowly (< 0.3 mL/min). Most clinicians inject between 0.2 and 0.4 mL per side. Because injecting the nasojugal groove can be extremely volume sensitive, it is important to initially treat conservatively to avoid overcorrection. Reevaluation in 2 to 4 weeks and touch-up treatment can be performed at that time if needed.

The Tyndall effect, which is visible material associated with a gray or blue color, is a side effect that may be detected at the injection site. This is a refractive phenomenon produced by superficially placed material. To minimize the occurrence of this phenomenon, filler must be injected in small amounts deep into the tissues.[83,84]

Postprocedure Care

No specific aftercare is required and patients can return to their usual routine right away. Bruising or swelling, if present, usually disappears in a few days.

2.3.3 Laser Skin Resurfacing

Fractional CO_2 laser resurfacing is an excellent nonsurgical treatment option for periorbital rhytids, fine lines, and lower lid laxity. This procedure should not be performed on patients with a poor lid distraction test. The senior author often treats the lower eyelids and crow's-feet with DeepFX CO_2 laser (Lumenis) at a setting of 17.5 mJ, 300 Hz, 15 to 20% density (▶ Fig. 2.6). ActiveFX can be performed on the upper and lower periorbital regions using a setting of 125 mJ, 100 Hz, Density.[3,4]

Postprocedure Care

An occlusive ointment is applied immediately after the procedure. Patients may gently wash the area three times a day, starting the morning after treatment, and then immediately reapply the occlusive ointment for at least 3 to 4 days. After healing is complete, an intense moisturizer may be used. Patients may use mineral makeup after the skin has healed, which is usually 5 days after the procedure.

2.3.4 Ulthera

Ulthera can be used for lifting and tightening of the brow skin. Treatment of the brow is usually performed in continuity with the face (▶ Fig. 2.7).

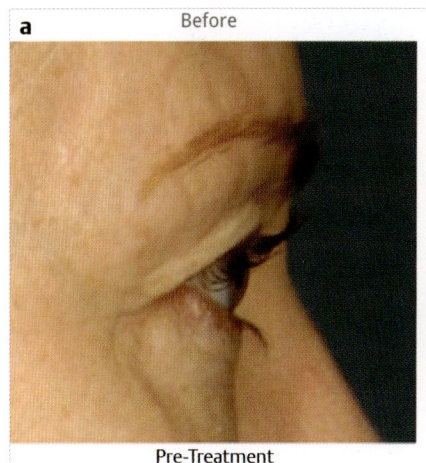
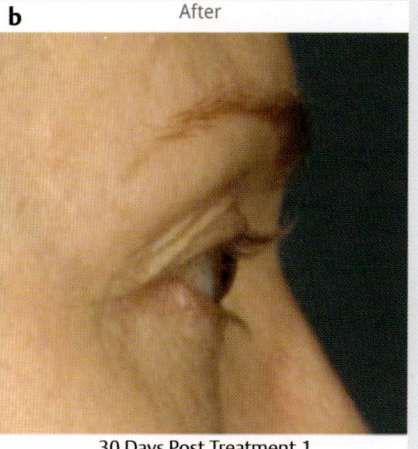

Fig. 2.7 (a) Before and (b) 30 days after Ulthera treatment of the brow.

Postprocedure Care

A light moisturizer and sunscreen is applied after the treatment. No specific aftercare is required, and patients can return to their usual routine right away. Immediately after the treatment, the skin feels tighter to patients. This initial response may shift to visible changes in 3 to 6 months.

2.4 Nonsurgical Perioral Rejuvenation

The aging lip is characterized by a decrease in vermilion show, blunting of Cupid's bow, and an attenuated white roll.[6,85] The repetitive actions of the circular orbicularis muscle can lead to vertical rhytids of the upper and lower lips. Marionette lines are characterized by vertical lines at the oral commissures, and are the result of depressor anguli oris (DAO) muscle hyperactivity (▶ Fig. 2.8). An increasingly deep nasolabial fold is formed by descent of the malar fat overlying the complex of the orbicularis oris, levator labii superioris, and zygomaticus major muscles. *Peau d'orange*, the French term meaning orange skin, describes a condition of dimpling of the skin over the chin, resulting from hyperactivity of the mentalis muscle.[6,86]

2.4.1 Treatment Plan and Results

Neuromodulators

In the lower face, the primary targets for facial rejuvenation with BoNTA are the oral commissures and lip lines. Treating the DAO muscle results in the improvement of the perioral appearance by softening the marionette lines and downturned oral commissures. Three units of Botox/Xeomin or Dysport equivalent injection per side at the point where the marionette line intersects with the mandible, which is approximately 1 cm inferior and lateral to the oral commissure, can attenuate these lines. It is imperative to avoid inadvertent injection into the lip depressors and orbicularis oris, which can lead to oral incompetence. The senior author treats the vertical perioral lip lines with 4 to 6 units of Botox/Xeomin or Dysport equivalent placed at the vermillion border of the upper and lower lips in multiple small aliquots. Hyperactivity of the mentalis muscle can be treated with a dose of 2 to 5 units of Botox/Xeomin or Dysport equivalent into target sites just below the prominence of the chin. One should avoid inadvertently injecting the orbicularis oris or depressor labii, which can cause lower lip depression.

Soft Tissue Fillers

In the lower face, the primary targets of soft tissue fillers include the nasolabial folds, lips, and oral commissures. For the nasolabial folds, the products can be injected superficially into the dermis to efface fine lines or deeper into the subdermal level to smooth the appearance of the nasolabial fold itself. Hyaluronic products or Radiesse are preferred to treat deep nasolabial folds (▶ Fig. 2.9). Serial puncture or linear threading techniques can be used. It is important to inject medial to the fold to avoid further cheek ptosis. For successful rejuvenation of this area, the triangle formed at the superior aspect of the fold by the junction of the nasal ala and cheek must be filled. To address the fine etched lines sometimes associated with the nasolabial fold, Belotero or Restylane Silk are effectively injected intradermally using a serial puncture technique.[6]

The upper lip should be approximately 75% of the volume of the lower lip, and the central lower lip should protrude slightly beyond the upper lip. Both the vermilion border and body of the lip can be treated. The senior author prefers Restylane in this area because of its relative firmness and its ability to contour the lip (▶ Fig. 2.10). The vermilion border is enhanced by the injection of Restylane into the potential space between the red and white lip. Frequently, this space can be entered with the needle, and the product can be injected along the entire length of the lip through hydrodissection, providing uniform placement of the product. Alternatively, a serial puncture technique can be used. The body of the lower lip is augmented by submucosal injection with a focus on the central one-third of the lower lip.[6]

Injection preparation for the oral commissures is similar to that for other areas of the face, using a topical anesthetic and ice. The fillers are placed in the subdermal plane in a triangle formed with its base at the lower lip. The corner of the mouth

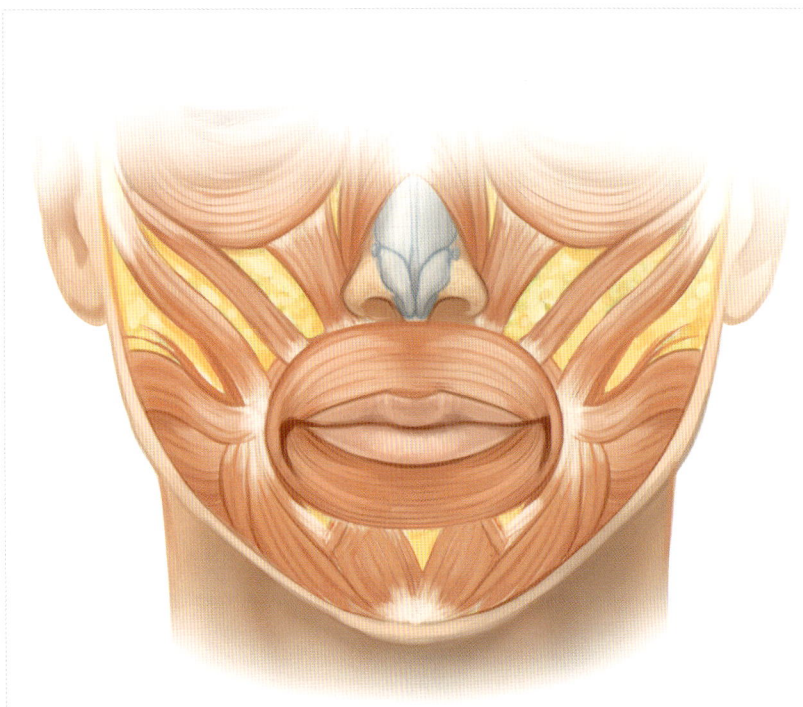

Fig. 2.8 Lower facial musculature pertinent to the treatment of marionette lines.

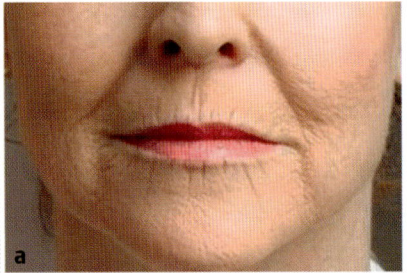
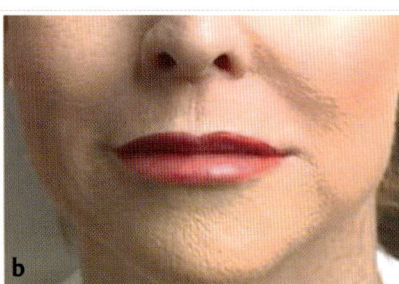

Fig. 2.9 (a) Before and (b) after Restylane injections to the nasolabial folds and lips along with fractional CO_2 laser skin resurfacing.

should be elevated during injection to raise sagging tissues. For the fine lines in this area, the senior author frequently uses Belotero and Restylane Silk.

Laser Skin Resurfacing

The senior author often performs fractional CO_2 laser skin resurfacing to treat the fine perioral rhytids in this area. DeepFX CO_2 laser with a setting of 20 mJ, 300 Hz, 15–20% density is often followed by ActiveFX using a setting of 125 mJ, 100 Hz, density.[3,4] It is important to blend the skin between the treated and untreated zones with the laser.

Halo (Hybrid Fractional Laser)

The Halo (Sciton, Inc.) hybrid fractional laser, which is a single laser platform, is based on evidence that a combined ablative/nonablative approach produces more robust results than ablative lasers alone but with similar or decreased postprocedural issues (i.e., pain, erythema, and petechiae [see Product Index (p. 181)]).[87] Prior to the Halo laser platform, our Institute would routinely combine 2940 nm resurfacing immediately prior to using a 1540 nm laser to achieve a more substantial resurfacing result for multicomponent facial/neck skin issues. This was a cumbersome process that required two different hand pieces, recalibration, and increased time for application. The Halo laser is a dual-wavelength platform, incorporating both 1470 nm for coagulation and 2940 nm for ablation. The 1470 nm can be adjusted for a depth of 200–700 microns to optimally target epidermal and dermal pigmented lesions, dermal elastosis, fine lines, texture, and pore size, whereas the 2940 nm can be adjusted for a depth of 0–100 microns to remove stratum corneum and epidermis. This allows for an optimal effect on both the superficial and deep layers of the skin, providing ablative results with nonablative downtime (**Videos 2.4** and **2.5**).

▶ Fig. 2.11 shows a 56-year-old patient with Fitzpatrick II skin with evidence of fine rhytids, dyschromia, and texture irregularities. She underwent single-pass Halo with intermediate settings (1470 nm: 400-micron depth, 30% density; and 2940 nm: 40-micron depth, 21% density). She is shown 2 weeks later with significant improvement (**Videos 2.13** and **2.14**).

Postprocedural Care

Postprocedural care for the products and devices used to treat this region is similar to that described previously.

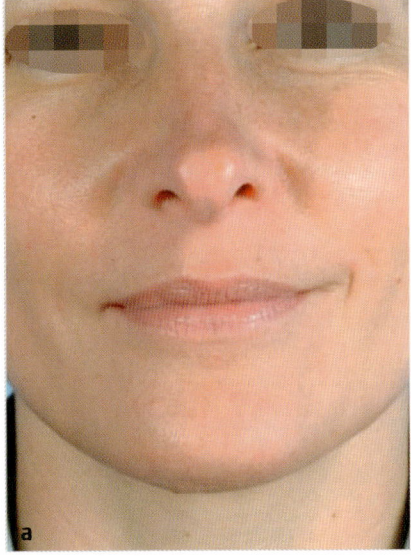
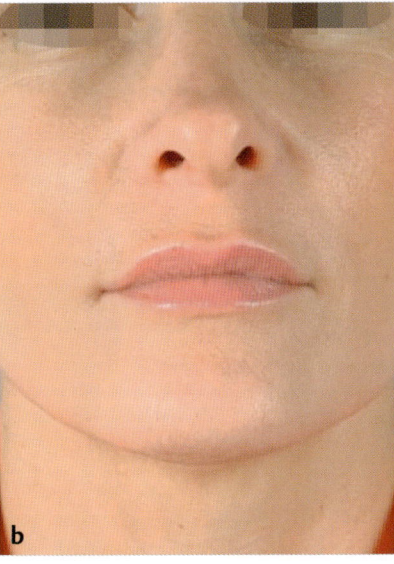

Fig. 2.10 (a) Before and (b) after microcheilia treated with Restylane injections.

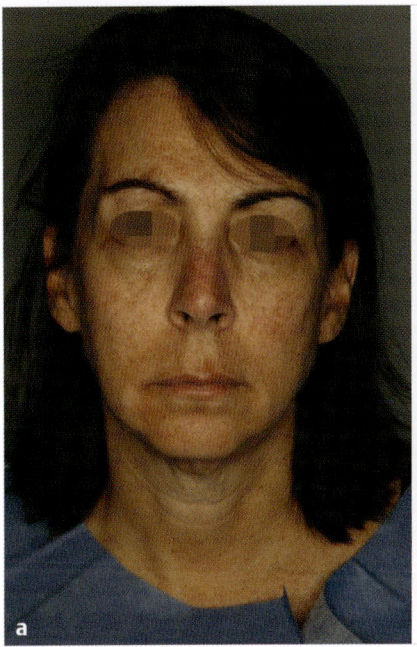
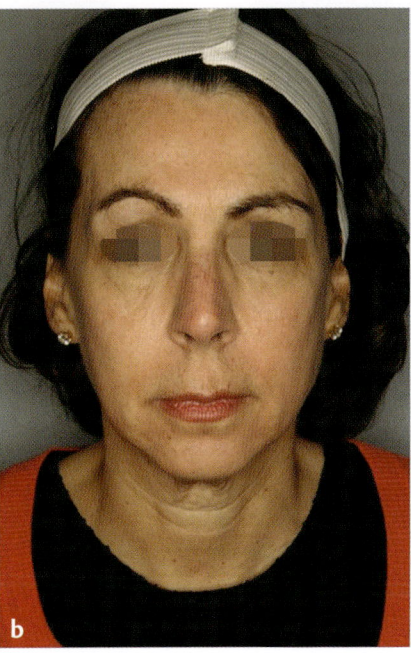

Fig. 2.11 (a) Pretreatment and (b) 2 weeks posttreatment using the Halo hybrid fractional laser.

2.5 Nonsurgical Midface and Malar Augmentation

The malar prominence descends inferomedially with aging to deepen the nasolabial crease and expose the lateral orbital rim. It is composed of a subcutaneous malar fat pad with underlying orbicularis oculi muscle. Deep to this is the suborbicularis orbital fat (SOOF), which is intimately associated with the periosteum of the infraorbital rim and the insertions of the zygomaticus major and minor muscles. When the midface structures are ptotic and the orbital rim is exposed, the juxtaposition of prolapsed orbital fat and the fallen SOOF creates a double contour. Attempts to erase this double contour with lower lid blepharoplasty and excessive fat removal result in a sunken, hollowed appearance.[88]

2.5.1 Treatment Plan and Results

When treating multiple areas of the midface with soft tissue fillers, malar/submalar augmentation should be performed first, because augmentation affects both the nasolabial fold and the tear troughs. Malar augmentation may lessen the volume of material required for nasolabial fold correction by taking up excess skin and lifting the midface region as a whole. This approach sometimes negates the need to treat the tear trough.

The goal in midface augmentation may range from restoring the loss of volume to dramatically changing the shape of the midface though placement of the fillers in noninherent locations. Many authors have described filler placement using Hinderer's lines.[89,90] With this method, the injection begins from the superior point of the malar eminence continuing onto the inferior maxillary zone. Injecting directly on top of the periosteum will lift up the superficial and deep fat pads. Injections are then continued medially to define the midface.[91]

The senior author, however, feels that midface volume loss is usually most evident in the anteromedial cheek because of descent of the malar fat pad. The first thing to do is to delineate a few key midface anatomic landmarks: the lower border of the cheek bone transversely down to the nasolabial fold; the upper border of the cheekbone and inferior orbital rim; the high point of the nasolabial fold; and the medial aspect of the bony zygomatic prominence. Filler is then injected predominantly in the upper two-thirds of the medial cheek (where the malar fat pad was previously located in youth), where most patients have the greatest degree of volume loss (▶ Fig. 2.12). Filler placement here will result in a more youthful and round midface. The injection is submuscular or deeper, and the techniques include fanning and cross-hatching of the product for uniform filling (**Videos 2.6**, **2.7**, **2.8**).

For the midface, it is important to use a product that has a higher G′, such as Juvéderm Voluma, Perlane (Restylane Lift), or Radiesse (▶ Fig. 2.13 and ▶ Fig. 2.14). Previous studies have shown that nearly half of the subjects with midface volume deficit who are treated with Juvéderm Voluma continued to see a clinical benefit for 24 months.[16,23]

2.6 Nonsurgical Face Lift

The aging face is characterized by the formation of rhytides by repetitive actions of facial muscles, elastosis of skin from sun damage, and progressive descent and loss of fat pads, combined with loss of skin elasticity.

2.6.1 Treatment Plan and Results

Soft Tissue Fillers

The primary areas of concern are the cheeks and the prejowl sulcus. As previously mentioned, Juvéderm Voluma or Radiesse in the midface is a good option. Treatment of mild jowling involves injection of the prejowl sulcus to camouflage the depression between the jowl and the mentum by creating a smooth transition between the two areas, rather than a relative concavity. Multiple injection techniques are possible including deep-dermal or dermal-subcutaneous junction injection between the two areas in a linear threading fashion. The needle is inserted within the skin of the jowl and/or within the skin of the mentum and threaded into the prejowl sulcus along the inferior border of the mandible. The jawline may be treated from the angle of the mandible to just posterior to the jowl, giving a nice lift and definition to the jawline.[92]

Ulthera

Ulthera treatment of the face may be performed alone or in continuity with a neck treatment. Typically, treatments are performed at a minimum of 2 depths with 1 pass of a 4 to 4.5-mm transducer and then retreating the area with a superficial 7 to 3.0-mm transducer. The first 2 depths may be followed with an advanced treatment protocol using the 10 to 1.5-mm transducer for dermal tightening (▶ Fig. 2.15 and ▶ Fig. 2.16). This multiple-depth treatment protocol is based on previous studies

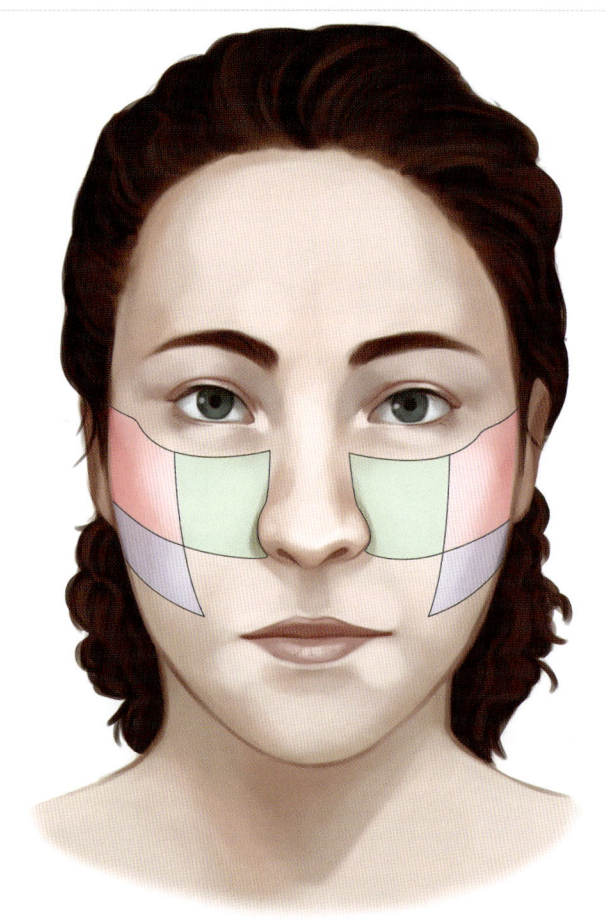

Fig. 2.12 Midface volume restoration. Key anatomic landmarks in midface volume restoration include the lower border of the cheek bone transversely down to the nasolabial fold; the upper border of the cheekbone and inferior orbital rim; the high point of the nasolabial fold; and the medial aspect of the bony zygomatic prominence. Filler is injected predominantly in the upper two-thirds of the medial cheek (green shading), where most patients have the greatest degree of volume loss. The injection is submuscular or deeper, and techniques include fanning and cross-hatching of product for uniform filling.

in which dual-depth treatments improved subjective outcomes on the upper face and midface.[45,93]

2.7 Nonsurgical Neck Rejuvenation (Lifting and Contouring)

The stigmata of the aging neck include hypertrophic or flaccid platysma muscles, skin excess, lipodystrophy, ptotic submandibular glands, and chronic sun damage (**Videos 2.9** and **2.10**).

2.7.1 Treatment Plan and Results

Ulthera

Similar to Ulthera treatment of the face, Ulthera neck treatments are performed at a minimum of 2 depths with 1 pass of a

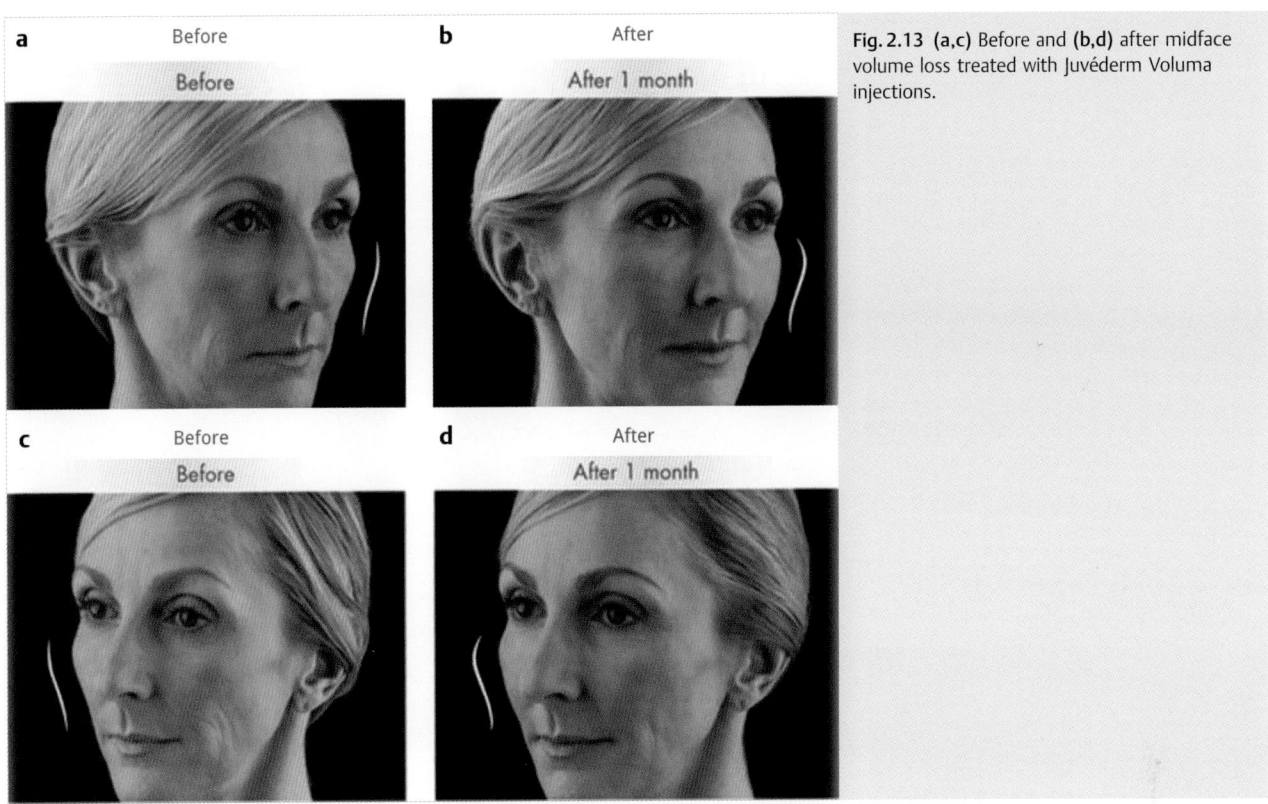

Fig. 2.13 (a,c) Before and (b,d) after midface volume loss treated with Juvéderm Voluma injections.

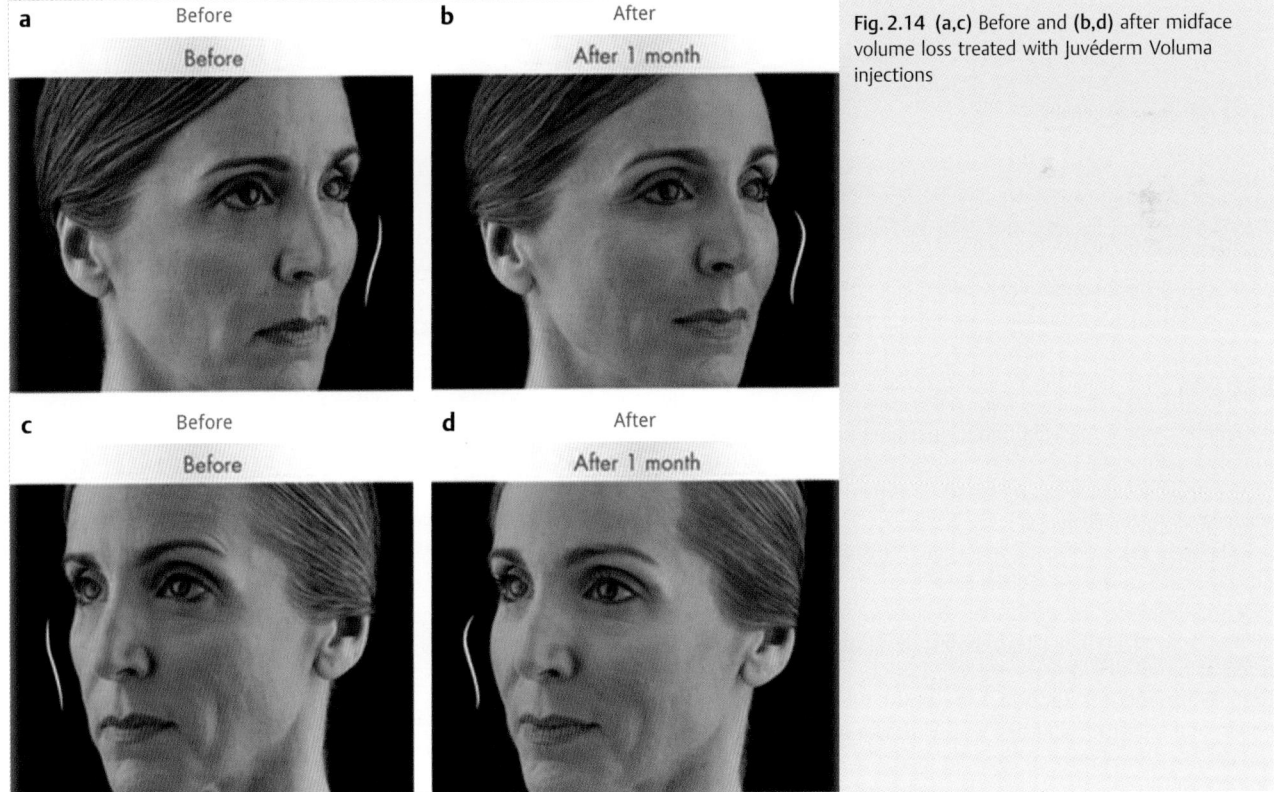

Fig. 2.14 (a,c) Before and (b,d) after midface volume loss treated with Juvéderm Voluma injections

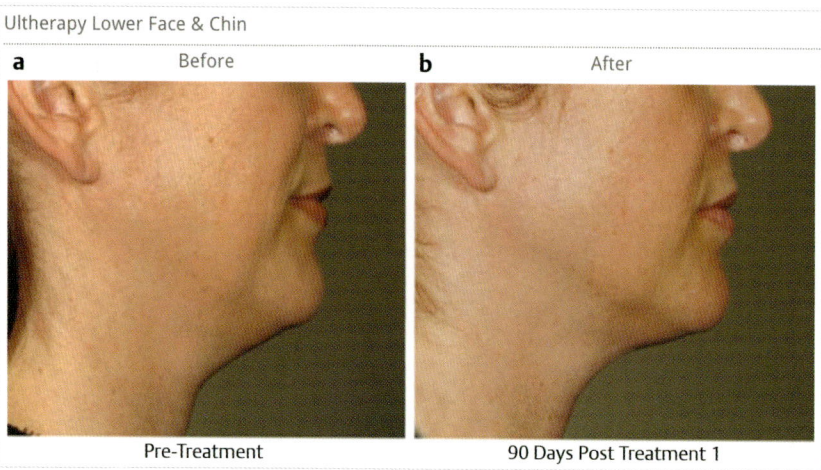

Fig. 2.15 (a) Before and (b) 90 days after Ulthera treatment of the lower face and chin

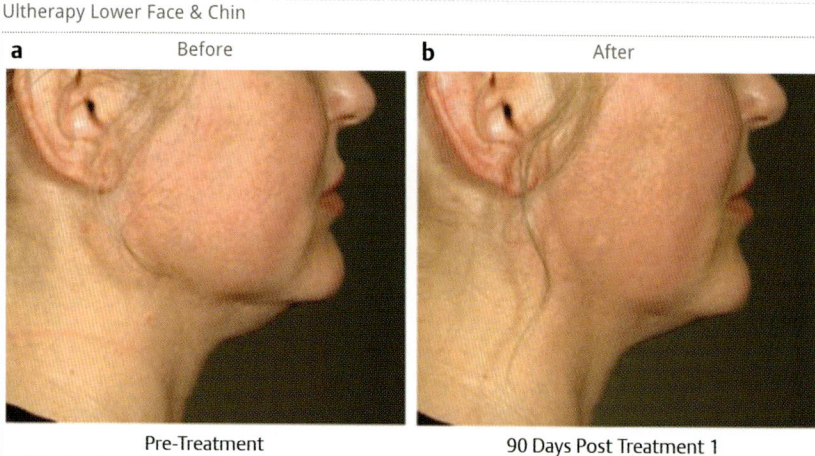

Fig. 2.16 (a) Before and (b) 90 days after Ulthera treatment of the lower face and chin.

4 to 4.5-mm transducer and then retreating the area with a superficial 7 to 3.0-mm transducer (▶ Fig. 2.17). The first 2 depths may be followed with an advanced treatment protocol using the 10 to 1.5-mm transducer for dermal tightening.[45]

Kybella

Kybella is a nonsurgical option for patients who do not want to undergo submental liposuction. It is indicated for improvement in the appearance of moderate to severe convexity or fullness associated with submental fat in adults.

Kybella is injected using a 30-gauge needle into subcutaneous fat tissue in the submental area. A single treatment consists of a maximum of 50 injections, 0.2 mL each (up to a total of 10 mL), spaced 1 cm apart. Up to 6 treatments may be administered at monthly intervals (▶ Fig. 2.18 and ▶ Fig. 2.19). Prior to each treatment, it is important to palpate the submental area to ensure sufficient fat and to identify subcutaneous fat between the dermis and platysma. To avoid injury to the marginal mandibular nerve, do not inject above the inferior border of the mandible or within a region defined by a 1.5-cm line below the inferior border (from the angle of the mandible to the mentum). Superficial injections into the dermis may result in skin ulceration. Postprocedure care includes wearing a chin strap for a few days after the procedure to minimize any swelling.

Neuromodulators

Younger patients with good skin elasticity and postoperative patients with residual neck banding are the ideal patients for neuromodulation in this area. The senior author injects 10 units of Botox/Xeomin or Dysport equivalent per band, mainly targeting the bands at the cervicomental area (▶ Fig. 2.20). Great care should be taken to avoid injection outside of the platysmal band, such as in the strap muscles, which can lead to complications of neck weakness, dyspnea, and ecchymosis (**see Video 1.1**).[15]

2.8 Nonsurgical Rhinoplasty

2.8.1 Treatment Plan

Fillers can be used to elevate the nose saddle, recontour the nasal tip, and inject filler at the base of the columella to lift the nasal tip as a whole. This is often useful in patients with aesthetic deformities too small to reliably refine with surgical correction or in patients who will not consider surgery.[92]

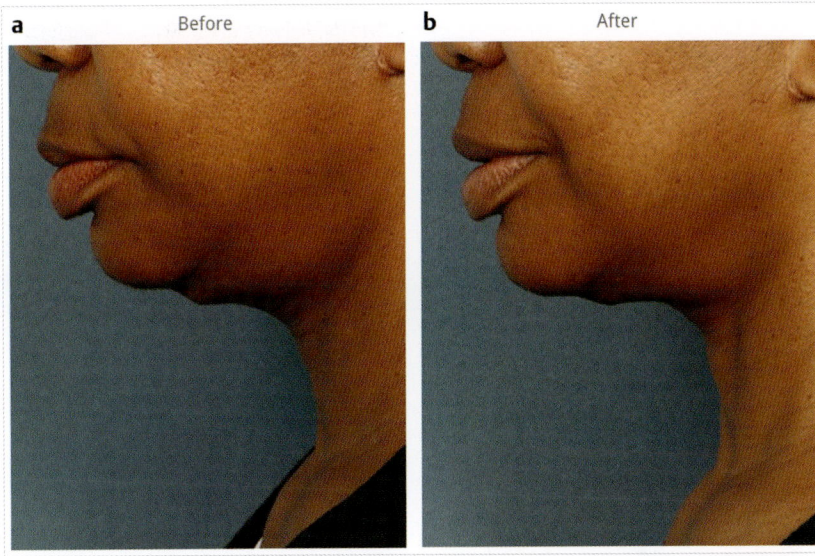

Fig. 2.17 (a) Before and (b) after submental fat treated with Kybella injections.

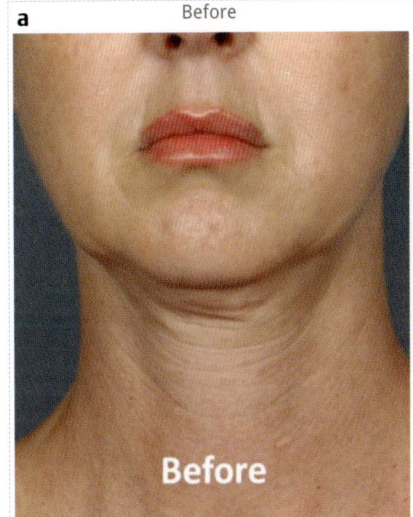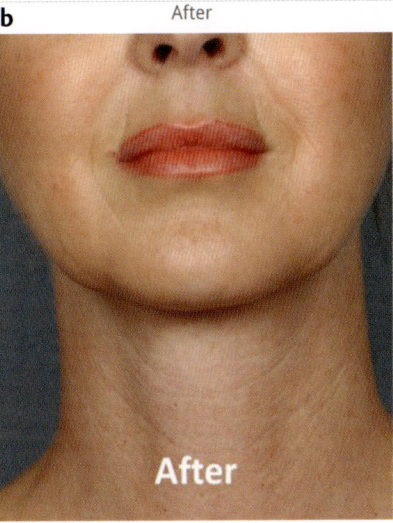

Fig. 2.18 (a) Before and (b) after submental fat treated with Kybella injections.

Injection is made in the deep dermis or subcutaneously in the tip and subcutaneously in the dorsum. Small amounts should be used with short linear threads or serial point injection. Molding or rolling can be used to smooth the material into the desired contour.

Caution is in order when performing injection rhinoplasty, because the nose is highly vascular with thin tissues under some pressure and tension against the underlying osseocartilaginous framework. Risks include intravascular injection with possible tissue loss in the nose, stroke or blindness, or vascular compromise due to compression with skin necrosis.[92]

2.9 Complications

2.9.1 Neuromodulators

Because the dosages used in cosmetic treatments are small, serious adverse events following BoNT are rare. Most adverse events are mild and temporary and include pain at injection sites, bruising, swelling, and flulike symptoms.[94] Advising patients to avoid medications that inhibit clotting for 2 weeks before treatment can decrease bruising. More significant complications are usually caused by poor injection techniques and unfamiliarity with muscle anatomy. Most of these result from diffusion of toxin into adjacent musculature, which can lead to unexpected muscle weakening. Periorbital complications include an overtreated frontalis, brow ptosis, eyelid ptosis, asymmetry, diplopia, ectropion, dry eyes, and decreased strength of eye closure. Brow ptosis can generally be avoided by injecting no more than 1 cm above the bony orbital rim in the midpupillary line and using lower doses in the frontalis.[84]

Upper eyelid ptosis most commonly occurs after BoNTA injections to the glabella, and can occur as early has 48 hours and as late as 14 days after injection (▶ Fig. 2.21). The duration rarely lasts more than 3 to 4 weeks. Most authors believe that the etiology of eyelid ptosis is diffusion of the toxin through the orbital septum into the levator palpebrae superioris muscle. However, the senior author feels that eyelid ptosis is related to

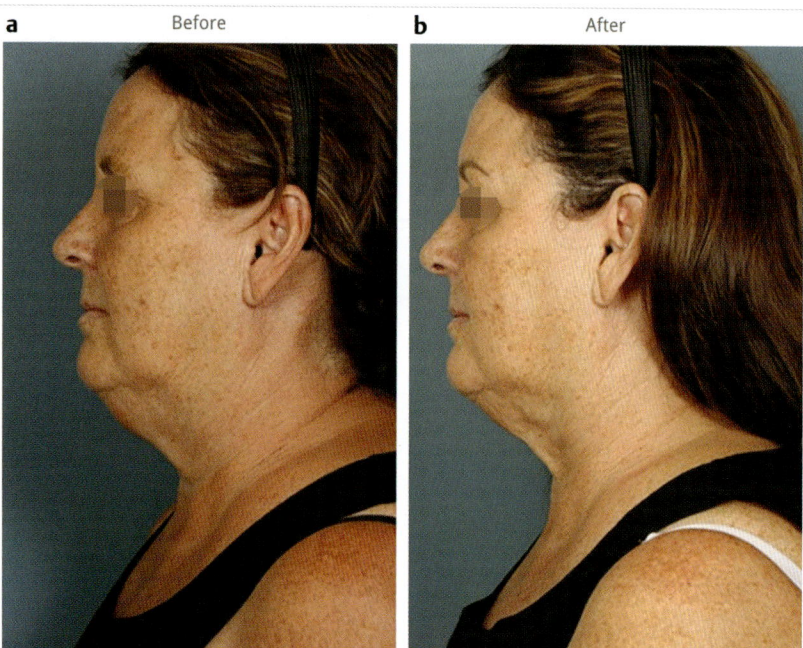

Fig. 2.19 (a) Before and (b) after submental fat treated with Kybella injections.

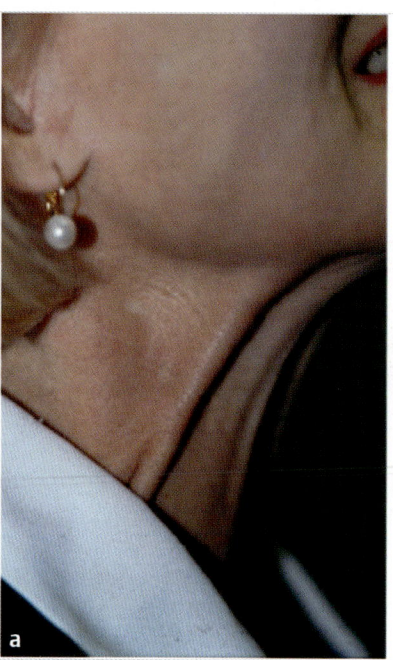 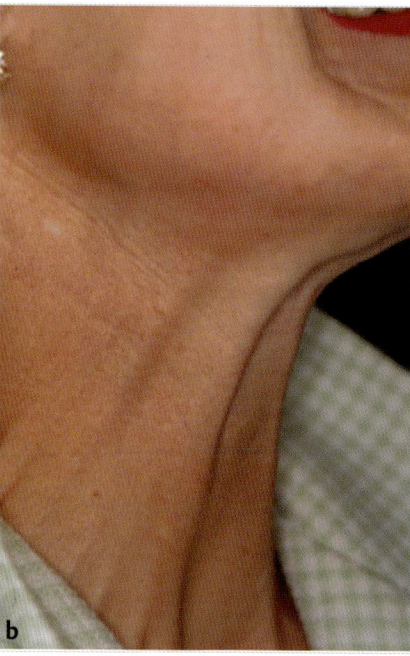

Fig. 2.20 (a) Before and (b) after platysmal bands treated with Botox injections.

hydrostatic pressure from injection or localized edema, with subsequent diffusion of product through the supraorbital and supratrochlear foramina (or notch) or the superior orbital fissure. Eyelid ptosis may be avoided by using a higher concentration (lower volume) of BoNTA and by applying low plunger pressure during injection.[84]

Lip asymmetries are seen in lower face injections. When performing botulinum toxin injections of the DAO muscle, injections should focus along the jawline inferior and slightly lateral to the oral commissure. Injecting too medially increases the risk for affecting the depressor labii muscle, causing asymmetric elevation of the lateral lip and an unfavorable functional outcome. Similarly, injection of the mentalis muscle should be directed near its origin at the mentum to prevent inadvertent paralysis of the more superiorly based depressor labii muscle.[15]

2.9.2 Soft Tissue Fillers

HA fillers have an excellent safety profile, and many complications can be avoided by using a careful injection technique. Though rare, the most serious complication associated with fillers is necrosis, which can occur when any filler is inadvertently

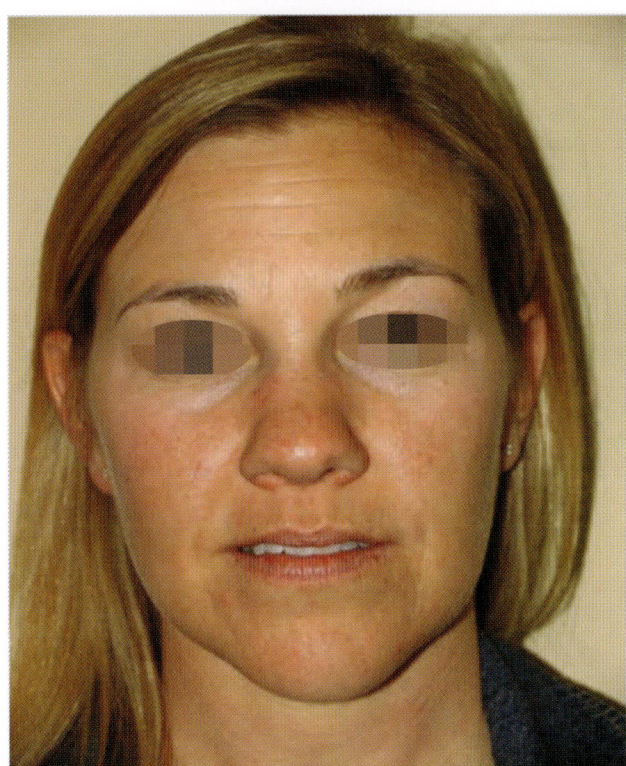

Fig. 2.21 Left eyelid ptosis after BoNTA injection.

injected intravascularly. Injectors must have a thorough knowledge of facial anatomy and blood supply. Slow injection (< 0.3 mL/min) with low pressure is particularly important for periorbital rejuvenation. If blanching and sudden pain occur, immediately stop and apply a topical vasodilator, because these are signs of possible blood vessel occlusion. Hyaluronidase should be given if an HA filler was used. Too superficial injection of HA filler can create visible ridges and an undesirable bluish tint known as the Tyndall effect. This is a well-known complication of HA injection into the nasojugal groove, which can be avoided by injecting into the subdermis. Other potential complications include arterial occlusion or embolization, which could result in blindness. Beading, clumping, and overcorrection are other potential complications. Massaging the area can help to distribute the filler. Finally, hyaluronidase can be used to reverse the unwanted effects of HA fillers. Other common complications include ecchymosis and edema.[17,84]

2.9.3 Kybella

Typical adverse events related to the use of deoxycholate (Kybella) have involved local, transient injection site reactions of mild to moderate intensity. The most common adverse events include pain, erythema, edema, ecchymosis, and numbness. Individual cases of marginal mandibular nerve injury were reported during clinical trials, all of which resolved spontaneously.[30,33,36]

The amount of postinjection inflammation and edema seems to be proportional to the amount of submental fat that is present. In the senior author's experience, patients with severe submental fat require a greater amount of deoxycholate and tend to experience more inflammation and edema after the treatment. Patients are encouraged to wear a chin strap for 1 to 3 days after treatment to reduce swelling.

2.9.4 Ulthera

Usually 2 to 3 hours of erythema is expected after the Ulthera procedure, but occasionally this may last 1 week or longer. This resolves spontaneously without intervention. Bruising is an infrequent but self-resolving complication. Sensory innervation to the treated areas reportedly occurs in up to 18% of patients.[40] Temporary numbness usually resolves without intervention in 2 to 3 weeks. Facial motor nerve injury has also been reported.[45] Full function of a near-total frontal-branch paresis returned by 6 months with observation alone.

2.9.5 Laser Skin Resurfacing

Mild complications of laser skin resurfacing include prolonged erythema, acne, milia, and contact dermatitis. Moderate complications include infection, pigmentary alteration, and eruptive keratoacanthomas. Severe complications include hypertrophic scarring and ectropion formation. Prolonged erythema is defined as posttreatment erythema that persists longer than 4 days with nonablative resurfacing and beyond 1 month with ablative treatment. It has been reported in < 1% of patients undergoing nonablative resurfacing and 12.5% of ablative laser–treated patients, although erythema typically resolves within 3 months in ablative laser–treated patients.[95,96] Fractional laser resurfacing treatments that use multiple laser passes or inadvertent stacking increase the risk of prolonged erythema.[78]

The rate of herpes simplex virus (HSV) infection, the most common type of infection that occurs after fractional laser skin resurfacing, has been reported in 0.3 to 2% of cases.[78,97] To minimize the risk of HSV reactivation, antiviral prophylaxis should be administered when a history of facial HSV is documented or if full-face ablative laser procedures are performed. Oral antiviral agents should be initiated 1 day before treatment and continued for 5 to 7 days. Bacterial infections are rarely observed after fractional skin resurfacing.[78,97] Because of the potential progression to scarring, broad-spectrum empiric antibiotics should be initiated and further adjusted based on culture results.

PIH is much less frequent with fractional laser skin resurfacing than with other ablative procedures, but it is observed in 1 to 32% of patients, depending on the system used, parameters applied, and skin phototypes treated.[78,98,99,100,101,102,103] Patients with darker skin phototypes (Fitzpatrick III-VI) have a higher likelihood of developing PIH, although hyperpigmentation often resolves without treatment, and in the senior author's experience has never been permanent. The application of topical steroids, bleaching, and peeling agents can hasten the resolution of PIH. Hypopigmentation is extremely rare, with a delayed onset (6 to 12 months postoperatively).[78]

Hypertrophic scarring is a rare complication of ablative skin resurfacing, and is usually caused by using excessively high energy densities, postoperative skin infection, and improper technique. The neck is especially susceptible to the development of scarring because of the small number of pilosebaceous units, and thin skin renders it more susceptible to thermal injury. Patients with a history of radiation or surgical procedures involving the neck or eyelids, or patients who have experienced postoperative wound infection, contact dermatitis, or keloid scarring, have the highest risk of scarring.[78] Early treatment of hypertrophic scarring involves the use of topical corticosteroids, silicone gel, and intralesional corticosteroid injections.[78]

2.10 Conclusion

Nonsurgical approaches for facial rejuvenation are in continuous demand by patients, and have evolved tremendously over the past several years due to the increasing development of new products and devices. It is crucial to understand the muscular anatomy and changes associated with the aging face to effectively treat patients. Just as important is the proper selection of products for patient goals, and well-thought-out and careful technique to optimize results and minimize complications. Perhaps the most critical key to success is proper patient selection and counseling. The limitations and indications of these treatments must be understood by the physician and patient to ensure the greatest possible satisfaction with minimally invasive facial rejuvenation. When the previously mentioned measures are taken, a true alternative to surgical intervention exists for many individuals.

2.11 Commentary

Julius W. Few Jr.

In this chapter, we see a scientifically supported approach to combining modalities to address age-related and nonaesthetic findings in the head and neck. In particular, multimodal approaches are based on currently available, U.S. FDA–approved modalities. As with much of technology, Juvéderm Volbella is currently approved for the treatment of perioral wrinkles and related deficiencies. The authors are to be commended for considering the future of available fillers and related novel technology.

We have found that the successful use of micro-focused ultrasound to treat the aging face and neck can lead to a rejuvenated neck but can also unmask platysmal banding that can be troubling to the patient, because this is a dynamic finding. We offer patients the use of a neuromodulator injection, typically 25 to 40 units of Botox or Xeomin or 50 to 80 units of Dysport injected along the course of the paramedian platysmal bands. For a more permanent solution, we offer closed platysmotomy first described in Brazil by Marcelo Daher.[104] The technique relies on the use of a sutures placed percutaneously around muscle band segments at three to six levels for each paramedian band, and then the suture is tightened or "used to saw" through the bands under local anesthesia injection. The muscle is then rendered inactive and the more lateral muscle can pull laterally unopposed.

Another solution to the more extensive submental platysmal band is a submental limited open corset platysmaplasty to the level of the thyroid cartilage with or without partial division, as shown in **Videos 2.11** and **2.12**, combined with simultaneous micro-focused ultrasound treatment to the upper face and lateral neck. This can be done under a simple local anesthetic, requires very little time for the surgical specialist to produce, and recovery is typically brief. (▶ Fig. 2.22 and ▶ Fig. 2.23).

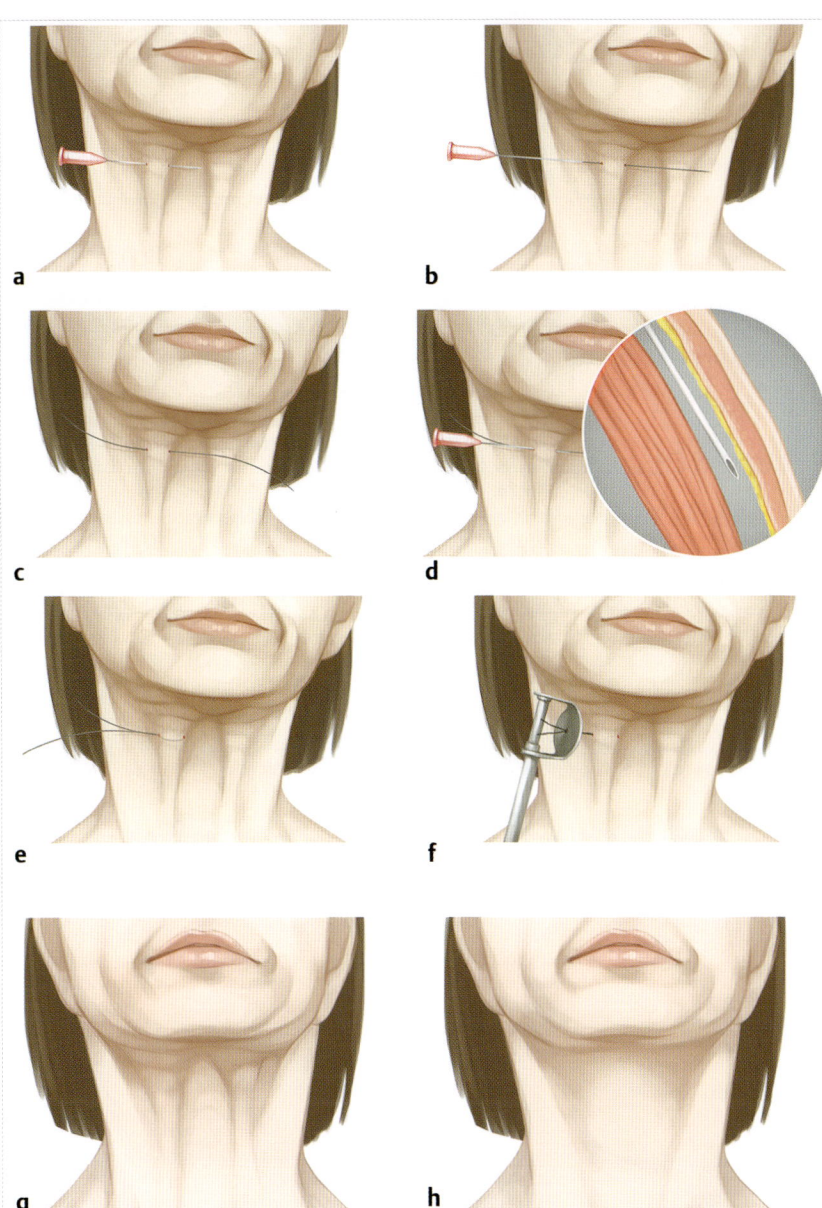

Fig. 2.22 The platysma band myotomy proceeds through the following schematic steps: (a) The needle transfixes the skin and passes behind the platysma band before emerging from the skin on the opposite side. (b) and (c) The steel wire is threaded through the needle, emerging from the opposite end. The needle is then removed, leaving the wire in position. (d) The needle is reinserted through the first entrance point. By digital maneuvering, a space is created between the dermis and the space around the platysma band until the end of the needle exits from the opposite hole. (e) The steel wire is folded over itself to form a loop whose point is introduced at the end of the needle emerging from the opposite side. The wire encircles the band in a loop, with the two ends together and outside the first entrance hole of the skin. (f) The platysmotome plate, supported on the skin, receives the two steel wires, which pass through the central hole of the plate. The wires go through the respective smaller holes of the rod and are rolled around it, after which the excess wire is cut. The "butterfly" blades on the inferior end of the hollow cylinder are turned, which forces the loop to section the muscle and exit through the initial entrance hole. (g,h) The appearance of the neck before and after sectioning of the platysma band. (Modified from Daher, JC: Closed Platysmotomy: A New Procedure for the Treatment of Platysma Bands Without Skin Dissection, Aesthetic Plast Surg. 2011 Oct; 35(5): 866–877)

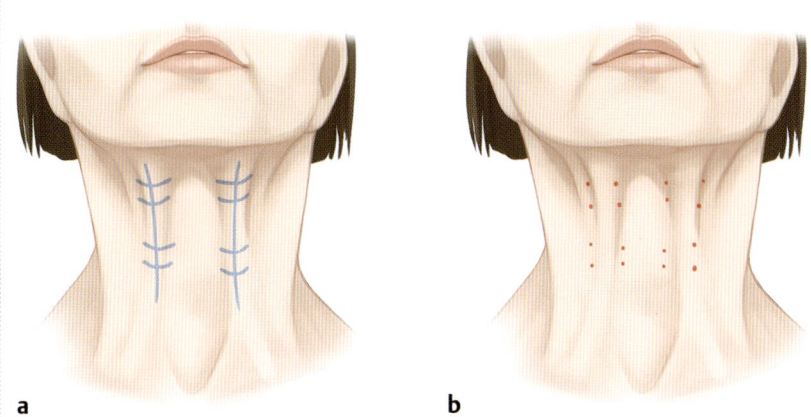

Fig. 2.23 (a) Frontal, close-up, preoperative view of a neck with two long, separate platysma bands marked for the bands to be cut at four levels. (b) Immediately after the procedure was performed to show the appearance of the skin, already described in the text. No facelifts or neck lifts were performed for this patient. (Modified from Daher, JC: Closed Platysmotomy: A New Procedure for the Treatment of Platysma Bands Without Skin Dissection, Aesthetic Plast Surg. 2011 Oct; 35(5): 866–877)

References

[1] Bapna S, Maas CS. Patient Selection, Counseling, and Informed Consent. In: Sadick NS, ed. Augmentation Fillers. New York: Cambridge; 2010:13–16

[2] Narins RS, Brandt FS, Lorenc ZP, Maas CS, Monheit GD, Smith SR. Twelve-month persistency of a novel ribose-cross-linked collagen dermal filler. Dermatol Surg. 2008; 34 Suppl 1:S31–S39

[3] Narins RS, Brandt FS, Lorenc ZP, et al. A randomized, multicenter study of the safety and efficacy of Dermicol-P35 and non-animal-stabilized hyaluronic acid gel for the correction of nasolabial folds. Dermatol Surg. 2007; 33 Suppl 2:S213–S221, discussion S221

[4] Eppley BL, Dadvand B. Injectable soft-tissue fillers: clinical overview. Plast Reconstr Surg. 2006; 118(4):98e–106e

[5] Reisman NR. Ethics, legal issues, and consent for fillers. Clin Plast Surg. 2006; 33(4):505–510

[6] Ali MJ, Ende K, Maas CS. Perioral rejuvenation and lip augmentation. Facial Plast Surg Clin North Am. 2007; 15(4):491–500, vii

[7] Engelman DE, Bloom B, Goldberg DJ. Dermal fillers: complications and informed consent. J Cosmet Laser Ther. 2005; 7(1):29–32

[8] The American Society of Plastic Surgeons (ASPS). Available at: http://www.plasticsurgery.org. Accessed November 30, 2015

[9] Scott AB. Botulinum toxin injection into extraocular muscles as an alternative to strabismus surgery. J Pediatr Ophthalmol Strabismus. 1980; 17(1):21–25

[10] Schantz EJ, Johnson EA. Botulinum toxin: the story of its development for the treatment of human disease. Perspect Biol Med. 1997; 40(3):317–327

[11] Schantz EJ, Johnson EA. Preparation and characterization of botulinum toxin type A for human treatment. In: Jankovic J, ed. Therapy with botulinum toxin. New York: Marcel Dekker; 1994:41–50

[12] Ramirez AL, Reeck J, Maas CS. Preliminary experience with botulinum toxin type B in hyperkinetic facial lines. Plast Reconstr Surg. 2002; 109(6):2154–2155

[13] Ramirez AL, Reeck J, Maas CS. Botulinum toxin type B (MyoBloc) in the management of hyperkinetic facial lines. Otolaryngol Head Neck Surg. 2002; 126(5):459–467

[14] Maas CS. Botulinum neurotoxins and injectable fillers: minimally invasive management of the aging upper face. Facial Plast Surg Clin North Am. 2006; 14(3):241–245

[15] Attenello NH, Sheu M, Maas CS. Neuromodulators in Facial Aesthetics. In: Papel I, ed. Facial plastic and reconstructive surgery. 4th ed. New York: Thieme; 2015

[16] Attenello NH, Maas CS. Injectable fillers: review of material and properties. Facial Plast Surg. 2015; 31(1):29–34

[17] Nettar K, Maas C. Facial filler and neurotoxin complications. Facial Plast Surg. 2012; 28(3):288–293

[18] Maas CS, Bapna S. Pins and needles: minimally invasive office techniques for facial rejuvenation. Facial Plast Surg. 2009; 25(4):260–269

[19] Carruthers JDA, Glogau RG, Blitzer A, Facial Aesthetics Consensus Group Faculty. Advances in facial rejuvenation: botulinum toxin type a, hyaluronic acid dermal fillers, and combination therapies–consensus recommendations. Plast Reconstr Surg. 2008; 121(5) Suppl:5S–30S, quiz 31S–36S

[20] Sundaram H, Cassuto D. Biophysical characteristics of hyaluronic acid soft-tissue fillers and their relevance to aesthetic applications. Plast Reconstr Surg. 2013; 132(4) Suppl 2:5S–21S

[21] Fagien S, Maas C, Murphy DK, Thomas JA, Beddingfield FC, III, Juvéderm Lips Study Group. Juvederm ultra for lip enhancement: an open-label, multicenter study. Aesthet Surg J. 2013; 33(3):414–420

[22] Callan P, Goodman GJ, Carlisle I, et al. Efficacy and safety of a hyaluronic acid filler in subjects treated for correction of midface volume deficiency: a 24 month study. Clin Cosmet Investig Dermatol. 2013; 6:81–89

[23] Jones D, Murphy DK. Volumizing hyaluronic acid filler for midface volume deficit: 2-year results from a pivotal single-blind randomized controlled study. Dermatol Surg. 2013; 39(11):1602–1612

[24] Hevia O, Cohen BH, Howell DJ. Safety and efficacy of a cohesive polydensified matrix hyaluronic acid for the correction of infraorbital hollow: an observational study with results at 40 weeks. J Drugs Dermatol. 2014; 13(9):1030–1036

[25] Lorenc ZP, Fagien S, Flynn TC, Waldorf HA. Clinical application and assessment of Belotero: a roundtable discussion. Plast Reconstr Surg. 2013; 132(4) Suppl 2:69S–76S

[26] Ahn MS. Calcium hydroxylapatite: Radiesse. Facial Plast Surg Clin North Am. 2007; 15(1):85–90

[27] Berlin AL, Hussain M, Goldberg DJ. Calcium hydroxylapatite filler for facial rejuvenation: a histologic and immunohistochemical analysis. Dermatol Surg. 2008; 34 Suppl 1:S64–S67

[28] Jacovella PF. Use of calcium hydroxylapatite (Radiesse) for facial augmentation. Clin Interv Aging. 2008; 3(1):161–174

[29] Kontis TC. Contemporary review of injectable facial fillers. JAMA Facial Plast Surg. 2013; 15(1):58–64

[30] Wollina U, Goldman A. ATX-101 for reduction of submental fat. Expert Opin Pharmacother. 2015; 16(5):755–762

[31] Rose PT, Morgan M. Histological changes associated with mesotherapy for fat dissolution. J Cosmet Laser Ther. 2005; 7(1):17–19

[32] Park EJ, Kim HS, Kim M, Oh HJ. Histological changes after treatment for localized fat deposits with phosphatidylcholine and sodium deoxycholate. J Cosmet Dermatol. 2013; 12(3):240–243

[33] Ascher B, Hoffmann K, Walker P, Lippert S, Wollina U, Havlickova B. Efficacy, patient-reported outcomes and safety profile of ATX-101 (deoxycholic acid), an injectable drug for the reduction of unwanted submental fat: results from a phase III, randomized, placebo-controlled study. J Eur Acad Dermatol Venereol. 2014; 28(12):1707–1715

[34] Reeds DN, Mohammed BS, Klein S, Boswell CB, Young VL. Metabolic and structural effects of phosphatidylcholine and deoxycholate injections on subcutaneous fat: a randomized, controlled trial. Aesthet Surg J. 2013; 33(3):400–408

[35] Salti G, Ghersetich I, Tantussi F, Bovani B, Lotti T. Phosphatidylcholine and sodium deoxycholate in the treatment of localized fat: a double-blind, randomized study. Dermatol Surg. 2008; 34(1):60–66, discussion 66

[36] Rzany B, Griffiths T, Walker P, Lippert S, McDiarmid J, Havlickova B. Reduction of unwanted submental fat with ATX-101 (deoxycholic acid), an adipocytolytic injectable treatment: results from a phase III, randomized, placebo-controlled study. Br J Dermatol. 2014; 170(2):445–453

[37] Rotunda AM, Weiss SR, Rivkin LS. Randomized double-blind clinical trial of subcutaneously injected deoxycholate versus a phosphatidylcholine-deoxycholate combination for the reduction of submental fat. Dermatol Surg. 2009; 35(5):792–803

[38] Fry WJ, Wulff VJ, Tucker D, Fry FJ. Physical factors Involved in ultrasonically induced changes in living systems: I. Identification of non-temperature effects. J Acoust Soc Am. 1950; 22(6):867–876

[39] Fry WJ. Intense ultrasound; a new tool for neurological research. J Ment Sci. 1954; 100(418):85–96

[40] Suh DH, Shin MK, Lee SJ, et al. Intense focused ultrasound tightening in Asian skin: clinical and pathologic results. Dermatol Surg. 2011; 37(11):1595–1602

[41] White WM, Makin IR, Slayton MH, Barthe PG, Gliklich R. Selective transcutaneous delivery of energy to porcine soft tissues using Intense Ultrasound (IUS). Lasers Surg Med. 2008; 40(2):67–75

[42] White WM, Makin IR, Barthe PG, Slayton MH, Gliklich RE. Selective creation of thermal injury zones in the superficial musculoaponeurotic system using intense ultrasound therapy: a new target for noninvasive facial rejuvenation. Arch Facial Plast Surg. 2007; 9(1):22–29

[43] Laubach HJ, Makin IR, Barthe PG, Slayton MH, Manstein D. Intense focused ultrasound: evaluation of a new treatment modality for precise microcoagulation within the skin. Dermatol Surg. 2008; 34(5):727–734

[44] Gliklich RE, White WM, Slayton MH, Barthe PG, Makin IR. Clinical pilot study of intense ultrasound therapy to deep dermal facial skin and subcutaneous tissues. Arch Facial Plast Surg. 2007; 9(2):88–95

[45] Brobst RW, Ferguson M, Perkins SW. Noninvasive treatment of the neck. Facial Plast Surg Clin North Am. 2014; 22(2):191–202

[46] Alam M, White LE, Martin N, Witherspoon J, Yoo S, West DP. Ultrasound tightening of facial and neck skin: a rater-blinded prospective cohort study. J Am Acad Dermatol. 2010; 62(2):262–269

[47] Kenkel J. Evaluation of the Ulthera system for improving skin laxity and tightening. Abstract presentation. ASAPS Annual Meeting. Vancouver, Canada, May 3–8, 2012

[48] Chan HH, Alam M, Kono T, Dover JS. Clinical application of lasers in Asians. Dermatol Surg. 2002; 28(7):556–563

[49] Tan J, Lei Y, Ouyang HW, Gold MH. The use of the fractional CO2 laser resurfacing in the treatment of photoaging in Asians: five years long-term results. Lasers Surg Med. 2014; 46(10):750–756

[50] Manstein D, Herron GS, Sink RK, Tanner H, Anderson RR. Fractional photothermolysis: a new concept for cutaneous remodeling using microscopic patterns of thermal injury. Lasers Surg Med. 2004; 34(5):426–438

[51] Tierney EP, Hanke CW. Ablative fractionated CO2, laser resurfacing for the neck: prospective study and review of the literature. J Drugs Dermatol. 2009; 8(8):723–731

[52] Avram MM, Tope WD, Yu T, Szachowicz E, Nelson JS. Hypertrophic scarring of the neck following ablative fractional carbon dioxide laser resurfacing. Lasers Surg Med. 2009; 41(3):185–188
[53] Geronemus RG. Fractional photothermolysis: current and future applications. Lasers Surg Med. 2006; 38(3):169–176
[54] Duplechain JK. Neck skin rejuvenation. Facial Plast Surg Clin North Am. 2014; 22(2):203–216
[55] Aslam A, Alster TS. Evolution of laser skin resurfacing: from scanning to fractional technology. Dermatol Surg. 2014; 40(11):1163–1172
[56] Waldorf HA, Kauvar ANB, Geronemus RG. Skin resurfacing of fine to deep rhytides using a char-free carbon dioxide laser in 47 patients. Dermatol Surg. 1995; 21(11):940–946
[57] Lowe NJ, Lask G, Griffin ME, Maxwell A, Lowe P, Quilada F. Skin resurfacing with the Ultrapulse carbon dioxide laser. Observations on 100 patients. Dermatol Surg. 1995; 21(12):1025–1029
[58] Fitzpatrick RE, Goldman MP, Satur NM, Tope WD. Pulsed carbon dioxide laser resurfacing of photo-aged facial skin. Arch Dermatol. 1996; 132(4): 395–402
[59] Alster TS, Garg S. Treatment of facial rhytides with a high-energy pulsed carbon dioxide laser. Plast Reconstr Surg. 1996; 98(5):791–794
[60] Alster TS. Comparison of two high-energy, pulsed carbon dioxide lasers in the treatment of periorbital rhytides. Dermatol Surg. 1996; 22(6):541–545
[61] Ross EV, Miller C, Meehan K, et al. One-pass CO2 versus multiple-pass Er: YAG laser resurfacing in the treatment of rhytides: a comparison side-by-side study of pulsed CO2 and Er:YAG lasers. Dermatol Surg. 2001; 27(8): 709–715
[62] Goldberg DJ, Whitworth J. Laser skin resurfacing with the Q-switched Nd: YAG laser. Dermatol Surg. 1997; 23(10):903–906, discussion 906–907
[63] Lupton JR, Williams CM, Alster TS. Nonablative laser skin resurfacing using a 1540 nm erbium glass laser: a clinical and histologic analysis. Dermatol Surg. 2002; 28(9):833–835
[64] Tanzi EL, Williams CM, Alster TS. Treatment of facial rhytides with a nonablative 1,450-nm diode laser: a controlled clinical and histologic study. Dermatol Surg. 2003; 29(2):124–128
[65] Lee MW. Combination 532-nm and 1064-nm lasers for noninvasive skin rejuvenation and toning. Arch Dermatol. 2003; 139(10):1265–1276
[66] Tanzi EL, Alster TS. Comparison of a 1450-nm diode laser and a 1320-nm Nd:YAG laser in the treatment of atrophic facial scars: a prospective clinical and histologic study. Dermatol Surg. 2004; 30(2 Pt 1):152–157
[67] Friedman PM, Jih MH, Skover GR, Payonk GS, Kimyai-Asadi A, Geronemus RG. Treatment of atrophic facial acne scars with the 1064-nm Q-switched Nd:YAG laser: six-month follow-up study. Arch Dermatol. 2004; 140(11): 1337–1341
[68] Doshi SN, Alster TS. 1,450 nm long-pulsed diode laser for nonablative skin rejuvenation. Dermatol Surg. 2005; 31(9 Pt 2):1223–1226, discussion 1226
[69] Wanner M, Tanzi EL, Alster TS. Fractional photothermolysis: treatment of facial and nonfacial cutaneous photodamage with a 1,550-nm erbium-doped fiber laser. Dermatol Surg. 2007; 33(1):23–28
[70] Alster TS, Tanzi EL, Lazarus M. The use of fractional laser photothermolysis for the treatment of atrophic scars. Dermatol Surg. 2007; 33(3):295–299
[71] Chrastil B, Glaich AS, Goldberg LH, Friedman PM. Second-generation 1,550-nm fractional photothermolysis for the treatment of acne scars. Dermatol Surg. 2008; 34(10):1327–1332
[72] Chan NPY, Ho SGY, Yeung CK, Shek SY, Chan HH. The use of non-ablative fractional resurfacing in Asian acne scar patients. Lasers Surg Med. 2010; 42 (10):710–715
[73] Jih MH, Goldberg LH, Kimyai-Asadi A. Fractional photothermolysis for photoaging of hands. Dermatol Surg. 2008; 34(1):73–78
[74] Jung JY, Lee JH, Ryu DJ, Lee SJ, Bang D, Cho SB. Lower-fluence, higher-density versus higher-fluence, lower-density treatment with a 10,600-nm carbon dioxide fractional laser system: a split-face, evaluator-blinded study. Dermatol Surg. 2010; 36(12):2022–2029
[75] Tierney EP, Hanke CW. Fractionated carbon dioxide laser treatment of photoaging: prospective study in 45 patients and review of the literature. Dermatol Surg. 2011; 37(9):1279–1290
[76] Preissig J, Hamilton K, Markus R. Current laser resurfacing technologies: a review that delves beneath the surface. Semin Plast Surg. 2012; 26(3):109–116
[77] Kaplan H, Gat A. Clinical and histopathological results following TriPollar radiofrequency skin treatments. J Cosmet Laser Ther. 2009; 11(2):78–84
[78] Metelitsa AI, Alster TS. Fractionated laser skin resurfacing treatment complications: a review. Dermatol Surg. 2010; 36(3):299–306
[79] Scheiner A, Baker SS. Laser Management of Festoons. In: Massry GG, Murphy MR, Azizzadeh B, eds. Master techniques in blepharoplasty and periorbital rejuvenation. New York: Springer; 2011:211–221
[80] Ahn MS, Catten M, Maas CS. Temporal brow lift using botulinum toxin A. Plast Reconstr Surg. 2000; 105(3):1129–1135, discussion 1136–1139
[81] Maas CS, Kim EJ. Temporal brow lift using botulinum toxin A: an update. Plast Reconstr Surg. 2003; 112(5) Suppl:109S–112S, discussion 113S–114S
[82] Finn JC, Cox S. Fillers in the periorbital complex. Facial Plast Surg Clin North Am. 2007; 15(1):123–132, viii
[83] Maas CS, Yu K, Egan KK. Neuromodulators and injectable soft tissue substitutes. In: Papel I, ed. Facial plastic and reconstructive surgery. 3rd ed. New York: Thieme; 2009:346
[84] Maas CS, Yu K, Nettar KD. Neuromodulators and fillers in periorbital rejuvenation. In: Massry GG, Murphy MR, Azizzadeh B, eds. Master techniques in blepharoplasty and periorbital rejuvenation. New York: Springer; 2011:289–296
[85] Maloney BP. Aesthetic surgery of the lip. In: Papel ID, ed. Facial plastic and reconstructive surgery. 2nd ed. New York: Thieme; 2002:344–352
[86] Loos BM, Maas CS. Relevant anatomy for botulinum toxin facial rejuvenation. Facial Plast Surg Clin North Am. 2003; 11(4):439–443
[87] Cohen JL, Ross EV. Combined fractional ablative and nonablative laser resurfacing treatment: a split-face comparative study. J Drugs Dermatol. 2013; 12(2):175–178
[88] Graham HD, Quatela VC, Sabini P. Endoscopic approach to the brow and midface. In: Papel ID, ed. Facial plastic and reconstructive surgery. 3rd ed. New York: Thieme; 2009:227–241
[89] Marianetti TM, Cozzolino S, Torroni A, Gasparini G, Pelo S. The "beauty arch:" a new aesthetic analysis for malar augmentation planning. J Craniofac Surg. 2015; 26(3):625–630
[90] Montes JR. Volumetric considerations for lower eyelid and midface rejuvenation. Curr Opin Ophthalmol. 2012; 23(5):443–449
[91] Shamban A. Customized approach to facial enhancement. Facial Plast Surg Clin North Am. 2015; 23(4):471–477
[92] Bass LS. Injectable filler techniques for facial rejuvenation, volumization, and augmentation. Facial Plast Surg Clin North Am. 2015; 23(4):479–488
[93] Sasaki GH, Tevez A. Clinical efficacy and safety of focused-image ultrasonography: a 2-year experience. Aesthet Surg J. 2012; 32(5):601–612
[94] Alam M, Dover JS, Klein AW, Arndt KA. Botulinum a exotoxin for hyperfunctional facial lines: where not to inject. Arch Dermatol. 2002; 138 (9):1180–1185
[95] Rahman Z, MacFalls H, Jiang K, et al. Fractional deep dermal ablation induces tissue tightening. Lasers Surg Med. 2009; 41(2):78–86
[96] Chapas AM, Brightman L, Sukal S, et al. Successful treatment of acneiform scarring with CO2 ablative fractional resurfacing. Lasers Surg Med. 2008; 40 (6):381–386
[97] Setyadi HG, Jacobs AA, Markus RF. Infectious complications after nonablative fractional resurfacing treatment. Dermatol Surg. 2008; 34(11):1595–1598
[98] Rokhsar CK, Fitzpatrick RE. The treatment of melasma with fractional photothermolysis: a pilot study. Dermatol Surg. 2005; 31(12):1645–1650
[99] Tanzi EL, Wanitphakdeedecha R, Alster TS. Fraxel laser indications and long-term follow-up. Aesthet Surg J. 2008; 28(6):675–678, discussion 679–680
[100] Chan HH, Manstein D, Yu CS, Shek S, Kono T, Wei WI. The prevalence and risk factors of post-inflammatory hyperpigmentation after fractional resurfacing in Asians. Lasers Surg Med. 2007; 39(5):381–385
[101] Hu S, Chen MC, Lee MC, Yang LC, Keoprasom N. Fractional resurfacing for the treatment of atrophic facial acne scars in asian skin. Dermatol Surg. 2009; 35(5):826–832
[102] Walgrave SE, Ortiz AE, MacFalls HT, et al. Evaluation of a novel fractional resurfacing device for treatment of acne scarring. Lasers Surg Med. 2009; 41 (2):122–127
[103] Rahman Z, Alam M, Dover JS. Fractional Laser treatment for pigmentation and texture improvement. Skin Therapy Lett. 2006; 11(9):7–11
[104] Daher JC. Closed platysmotomy: a new procedure for the treatment of platysma bands without skin dissection. Aesthetic Plast Surg. 2011; 35(5): 866–877

3 Background of Noninvasive Technology: Evolving Patient Selection

Julius W. Few Jr.

Summary

This chapter discusses the ability to incorporate nonsurgical technology into a clinical practice and how powerful that enhancement can be. However, there are risks, and patient selection and an expanding patient base are at the forefront. As technology continues to evolve and grow, we are seeing more and more near-surgical outcomes without the surgery. As a result, we are seeing exponentially more patients seeking nonsurgical treatment options. Although surgical intervention remains the gold standard for cosmetic enhancement, we are now realizing that there are a variety of ways to achieve our patients' goals without surgery.

Keywords: invasive, noninvasive, risk, microfocused ultrasound, fillers, toxins, photorejuvenation, intense pulsed light (IPL) treatments

> **Key Points**
>
> - Patients can be happy with their results without necessarily achieving surgical perfection.
> - Some patient groups who have traditionally not been candidates for surgery, such as patients of color, may be good candidates for minimally invasive procedures.
> - As technology continues to evolve and grow, we are seeing more and more near surgical outcomes without surgery and hence an increase in our patient base.
> - In addition, patients who get an improvement with nonsurgical cosmetic care may pursue surgical cosmetic care in the future.

3.1 Introduction

If you had asked me what I wanted to do in medical school, the answer was "ophthalmic surgeon" in my second year and "heart surgeon" in my third year. This is particularly important to the evolution I will highlight below.

The birth of The Few Institute came 8 years after I was at a major metropolitan academic medical center, Northwestern Memorial Hospital in Chicago. I was the fourth plastic surgeon to join the practice after spending time learning about oculoplastic surgery. I was fortunate to be given a lot of freedom in the beginning, and I focused on a traditional academic plastic surgery practice. I taught the residents from Northwestern University and did active clinical research, while growing a very busy reconstructive and cosmetic practice. As I continued to treat a very sophisticated group of patients while doing research with the dermatology department next door, it became very apparent that less invasive cosmetic modalities were desirable. In addition, major concerns about injectable treatments in patients with pigmented skin led me to do the first clinical study focused on hyaluronic fillers in skin of a color, such as Restylane.[1] This study not only proved that injectable fillers could be used safely in skin of color, but also it highlighted the important fact that people of color are just as interested in cosmetic enhancement as people with nonethnic skin. This realization helped me to really ask the question, "What are the barriers to cosmetic surgery?" A principle barrier is the perception of risk, risk of complication, risk of loss in identity, permanent changes, "looking fake," etc. As I looked closer, it became apparent that the ability to offer a nonsurgical option in a patient with a history of keloids or a patient who is averse to surgery in general, was widely embraced, and I could witness the birth of cosmetic ethnic medicine on a larger scale.[2]

In the late 1990s, the advent of filler and botulinum toxin created a quiet revolution.[3] I remember sitting in a national American Society of Plastic Surgeons (ASPS) meeting and having various surgeons state that this was a fad that will pass, just like skin-only facelifts, because the general belief at the time was that "lesser invasiveness means lesser results." According to statistics from the major dermatologic and plastic surgery organizations,[4] there is more than a tenfold dominance, which is increasing, for injectable treatments compared to aesthetic surgery.

As an early adopter of the use of fillers and neurotoxins, I learned many things about the larger population of patients wanting minimally invasive cosmetic enhancement. An important misconception for us as plastic surgeons is the one definition for successful rejuvenation of the face and neck: "surgical perfection." Although surgical intervention remains the gold standard for cosmetic enhancement, I am now realizing that there are a variety of ways to achieve our patients' goals without surgery. I began to learn that making a heavy frown line, or "parenthesis," softer around the mouth through a nonsurgical technique could make a woman feel instantly better, sometimes several magnitudes greater than the happy surgical patient. The difference was that it was much easier to get the desired result, and the recuperation time was shorter and easier by comparison. I learned that the experience for the cosmetic patient was often as important as (in some cases more important than) the result, assuming there was visual improvement. This was the "Eyes Wide Shut" moment for me as a plastic surgeon. As my experience grew, especially in certain groups of patients, such as certain ethnic patients, who were traditionally not candidates for surgery, I learned that these patients were candidates for minimally invasive treatment. This rapid increase in the patient base opened the door to developing strategies in minimally invasive procedures, such as light- and energy-based treatments, and injectable treatments.

3.2 More Than Skin Deep

According to Dr. Dayan,[5] it turns out that looking happy and healthy is more than just a superficial enhancement. It can lead to better pay at work, improved subjective mood, and more.

The use of botulinum toxin type A (Botox) to treat glabellar frown lines has been shown to improve major depressive symptoms in susceptible patients, according to a blinded, placebo-controlled study.[5] This is particularly important as we look at the growth of cosmetic medicine and the barriers that patients have in seeking treatment.

Motivation for a given appearance can be a powerful tool to overcome fear of a procedure. If the rewards are high enough, as science is showing us, then those relative risks become less of a concern to our consumer. As technology continues to evolve and grow, we are seeing more and more near-surgical outcomes without the surgery. As a result, we are seeing exponentially more patients seeking nonsurgical treatment options.

Why would someone accept a less-than-ideal enhancement to their appearance? If we look at the science, some improvement is better than none, because it does affect one's persona, and the way the outside world relates to these changes can be dramatic in terms of both one's personal and professional life. I have had many patients come back to me after cosmetic intervention and indicate that they got a major promotion at work and/or found that special someone they never thought they would find. This type of event leads the cosmetic patient to say, "This was the best investment I have ever made." This feeling for the patient is enhanced when the patient did not have to miss a day of work and suffered very little discomfort. The power of such an experience has dramatically built a cosmetic following that exceeds any other component of my practice.

3.3 History Does Repeat Itself

As previously mentioned, I had a strong interest in cardiothoracic surgery. I did research in this area, and one of my most trusted advisors specialized in this area. If we look at the history of cardiac surgery, there are many parallels to current plastic surgery. Cardiac surgery is a dramatic surgery with dramatic effects. Cardiology was largely diagnostic 25 years ago, when it was a distant second to the definitive nature of cardiac surgery treatments, and relegated largely to supporting patients after their surgery. This paradigm has dramatically changed. Cardiac surgery can largely be avoided by minimally invasive approaches performed by the interventional cardiologist. Long ago, there was only a handful of cardiac surgeons who embraced minimally invasive approaches and innovated in the area of circulatory medicine. I believe the same holds true for plastic surgery. As technology continues to evolve and we see more applications that allow for results without an incision or just a minimal one, we will see the base of patients grow and the demand for invasive procedures drop, as we did with cardiac surgery. Will we look at the facelift 10 years from now like we do the open patent foramen ovale surgical repair now? With the current technology, one can only imagine what the future will hold (▶ Table 3.1).

Table 3.1 Surgical and Nonsurgical Pros and Cons

PRO	CON
More defined but more involved	Longevity is less without maintenance
Predictable but very technical	Degree of improvement can be less if the patient is not a good candidate
More permanent, whether a good or bad result	Progressively improving result with time, which can be a positive for the patient fearing drastic alterations
May be more cost-effective in severe cases	Less risk
More control of bone and soft tissue combined	Less recovery
Historic gold standard	Duration

3.4 Practical Considerations

In 2008, I considered the acquisition of the new Ulthera (Ulthera, Inc.) platform (microfocused ultrasound), for nonsurgical browlift and facelift, primarily due to the concern of the declining U.S. economy and an assumption that patients would want a nonsurgical, less expensive alternative to facelifting (see Product Index (p. 176)). In 2009, I made the purchase. I quickly realized that the patient appreciated a less-than-facelift result and returned wanting to do other nonsurgical applications, such as those with lasers and fillers, because they liked the Ulthera model. This lead to the "stackable treatment,"[6] an approach that purely looked at potential synergies in blending and combining noninvasive and minimally invasive approaches (see Video 1.1). A more detailed review of blending strategies will be reviewed in later chapters.

The second point of evolution was the use of energy-based technology, such as radiofrequency and magnetic field generation, to aid in the resolution of swelling and skin tightening in the postliposuction patient, and patients undergoing traditional, ultrasonic, and laser liposuction. Patients appreciated the proactive approach. There was no disposable cost, and it fit nicely into our value-added model, justifying a differential cost model. Patients are much more accepting of a treatment that costs more if there is little pain and minimal downtime involved, as long as there is enough of an improvement.

The advantages are numerous when looking at nonsurgical cosmetic procedures. Fillers and toxins represent the perfect example. They are readily available, and the results are relatively predictable but can be largely reversible and are not permanent in nature. Fillers and toxins can be combined in all kinds of creative ways and are largely amenable to customization. For patients who are uncertain as to what approach they wish to consider, the nonsurgical approach is often more palatable and allows the potential surgical patient to gain confidence in advancing to a surgical application, if it is in his or her best interest. The so called "7/47" effect has been referenced by the injectable industry through internal surveys and holds great reality for the plastic surgeon and nonsurgeon alike.[7] The survey finds that 7% of the general population will go to a non-surgeon for plastic surgery. This number increases to 47% if a patient has a good outcome from a nonsurgical treatment provided by the nonsurgeon. The clear message is that patients who get an improvement with nonsurgical cosmetic care will pursue surgical cosmetic care. This is the definition of a continuum of beauty, in which a rainbow of options exists for the patient who wants wrinkled, tired-appearing skin to look better, from injectables to facelifting with or without skin resurfacing.

3.5 Pretreatment Planning

When looking at minimally invasive and noninvasive cosmetic medical treatments, I note that there a number of variables to consider and present to the patient. Timing is crucial, especially as it relates to treatment options. When looking at neurotoxin therapy, such a Botox injection, I typically advise patients to have their treatment at least 2 weeks in advance of an important event. This can be accompanied by filler to deficient fat pockets of the face, such as the cheeks. While botulinum toxin treatment will typically be effective for 3 to 6 months, fillers are affective for 1 year or more, making the timing of treatments important to plan for the patient in terms of scheduling and financial considerations.

It is therefore easy to carry over this concept to the use of the energy-based applications. For example, the use of microfocused ultrasound platform (Ulthera) typically gives a roughly 2-year enhancement for face and neck treatments. Patients will typically do their second treatment at 18 months, and we time this with their filler and toxin treatment so that only one trip is needed, maximizing efficiency for the patient. In addition, similar to taking care of an automobile, patients are given a general budget of the expenses for their given care plan so that they are able to break down the cost on a monthly basis instead of thinking about the expenses of the cosmetic treatments in large lump sums. This also allows the patient to look at surgical alternatives.

When comparing treatment alternatives, a patient can put a facelift, blepharoplasty, and ablative laser resurfacing next to filler, botulinum toxin injection, microfocused ultrasound, and a series of intense pulsed light (IPL) photorejuvenation treatments. One can look at the time off work and the financial impact of lost productivity versus the time taken to visit a given medical office. One must also look at longevity as well. If a series of noninvasive treatments ends up delivering a result that ultimately costs the same and has more maintenance involved, the patient may opt for the surgery because of its ease and predictability. Patients can also take a hybrid approach, in which they do a submental necklift in the office under local anesthesia and combine it with fillers and laser or microfocused ultrasound to the upper face or radiofrequency-based skin tightening therapy. In this hybrid approach, the patient weighs in a very strategic way the tolerance for recovery, the affordability, and the greatest result or degree of improvement that can be achieved through each treatment option. If one does not look at the minimally invasive approach in this way, the patient will be confused and it will be unlikely that the patient will end up with the most ideal outcome (**see Video 2.11**). In reality, I have seen patients who have a truly amazing result from their filler, but they were terribly upset because they were bruised for 10 days and felt that surgery would have been easier. When reviewing the options, these examples are very helpful to allow the cosmetic patient to make the most informed decision, minimizing the likelihood for an unhappy patient.

3.6 Acquisition of Novel Technology

When considering the acquisition of new technology, one must first look at the pool of patients available. It is a common mistake to buy a technology, like the latest edition laser, thinking it will bring in all sorts of new laser patients. While this is possible, it is incredibly risky as an investment. It is far wiser to develop a more formal business plan in which there is an inventory of potential candidates that currently reside in your practice, and to assess what this could mean in terms of actual patient treatment days, which is the number of patients per day plus the net financial outcome. For fillers and neurotoxins, the risk is lowest, given the relative predictability of overhead, the assessment of actual consumers, the ease of acquiring, and the long shelf life with the ability to grow other parts of the aesthetic business. As one moves into energy-based technology, the assessment becomes much more complicated:

- Is the device a laser, lifter, smoothing, or tightening device?
- What is the current base of patients in your practice?
- Have you taken a poll for the potential interest if the new offering were available?
- Have you taken a poll for the cost tolerance by your clients?
- Are you able to bundle your new offering with something else?
- What is your backup if patients are not accepting of the treatment result?
- Are there disposables?
- If so, how does the disposable affect the treatment cost?
- Is there room to make the treatment financially effective for your practice compared to other offerings?

These are some of the vital questions one must ask before acquiring a new technology. It is very easy to get overwhelmed by the hype and marketing of a new technology. Making such an important capital decision on emotion alone is a major mistake, and one that can be devastating to a clinical practice.

> **Basic Considerations for Acquiring New Technology**
>
> 1. Can the practice afford it? It is critical to review the financial implications of making a corporate loan or using vital business reserves to acquire a new technology. This basic question must be answered, because purchasing a new technology that the practice cannot afford leads to desperate behavior that clouds good clinical judgment, and both the patient and practice will suffer the consequences.
> 2. Have you created a business plan? Again, a good accountant can help with this effort. Some of the more sophisticated companies have already done some of this work for you, based on your demographics. You must look at the amount of internal interest you have for new applications, the financial return of the new technology versus the cost of overhead, the potential to draw new clients (this is usually where the exaggerations occur, because you never get as many new clients as you think), the time to payoff, the service plan cost, the annualized cost to operate the device, and the cost to drop the technology if needed. The annualized cost is one of the most elusive points. One must look at the cost of the hardware, the cost of staffing (and pulling staff away from other money-generating activities), the annual service contract cost, and the interest cost to finance the new technology. Does the novel technology have the ability to increase the utilization of an existing technology? This finding has been very powerful in our practice. For example, when we offered in-office laser liposuction, our utilization of nonsurgical skin tightening increased by more than 50%. There are some technologies that have hidden value, ones that pique the interest of our clients. Cryolipolysis is an example. This is a technology that is well known across our population, and the offering of such a service can have a major appeal to new clients.
> 3. Market saturation. Are you literally going to be the last person in your community to acquire a given technology? If so, you must rely completely on internal appeal, which means that your existing clients will see the new acquisition as value-added for them, because you brought the technology in so that they do not have to leave your practice. This can be very powerful and defy the typical logic of purchase planning. In general, if the market is saturated, one must move cautiously and put the burden of proof on the manufacturer.
> 4. Trial period. It is often beneficial to trial a new technology, "test drive it" to get staff feedback and envision it in your practice. This is typically something you have to ask for, and the period of time varies, depending on availability and how in demand the technology is. Even if you have to pay for the disposable cost, this opportunity is invaluable.
> 5. Do you have physical room for the technology? If you are in a big city like I am, raw space comes at a premium. If you are looking to acquire a new technology that is physically large, you must look at the available space. What will you have to displace to make room for the new item? Are you putting a new technology in place at the expense of a more profitable offering in your practice? Will the new item generate enough to make it appropriate for the clinic, looking at the cost for a given space?

3.7 Conclusion

The ability to incorporate nonsurgical technology into a clinical practice can be a powerful enhancement when applied logically. One must look at science, business, and practicality when considering the addition of nonsurgical technology. For the surgeon, it may be a very foreign concept, because surgeons are conditioned to look for a specific type of result—the surgical result—which is part of the continuum of beauty[8] (▶ Fig. 3.1 and ▶ Fig. 3.2).

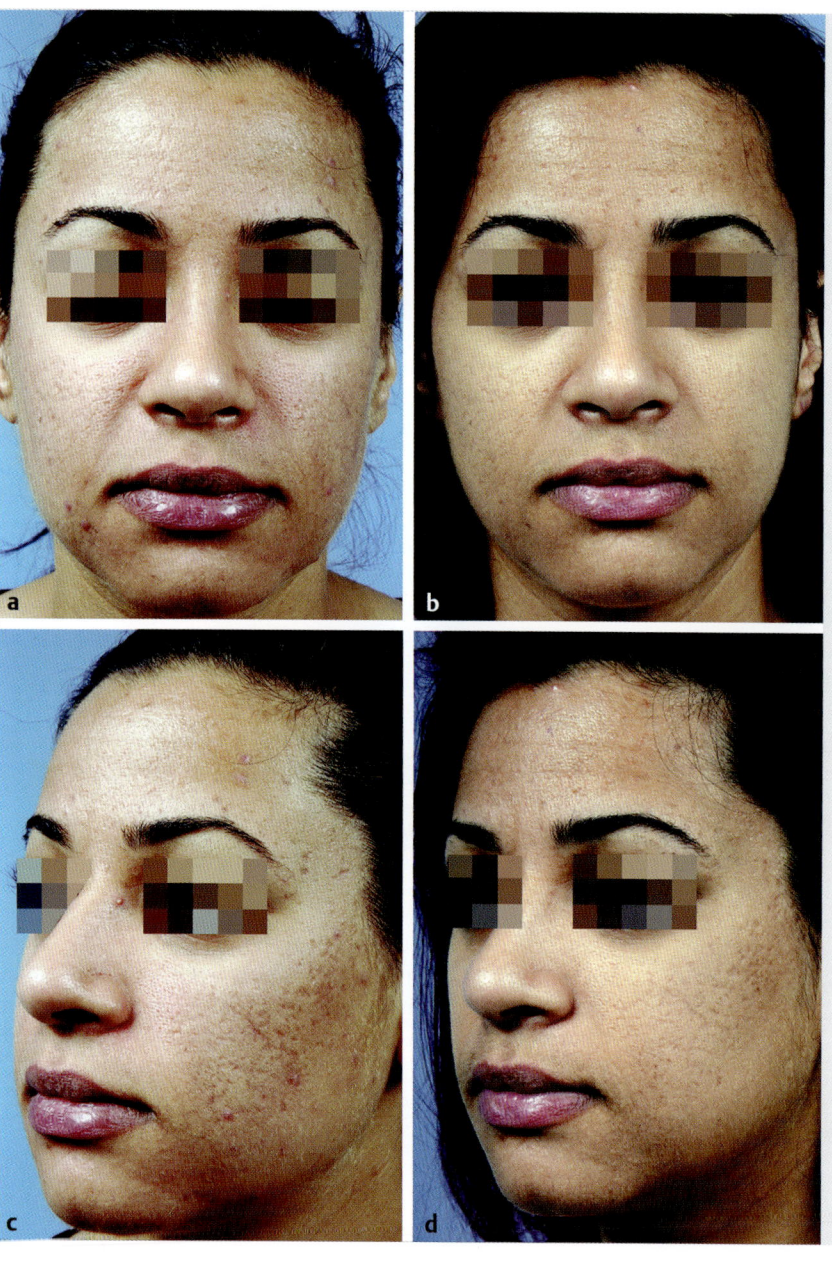

Fig. 3.1 (a,c) This woman with Fitzpatrick type IV skin requested treatment of her active acne and related scars. Her acne scars were initially treated with three rounds of dermabrasion. Once the acne was brought under control, a combination of nonablative and ablative laser resurfacing was performed (Palomar fractional erbium laser system). **(b,d)** The postoperative results at 6 months are shown. (Reproduced with permission from Nahai F. The Art of Aesthetic Surgery: Principles and Techniques, 2nd ed. Vol. 1, Thieme Publishing, 2010)

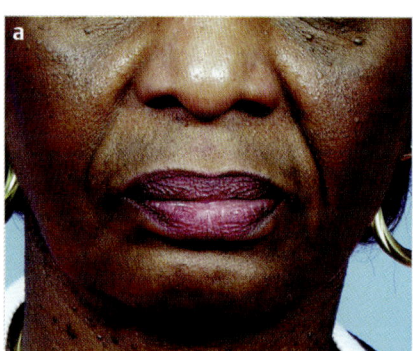
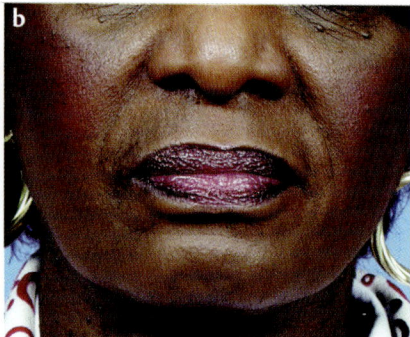

Fig. 3.2 (a) This 60-year-old woman with Fitzpatrick type V skin underwent "liquid facelift" using two syringes of Restylane to her nasolabial folds, marionette lines, and prejowl sulci. **(b)** Follow-up at 1 year. (Reproduced with permission from Nahai F. The Art of Aesthetic Surgery: Principles and Techniques, 2nd ed. Vol. 1, Thieme Publishing, 2010)

References

[1] Odunze M, Cohn A, Few JW. Restylane and people of color. Plast Reconstr Surg. 2007; 120(7):2011–2016

[2] Few JW Jr. "Facial Aesthetic Surgery in Skin of Color." The Art of Aesthetic Surgery Principles & Techniques. 2nd ed. 2011:88–113

[3] Carruthers J, Carruthers A. The adjunctive usage of botulinum toxin. Dermatol Surg. 1998; 24(11):1244–1247

[4] The American Society for Aesthetic Plastic Surgery. Cosmetic Surgery National Data Bank STATISTICS, 2014. http://www.surgery.org/sites/default/files/2014-Stats.pdf

[5] Dayan SH. Mind, Mood, and Aesthetics. Aesthet Surg J. 2015; 35(6):759–761

[6] Few JW. Continuum of Beauty: Blending of Surgical and Nonsurgical Cosmetic Medicine. Treat Strateg Dermatol. 2012; 2(1):29–31

[7] Boundless. "Basic Principles of Operant Conditioning: Thorndike's Law of Effect." Boundless Psychology. Boundless, 08 Aug. 2016. Retrieved 01 Dec, 2016 from https://www.boundless.com/psychology/textbooks/boundless-psychology-textbook/learning-7/operant-conditioning-47/basic-principles-of-operant-conditioning-thorndike-s-law-of-effect-196–12731/

[8] Nahai F. The Art of Aesthetic Surgery: Principles and Techniques. 2nd ed. Vol. 1, Thieme Publishing; 2010

4 Blending and Sequencing Considerations

Daniel R. Butz and Julius W. Few Jr.

Summary

This chapter addresses the benefits of combining three modes of noninvasive treatments (focused ultrasound, volume restoration, and laser resurfacing) to achieve optimal results. In the ideal patient, the results of this combination often resemble surgical results.

Keywords: focused ultrasound, volume restoration, laser resurfacing, ptosis, stacking, Fitzpatrick skin type, autologous, synthetic

> **Key Points**
> - The results of noninvasive approaches can approach surgical outcomes by targeting the three primary components of aging: volume loss, facial anatomy ptosis, and skin elasticity loss.
> - It is vital to address at least two of these three primary components of aging for optimal nonsurgical blending to create a true synergy.
> - When one combines the three modes of noninvasive treatment, one can apply less fluence with laser resurfacing and less volume with the given filler to achieve optimal results that are often close to those of surgery in the ideal patient.
> - The ideal patient for stackable treatments to the face and body represents the man or woman in good shape with early aging changes, nonobese, and with at least one of the three aging components.

4.1 Introduction

Comprehensive care of the aesthetic patient relies on targeted treatment of all the given components that take away from a given individual's aesthetic balance. Regardless of surgical or nonsurgical treatment, the goal remains the same: a balanced natural result. When we look at stacking nonsurgical therapeutic modalities, we approach it surgically to isolate the given component and find the best possible matching treatment. The use of focused ultrasound alone can deliver less-than-dramatic results, but the combination of facial fillers and laser resurfacing gives the patient a result that is relatively immediate. Also, given the lesser fluence required for laser therapy, the downtime is significantly less than that of tradition ablative laser resurfacing.[1] The ability to create fine-tuned detail in the treatment of facial aging with combined nonsurgical modalities is very appealing to the discerning cosmetic patient, because treatments can be repeated as indicated to further enhance an already good improvement.

When looking at the sequence for the given treatments, we have found that the following sequence works well. We tend to do the focused ultrasound or related lifting technique first, followed by volume restoration, and then resurfacing, even if it is all done on the same day. The rationale relates to placing energy first, and then volume to "stretch" ptotic skin, which makes the laser resurfacing easier. In addition, regardless of synthetic or autologous filler substances, there is lidocaine present in the filler, making laser work less uncomfortable in the office setting. These treatments are readily tolerated with little or no oral sedation, and the typical treatment time is less than 2 hours for combined treatments. The ability to offer these treatments in the office means that patients can do so without the support of friends or family, so it is another level of discretion and privacy that the patient can really appreciate.

The major disadvantage of the nonsurgical approach has been the lack of "surgical longevity." Although the given nonsurgical approaches typically last 18 to 24 months, the combination or stacking of therapies results in a longer-longevity that approach surgical outcomes in some cases.[2] In addition, patients do not find the idea of upkeep difficult in most cases, because the interval is long between enhancement, given the long life of fillers, such as Juvéderm Voluma (Allergan, Inc.), and autologous fat (**See Video 2.1**). The use of an ablative laser adds to this package by having long-standing efficacy for facial resurfacing (see Product Index (p. 176)).

For stacking principles on the body, we have found the ability to use cryolipolytic fat reduction with skin-tightening radiofrequency technology to be highly synergistic in certain patients, especially those with significant loss in skin elasticity. The treatments are typically spaced out in their application by 2 to 4 weeks after the initial cryolipolysis session. The ability to use combined modalities for body contouring offers a legitimate alternative to the potential liposuction patient. This approach can even be utilized in the postliposuction patient with residual fat and/or skin laxity, allowing the plastic surgeon great fluidity in the comprehensive treatment of the cosmetic patient.

Cosmetic medicine is as much an art as it is science. One can use principles that are presented in the following text to combine other modalities in a safe, effective manner to deliver heightened results to the cosmetic patient.

4.2 Patient Selection

As with all patients in the plastic surgeon or dermatology practice, patient selection is the golden key in cosmetic medicine. The same is true for combination/stacking approaches to the cosmetic patient. To begin, patient expectations must align with the given combination. Patients must be willing to accept some uncertainty to the level of result and the prerequisite time to achieve a given result, which is typically 90 days or more. In addition, patients who do best with the stackable approach are those who are mild to moderate in their level of deficiency. For patients with more severe or end-stage change, the limits of nonsurgical treatments can be found, which we have learned this through our more severe patients who will only accept a nonsurgical solution regardless of the degree of gain.

The ability to add different modalities reduces the risk of not getting a response, which is sometimes seen with most non-surgical modalities in isolation. The "nonresponder" rate for a given nonsurgical modality is a particularly difficult concept for the plastic surgeon and an important consideration for patient selection. One reason why the "nonresponder" rate is difficult is that it may be much better for a patient to go to surgery if the plastic surgeon wants a degree of control and predictability while being willing to accept the surgical risk. The key is not "talking" the patient into a given approach but rather giving a spectrum of options for the patient to consider, from nonsurgical to surgical and everything in between. The patient is then able to look at the longevity of a given result, versus the risk, versus the predictability and efficacy. One can often be surprised by the level of patient satisfaction with a given combined surgical and nonsurgical result. We have all had patients after a very powerful surgical result who express only moderate satisfaction; although the same response can be true for a nonsurgical patient, it can also be the exact opposite. The nonsurgical patient may achieve 90% of the ideal result and be much more excited about their outcome than a different surgical patient who has 95% of their goal achieved, simply due to the level of commitment the patient has given to the process.

4.3 Technical Steps/Treatment Plan

The technical process begins with an assessment of the aging components, skin, volume, and ptosis:
- Skin
  1. Fitzpatrick skin type.
  2. Solar damage.
  3. Wrinkle severity score.
  4. Pigmentation irregularity.
  5. Pre-existing lesions.
- Volume
  1. Facial fat compartment volume loss.
  2. Restoration vs. enhancement.
  3. Autologous vs. synthetic.
- Ptosis
  1. Facial.
  2. Cervical.
  3. Periorbital.
  4. Perioral.

4.3.1 General Sequence: Face

1. Lift ptotic tissue before adding volume:
   - Allows more effective, anatomic placement of filler.
   - Avoids premature breakdown of filler or toxin by heat.
2. Fill volume deficit before skin resurfacing:
   - Allows more effective resurfacing with lasers.
3. Lift ptotic tissue before or during resurfacing of the skin.

4.3.2 General Sequence: Body

1. Remove unwanted fat before using skin-tightening technology:
   - Can be done in the same setting or in sequence.
   - Allows for augmented skin redraping as the underlying soft tissue redrapes.
   - Focused ultrasound and radiofrequency represent the current preferred tightening technologies.
2. Remove unwanted fat before using cellulite-eliminating technology:
   - Breaks down and smooths some of the cellulite tissue.
   - Can be done using surgical or nonsurgical strategies, such as laser lipolysis and cryolipolysis, respectively.
   - Preferred cellulite management is through currently USFDA-approved modalities of laser-assisted or energy-assisted subcision, done concurrently or staged in two settings.
3. Use cosmeceutical to aid in surface management of fine lines, wrinkles, and pigment:
   - Lasers can be used as part of this strategy.
4. Postsurgical edema reduction and skin tightening can be enhanced by combined multipolar radiofrequency and magnetic field generation.

All stacking treatments are individualized. Ultrasound treatments target the submental area and jowling. Patients are instructed to take an oral sedative and a nonsteroidal anti-inflammatory drug (NSAID) prior to treatment. All patients are given the option of having a regional block performed 10 minutes prior to treatment. Full-face and lower-face treatments are performed over approximately 60 minutes (**see Videos 2.9** and **2.10**). Patients are treated with hyaluronic acid fillers, botulinum toxin, laser, or liposuction (**see Video 1.1** and **Video 2.3**).

Volume deficits are corrected to 85%. Laser resurfacing is typically performed at 80% of the usual fluence. The resultant skin tightening and volume correction work synergistically to achieve a natural aesthetic result. Laser resurfacing consists of a deep and superficial component with feathering in certain areas for less advanced signs of aging or thin skin (upper/lower eyelids, neck).

The stackable technologies we most frequently use are the radiofrequency (Venus Freeze, Venus Concepts), Microfocused Ultrasound (Ultherapy, Ulthera, Inc.) and Cryolipolysis (CoolSculpting, ZELTIQ Aesthetics, Inc.) (see Product Index (p. 176)). Venus Freeze uses radiofrequency to heat the epidermis and dermis to cause thermal contraction. After cleaning the area, you take a baseline temperature. You then apply a thin layer of glycerin gel. The length and temperature used is based on the area being treated. The end temperature should be 39–45 °C. For optimal results, patients require 6 to 8 treatments spaced 1 to 10 days apart, and they frequently need maintenance treatments 3 times per year.

Microfocused ultrasound can heat the dermal layers and the SMAS layers of the face to cause contraction and skin tightening. Once the areas we are targeting are selected, the appropriate transducer is selected, based on the various areas of the face. The treatment area is cleaned and then marked using the transducer template. Ultrasound gel is applied, and the treatment is performed using Ulthera's "amplify" settings as a guideline. Treatment sessions take 1 to 2 hours depending on the extent of the treatment. A single session typically gives results that last for 1 to 2 years.

CoolSculpting uses cooling technology to freeze fat cells and cause cell death. After discussing with the patient the areas they would like to target, you clean those areas and mark the

Blending and Sequencing Considerations

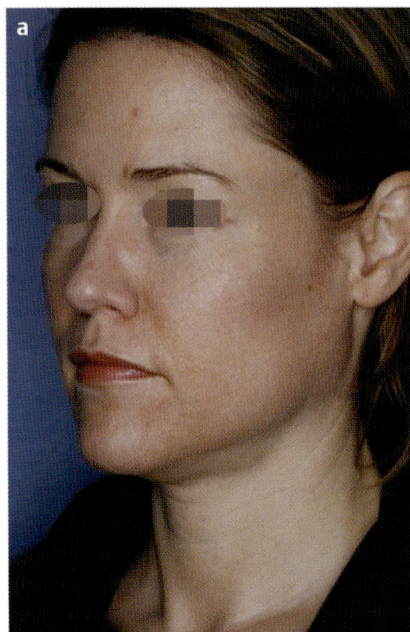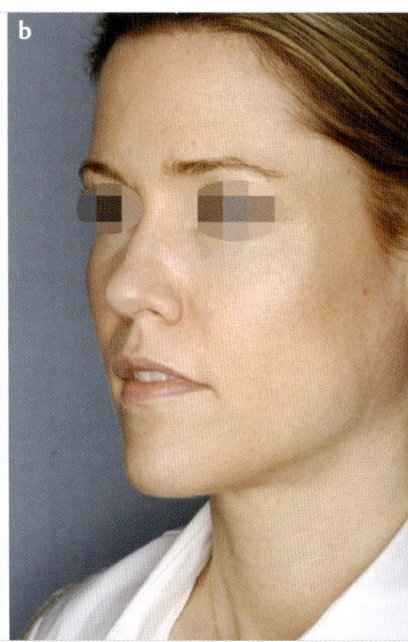

Fig. 4.1 (a) Before and (b) after photographs a patient who had stackable treatment including Ultherapy, laser, filler, neurotoxin, and upper blepharoplasty.

middle portion of the adipose mound (see Product Index (p. 180)). The CoolSculpting templates are placed on the areas with the marks in the center. The temperature settings are adjusted to 60–75–60. A gel pad is applied to the area to protect the skin. Once the appropriate applicator is applied and the vacuum is turned on, the treatment lasts 1 hour or 1 hour and 15 minutes for the outer thighs. The vacuum is then turned off and the applicator is removed. The area should then be massaged for 2 minutes to help break down more fat cells. This treatment can provide a 20 to 25% reduction in adipose cells in the targeted area.

4.4 Results

The following are case examples of how stackable treatments can be utilized and some of the outcomes we have achieved.

4.4.1 Case Example 1

This 44-year-old woman desired facial rejuvenation to address undesirable neck fullness and periorbital region aging (▶ Fig. 4.1). She underwent a stackable treatment including Ultherapy, laser, filler, neurotoxin, and ultimately upper blepharoplasty. In younger patients, we find that the use of double deep passes to the submental central region can be very effective to shrink unwanted small collections of fat, as seen in this patient (**Videos 4.1** and **4.2**). In addition, her sequence began with neurotoxin to maintain the glabella, crow's-feet, and forehead. We then initiated Ultherapy for the full face and neck rejuvenation combined with revolumization to the midface, anteromedial area, and zygomaticomaxillary area. The same-day process was completed with full-face 2940 ablative laser resurfacing. One year later, the patient elected to undergo in-office, primarily upper blepharoplasty for nasal fat reduction and dermatochalasis. For the nonsurgical portion of her rejuvenation program, she missed a half day of work. She is seen 18 months after her complete rejuvenation process.

4.4.2 Case Example 2

This 76-year-old woman with Fitzpatrick skin type VI desired facial rejuvenation. She underwent full-face Ultherapy combined with facial fat grafting to the midface, nasolabial folds, and marionette lines (▶ Fig. 4.2). She is seen more than 2 years after her stackable rejuvenation program. There was negligible recovery and downtime, according to the American Society for Aesthetic Plastic Surgery (ASAPS) Guidelines.[3]

4.4.3 Case Example 3

This 62-year-old woman with Fitzpatrick skin type II presented with facial volume loss, ptosis, and fine rhytides (▶ Fig. 4.3). The patient underwent stackable treatment with Ultherapy, Juvéderm Voluma into the malar region, full-facial intense pulsed light treatment, and neurotoxin injections (**See Video 2.2**). The rejuvenation process began with neurotoxin to the glabella and crow's-feet. Full-face and neck Ultherapy followed with Juvéderm Voluma injection to the anteromedial and zygomaticomaxillary regions of the midface (**Video 4.3** and **see Videos 2.6, 2.7, 2.8**). A 4-session series of in-office intense pulsed light skin resurfacing followed, with no recovery time. The patient had no adverse events and did not miss any work. Her results are seen 1 year later.

4.4.4 Case Example 4

This 38-year-old woman with an unfavorable abdomen contour was postpartum and desired adipose reduction and skin tightening (▶ Fig. 4.4). She underwent CoolSculpting treatment of the abdomen followed by 6 Venus Freeze radiofrequency

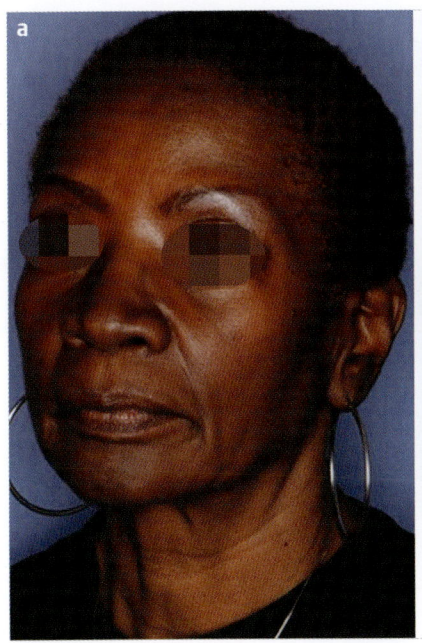 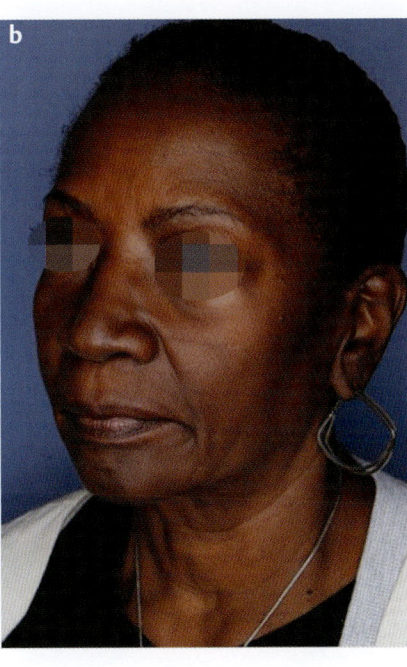

Fig. 4.2 (a) Before and (b) after photographs of a patient who had Ultherapy combined with facial fat grafting.

treatments with magnetic field generation. Her results are seen 6 months later.

4.5 Postoperative Care

Postoperative care is a combination of recommendations based on the treatments received. We encourage all of our facial rejuvenation patients to begin general skin care treatment that includes sun avoidance/aggressive protection and tobacco cessation.

Laser treatments are the most disruptive to the superficial skin and require the most postprocedural care. Patients undergoing laser treatments are told to avoid direct sun exposure and/or artificial tanning and to begin using a daily sunscreen, with an SPF of 30 or higher. If they are on aspirin, we ask them to withhold taking it for 7 days before the procedure to decrease the risk of bruising. We also have them avoid St. John's wort and vitamin E. All patients receiving perioral laser treatment take prophylactic antiviral therapy for 4 weeks, beginning on the morning of their treatment.

Postoperatively, we have patients use cool, moist compresses made with soft gauze for the first 12 hours after laser treatment. For the first 3 to 5 days following treatment, patients must keep their skin protected and moist by washing the skin twice a day with a gentle cleanser such as Cetaphil and applying a topical barrier balm three times per day. After the skin begins to heal after 3 days, it will be dry and tight. Patients are encouraged to apply moisturizing cream during the day, and they must wear a sunscreen with an SPF of 30 or higher at all times. They are not allowed to wear makeup until full re-epithelization has occurred, and they need to avoid direct sunlight until all of the redness has resolved. Finally, they should avoid any irritating creams, such as Retin-A (tretinoin, Valeant Pharmaceuticals International, Inc.), retinol, antihyperglycemic agents (AHAs), or scrubs for at least 4 weeks. They typically only require acetaminophen for pain control.

Patient receiving neurotoxins and/or injectables are told to avoid massaging the area and to avoid strenuous activity for 4 hours after getting the injections. They should also avoid aspirin and NSAIDs for 3 to 4 days to minimize bruising.

If patients only undergo Ultherapy and fillers, they require less postprocedural care. After the treatment, the skin may be slightly pink or red in those areas, and they should avoid hot water when washing or showering until the "blush" has subsided. This is normally only a few hours. They should avoid any exfoliation for at least 1 week or until all sensitivity in the treatment area has subsided. However, makeup may be applied immediately after the procedure, and soothing nonirritating creams or moisturizers should be used.

4.6 Complications and Shortcomings

The most common complications with stackable treatments include those common to all procedures, most commonly bruising and swelling.[4] The degree of bruising is directly related to the use of needles and to a lesser extent microfocused ultrasound. The level of bruising is typically much less than that seen with surgery. In addition, the use of a blunt tip cannula for filler injection largely avoids the risk of bruising. Although the complications seen with the combined approach have been minimal, things such as delayed erythema and/or swelling from the use of a laser can be seen in certain patients, especially those with rosacea or other predispositions to erythema. The risk of bacterial infection exists for any treatment that violates the epidermis, but the risk is minimal with good clean technique. In susceptible patients for herpetic infection, it is important to utilize viral prophylaxis when using energy or injectable treatments around the mouth.

With microfocused ultrasound or radiofrequency-based lifting of tissue, neuropraxia has been reported, but no cases of

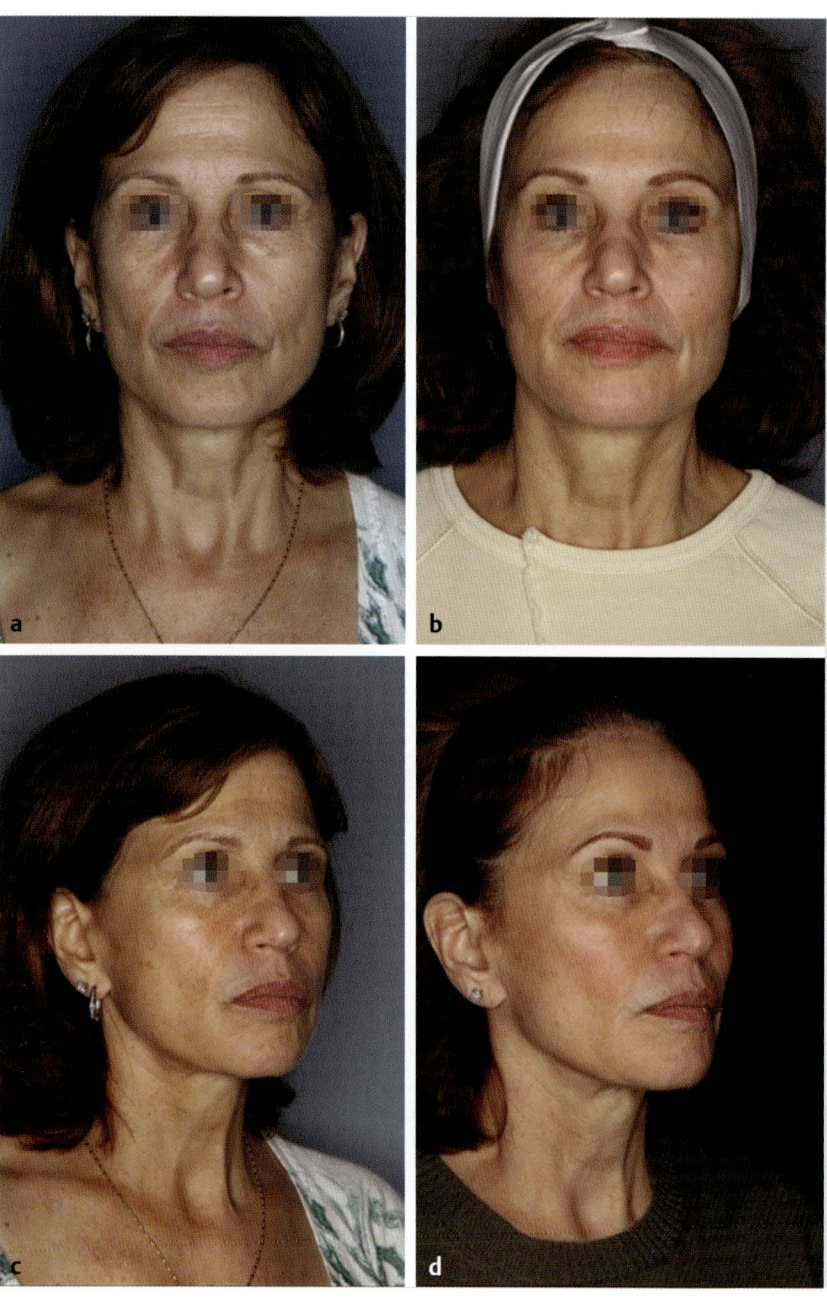

Fig. 4.3 (a,b) Before and (c,d) after photographs of a patient who had CoolSculpting followed by Venus Freeze radiofrequency with magnetic field generation of the face.

permanent loss have been reported. With the use of fillers, one must be concerned of the dreaded intravascular event and the potential management of sequelae. We have found that the use of blunt tip cannulas lessens that risk and are the primary indication for most filler applications in our practice.

The single greatest risk one must be prepared for is lack of response.[5] No matter how aggressive one is with nonsurgical approaches, there will be the occasional nonresponder. In most cases of nonresponse, we are willing to give the patient the following options:
- Attempt a second round of treatment at no additional cost
- Give a monetary credit to his or her account to allow for other offerings
- Offer a surgical substitute

In our practice, we have managed to keep the nonresponse rate to less than 5%. It is possible to have a lower nonresponder rate, but the provider must be willing to turn more patients away from stackable treatments. In addition, the response to subsequent treatments is greater than the response to the initial treatment.

4.7 Conclusion

The ability to combine noninvasive and minimally invasive cosmetic modalities has major synergistic potential, minimizing the "nonresponse" rates for standalone treatment modalities. In addition, one can target, with surgical precision, areas of aging or cosmetic change to illicit an enhancement that requires little

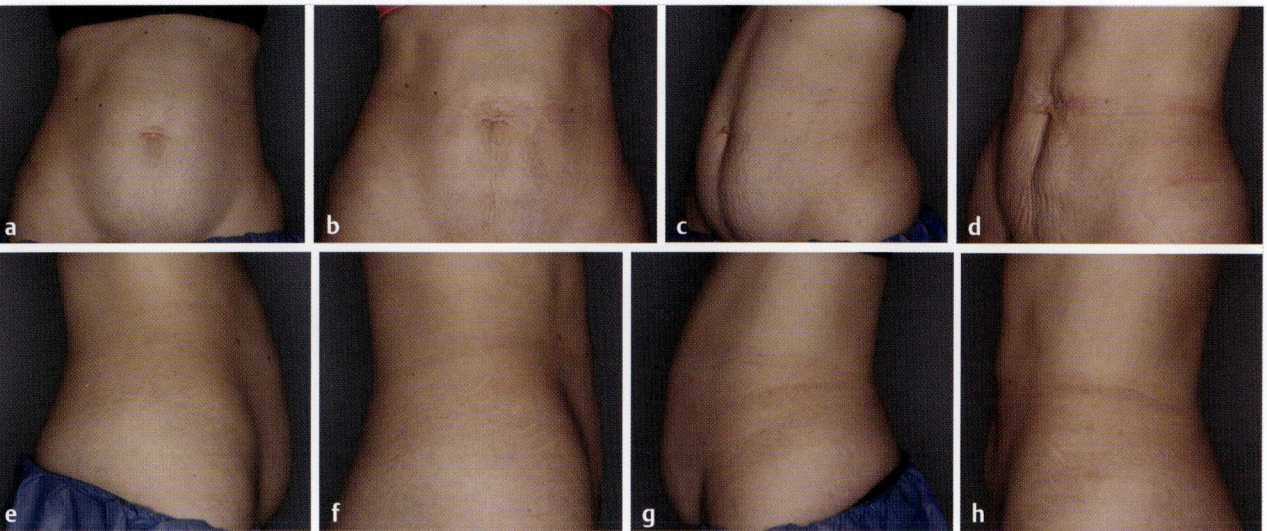

Fig. 4.4 (a-h) Before and after images of a case involving CoolSculpting followed by Venus Freeze radiofrequency with magnetic field generation of the abdomen.

to no downtime. The use of stackable technology can be applied to new patients to aesthetic medicine or to the patient who has undergone past cosmetic surgery and is looking for maintenance. The principles presented can easily be expanded and effectively molded to the needs of any modern cosmetic practice.

4.8 Acknowledgement

The authors thank Shay Moinuddin, Diane Cordon, and Diana Berman, staff and research assistants at The Few Institute.

References

[1] Kulick MI. Back to basics: Understanding the terminology associated with light- and energy-based technology. Aesthet Surg J. 2011; 31(8):984–986

[2] Beer KR. Combined treatment for skin rejuvenation and soft-tissue augmentation of the aging face. J Drugs Dermatol. 2011; 10(2):125–132

[3] The American Society for Aesthetic Plastic Surgery. Cosmetic Procedures, Skin Resurfacing. http://www.surgery.org/consumers/procedures/. Accessed 1/2017

[4] Hassouneh B, Newman JP. Lasers, fillers, and neurotoxins: avoiding complications in the cosmetic facial practice. Facial Plast Surg Clin North Am. 2013; 21(4):585–598

[5] Oni G, Hoxworth R, Teotia S, Brown S, Kenkel JM. Evaluation of a microfocused ultrasound system for improving skin laxity and tightening in the lower face. Aesthet Surg J. 2014; 34(7):1099–1110

5 Diverse Skin Type Considerations and Applications for Nonsurgical Combinations

Valerie D. Callender, Moneé Thomas, and Susan C. Taylor

Summary

Diverse skin types have qualities with implications on noninvasive cosmetic procedures. Considerations when treating skin of color include skin type, ethnic background, the indication for the procedure, and realistic treatment goals. Nonsurgical combination therapies can be safely and effectively used for rejuvenation of the facial skin of patients with skin of color.

Keywords: skin of color, ethnic skin, acne scarring, hirsutism, melasma, chemical peels, neuromodulators, fillers, postinflammatory hyperpigmentation, keloids

Key Points

- Currently, the United States population is approximately 300 million and those with darker skin represent 30% of the population, many of whom desire noninvasive cosmetic procedures.
- The most conclusive data regarding the differences in the structure, function, and biology of skin of color included a greater number of stratum corneum layers with possible increased resistance to irritants, increased size and density of melanosomes, and a more compact dermis. These differences have implications related to noninvasive cosmetic procedures performed in this population.
- Factors to consider when selecting an aesthetic procedure in the patient with skin of color include the patient's skin type, his or her ethnic background, the indication for the procedure, and realistic treatment goals.
- The most common cosmetic concern of the patient with skin of color is dyschromia including melasma, postinflammatory hyperpigmentation (PIH), and UV-induced hyperpigmentation. Additionally, age-associated solar lentigines is concerning in Asians, and dermatosis papulosa nigra (DPN) is concerning in those of African descent.
- Additional cosmetic concerns for the population of patients with skin of color include acne-induced scarring, facial hair growth, keloidal scarring, and loss of volume of the midface with sagging and facial frown lines.
- Combination therapies used to address dyschromias include topical skin lightening agents combined with microdermabrasion, chemical peels, microneedling, or laser therapy.
- Nonsurgical combination therapies, neuromodulators, and fillers, as well as skin-tightening technology, are safely and effectively used for rejuvenation of the facial skin of patients with skin of color.
- Patients with darker skin types have an increased risk of developing adverse events to topical antiaging medications and common aesthetic procedures such as postinflammatory hyperpigmentation and hypopigmentation as well as hypertrophic and keloidal scarring.

5.1 Introduction

The concept of beauty is global, and people with ethnic skin comprise a large portion of the world's population. Individuals from all racial and ethnic groups are interested in aesthetic procedures to address their cosmetic concerns as well as the unique aspects of their aging skin. In fact, the American Society of Aesthetic Plastic Surgery's (ASAPS) 2015 statistics on cosmetic surgery reported that there were approximately 12.8 million surgical and nonsurgical cosmetic procedures performed in the United States, and the number of cosmetic procedures over the 5 years beginning in 2011 increased by 39%, with a 44% increase in nonsurgical procedures compared to an increase of 17% in surgical procedures.[1] This striking difference is a direct result of the preference for nonsurgical procedures that are presumed safer, are less invasive, have a speedier recovery, and are more financially affordable.

Women reportedly had 11.5 million (90.5%) cosmetic procedures performed in contrast to the 1.2 million (9.5%) that occurred in men. Among all cosmetic procedures, 25% were performed on those classified as racial or ethnic minorities, up 3% from last year[1] (**see Text Box** below).

2015 American Society for Aesthetic Plastic Surgery (ASAPS) Cosmetic Demographics: Percentage of Racial and Ethnic Minorities

- Hispanics: 9.7%
- African Americans: 7.7%
- Asians: 6.2%
- Other non-whites: 1.3%

Reproduced with permission from ASAPS. www.surgery.org. Accessed 4/30/2016

The most common nonsurgical procedures include botulinum toxin type A injections, soft tissue filler injections (primarily hyaluronic acid), laser hair removal, facial chemical peels, and microdermabrasion. These procedures are frequently combined to provide the optimum results for each patient. Although each of these procedures is routinely performed in individuals of all races and ethnicities, special consideration and application techniques must be recognized and implemented in patients with darker skin types. Additionally, an understanding of the structure and function of ethnic skin is important, especially when considering combining these procedures in patients with darker skin tones. Adverse events may be unique in patients with darker skin tones. For example, dyschromia as a result of disruption of the epidermal barrier or stimulation of melanocytes, is a known adverse event that can occur postprocedurally in patients with skin of color. Additionally, the incidence of keloids and hypertrophic scarring in patients with skin of color ranges from 4.5% to 16% compared to less than 1% in Caucasians[2]; therefore, special attention must be given to this potential complication.

This chapter will focus on the aesthetic patient with skin of color and include common cosmetic concerns, nonsurgical aesthetic procedures (particularly those that are utilized in combination to treat those concerns), and the management of potential complications that may occur in this group of patients.

5.2 Structure and Function

Data in the medical literature regarding racial and ethnic differences in the structure and function of skin are sparse and often inconclusive. Each of the studies that have been performed include only a small number of subjects, the methodology varies from study to study, and the results are often contradictory. A close review of the literature reveals differences in stratum corneum structure, lipid content, and melanin production and dispersion. Dermal differences have likewise been demonstrated and include variations in fibroblasts, collagen, elastin, and mast cells. These identified differences in skin structure and function are likely responsible for the increased occurrence of the adverse events seen as a result of cosmetic procedures, keloidal scars, and dyschromias in patients with skin of color.

The stratum corneum is the outermost layer of the skin and is responsible for acting as a skin barrier and providing resistance to the outside environment. Its unique composition of corneocytes, lipids, and proteins permit water to be retained within the skin and prevents the loss of water across the epidermis, called *transepidermal water loss* (TEWL). Regarding the stratum corneum structure, although the thickness of the stratum corneum has been determined to be similar between white and black skin, there is a greater number of cell layers in black skin compared with white skin.[3,4,5,6,7,8] Hence, the stratum corneum in black skin is believed to be more cohesive, more compact, and has better epidermal barrier function than white skin. The superiority of the barrier was demonstrated in subjects with darker skin phototypes V and VI, regardless of race, who were demonstrated to have more compact cell layers as compared to those with lighter skin phototypes II and III.[6]

These findings would suggest less susceptibility to irritants that may be found in antiaging products as well as ingredients in chemical peeling agents. However, studies evaluating if darker skin is more or less susceptible to irritants have been found to be contradictory. A study in black, white, and Asian subjects by Kompaore et al[9] showed an increase in baseline TEWL in Asian and black patients, indicating that they have a more compromised barrier function and an increased susceptibility to irritants.

A more recent study by Hicks et al[10] evaluating irritant contact dermatitis using confocal histopathology in vivo demonstrated more severe irritant reactions in white skin. In addition, when comparing reactions to sodium lauryl sulfate, white skin reacted more than black skin. These results suggest that black skin is more resistant to irritants and has a more intact and stronger stratum corneum. Based on this study, black skin should be able to tolerate stronger peeling agents. However, stratum corneum barrier function is only one factor in the complex structure and function of the skin.

Differences in melanocyte synthetic activity and melanosomes among individuals with skin of color likely accounts for a lower tolerability to procedures and to the frequently occurring adverse event of dyschromias produced by chemical peel and laser procedures. Although the number of melanocytes is constant among races, the activity of the melanocytes varies among the races.[11,12,13] Pigmentation of the skin is directly related to the type of melanosomes produced and the melanin content of the melanosome.[14,15,16] Differences in melanosome size, density, and aggregation correlate with skin color, with immature, small, stage I or II melanosomes aggregated in groups being seen in white skin. In contrast, large individually dispersed, nonaggregated stage IV melanosomes are seen in darker people of African descent. A study confirmed that more melanosomes were transferred into basal keratinocytes in the skin of subjects of African descent, with fewer transferred in Caucasian skin.[17] Likewise, the enzyme tyrosinase is more active in darker skin and with higher total melanin content as determined through melanocyte cultures.[15]

There are likely differences at the cellular level between the dermis of black and white individuals. Our primary focus is on the dermal fibroblast cells that produce collagen, the building block for keloidal scars. When the fibroblasts in blacks and whites were compared, it was determined that the fibroblasts in blacks were larger, contained either two or more nuclei and were of greater quantity than those fibroblasts isolated from white female facial skin.[18] Furthermore, the size, array, and orientation of collagen fiber bundles differed in black skin, where they were smaller, packed together very closely, and arranged in a parallel array. Between the collagen bundles, there were more collagen fibrils as well as glycoprotein fragments in black skin as compared to white skin. The reactivity of the fibroblast cell is the result of a poorly understood interaction between mast cells, cytokines, and fibroblasts. Although the number and size of mast cells, which play a role in fibroblast hyperactivity, was the same between whites and blacks, there has been demonstrated decreased collagenase in black skin.[18] The propensity for less breakdown of collagen in black skin may partially explain the increased risk for keloid formation in black patients and those patients with darker skin tones. Hence, patients with skin of color undergoing procedures must be evaluated for the potential of keloidal scar formation. Additionally, the arrangement of collagen bundles could have implications for procedures that involve injections.

Finally, there are functional and biological differences in the skin of individuals with skin of color. The increased amount and dense concentration of melanin in darker skin, along with melanin's distribution throughout the epidermis, provide the benefit of photoprotection, resulting in less pronounced photoaging and fewer skin cancers. Although the melanin content in patients with skin of color provides protection from UV radiation, pigmented skin is not immune from damage. A study from Thailand, among other studies, demonstrated that darker-skinned individuals had the ability to experience significant photodamage, including atypia, atrophy, collagen and elastin damage, and hyperpigmentation.[19,20] Improvement in the hyperpigmentation associated with photodamage and aging is indeed a primary concern that drives individuals of color to seek cosmetic treatments.

Diverse Skin Type Considerations and Applications for Nonsurgical Combinations

Table 5.1 Skin Type Classifications

Skin Type Classifications	Objective Measurement and Utilization in Practice
Fitzpatrick skin types[22]	Phototype (FST), the ability to burn or tan, skin color, phototherapy, skin cancer risk
Kawada skin types[23]	Phototype in Japanese individuals (JST)
Glogau Scale[24]	Photoaging in Caucasians
Lancer Ethnicity Scale[25]	Ancestry and FST, laser surgery, chemical peels
Goldman World Classification of Skin Types[26]	Skin color, response to burning or tanning, PIH
Fanous Classification[27]	Race and genetics, laser resurfacing, chemical peels, dermabrasion
Willis & Earles Scale[28]	People of African descent, skin color, UV light reaction, pigmentary disorders
Taylor Hyperpigmentation Scale[29]	Skin color, dyschromias
Roberts Skin Type Classification System[30]	Phototypes, pigmentation, photoaging, scarring

FST = Fitzpatrick skin type; JST = Japanese skin type; PIH = postinflammatory hyperpigmentation; UV= ultraviolet.

In summary, the most conclusive data regarding the differences in the structure, function, and biology of skin of color included a greater number of stratum corneum layers, with possible improved resistant to irritants, increased size and density of melanosomes, and a more compact dermis with closely stacked collagen bundles and prominent and numerous fiber fragments. These differences have implications related to non-invasive cosmetic procedures performed in this population.

5.3 Skin Type Classifications

Currently, the United States population is approximately 300 million, and those with darker skin (non-white) represent 30% of the population. The U.S. Census Bureau predicts that the population of people with skin of color will represent > 50% of the U.S. population by 2060.[21] This increase in diversity will bring more diversity to our practices; therefore, understanding the individual skin type of a patient becomes clinically relevant.

One classification of skin type presents a myriad of challenges, and several systems have been developed. The original classification of skin types was based on the skin's ability to either tan or burn when exposed to ultraviolet light. Other systems were based on genetic factors, the reaction of the skin to sun exposure, and the hallmarks of aging. With time, these skin classification systems evolved to include other important factors such as the skin's response to procedures.

▶ Table 5.1 lists several of the current skin type classifications commonly used in clinical research, published literature, and clinical practice.[22,23,24,25,26,27,28,29,30] However, the skin type classification system used most often today is the Fitzpatrick Skin Type (FST), which remains the gold standard.[22] The FST classification was developed in 1975 by Thomas B. Fitzpatrick,[22] a Harvard dermatologist, to document the response of different skin types to UV radiation, and was mainly used to guide dosing levels for phototherapy and the potential risk of skin cancer (see Fitzpatrick Skin Types Text Box). It has been adapted as a proxy for skin color and by extension to describe a range of racial and ethnic skin types. Because this skin type system is widely known and has been used across all medical and surgical specialties, this chapter will focus on the safety and efficacy of various procedures in patients with FST IV-VI.

Fitzpatrick Skin Types

- Skin Type I – Always burns, never tans (pale white skin)
- Skin Type II – Burns easily, tans minimally (white skin)
- Skin Type III – Burns moderately, tans uniformly (light brown skin)
- Skin Type IV – Burns minimally, always tans (moderate brown skin)
- Skin Type V – Rarely burns, tans profusely (dark brown skin)
- Skin Type VI – Never burns (deeply pigmented dark brown to black skin)

5.3.1 Aesthetic Consultation

In the author's experience and the findings of a variety of practice surveys, the most common cosmetic concern of the patient with skin of color is dyschromia[31,32,33,34,35] (▶ Fig. 5.1). The

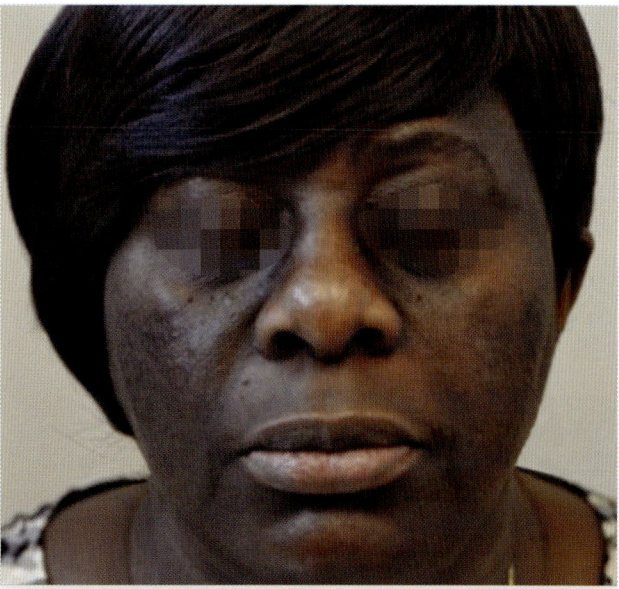

Fig. 5.1 Dyschromia and facial hyperpigmentation.

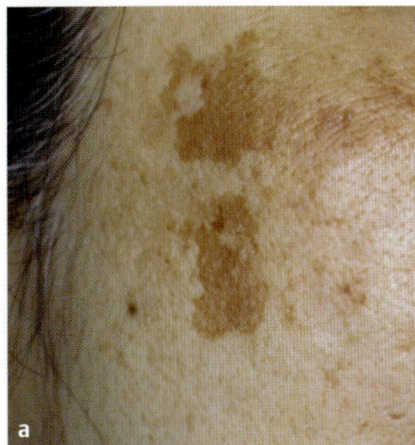
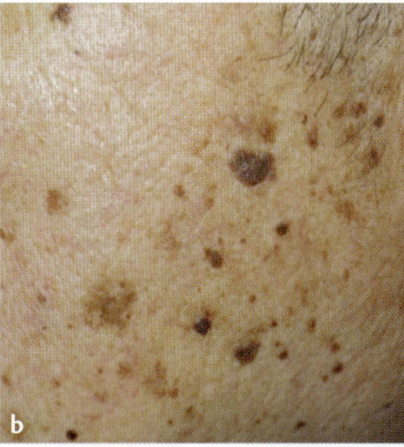

Fig. 5.2 Hyperpigmented lesions with hyperkeratosis in Asians. (a) Solar lentigo. (b) Seborrheic keratoses. (Reproduced with permission from Pu LLQ: Aesthetic Plastic Surgery in Asians: Principles and Techniques, 2015, Thieme Publishing Group)

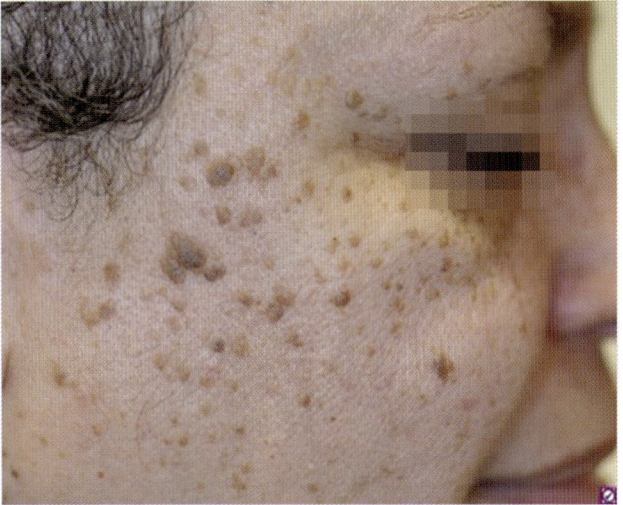

Fig. 5.3 Dermatosis papulosa nigra (DPN) in a woman of African descent.

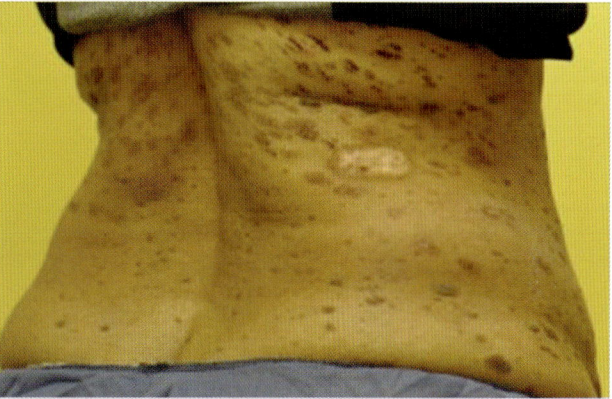

Fig. 5.4 Adverse events in a patient with skin of color after having cryotherapy.

dyschromias include melasma, postinflammatory hyperpigmentation (PIH), and UV-induced hyperpigmentation. These disorders impact negatively on the quality of life of patients with skin of color. In addition, age-associated solar lentigines frequently develop in Asians[36] (▶ Fig. 5.2), and dermatosis papulosa nigra (DPN) develop in patients of African descent (▶ Fig. 5.3). The protective effects of melanin in patients with darker skin delays the onset of facial rhytids to a later age. Hence, the aging face in the patient with skin of color has a different appearance as compared to those with lighter skin (▶ Fig. 5.4).

Furthermore, patients with darker skin types have an increased risk of developing adverse events to topical antiaging medications as well as aesthetic procedures. These adverse events include postinflammatory hyper- and hypopigmentation, as well as hypertrophic and keloidal scarring. These may occur after common procedures including chemical peels, microdermabrasion, laser surgery, electrodessication, and cryotherapy (▶ Fig. 5.5).

Obtaining a detailed patient history, performing a thorough physical examination, performing on test areas, and proceeding cautiously prior to initiating the full procedure will all minimize potential complications in patients with skin of color. Clinicians should not only document the patient's skin type (FST I-VI) but also perform an extended history including the patient's ethnic origin, relevant cultural concerns, alternative products used, and history of skin reactions or allergies. Clinicians should also perform a complete skin examination looking for PIH as well as atrophic, hypertrophic, or keloidal scarring, followed by obtaining clinical photography.

5.4 Nonsurgical Procedures

5.4.1 Melasma

Melasma is a very common disorder of hyperpigmentation that predominantly affects individuals with darkly pigmented skin (▶ Fig. 5.6). Although extensive research regarding treatments for melasma exists, treatments are not optimal because of the relapsing nature of the disease and the increased risk of PIH associated with treatment options. Given these frustrations for both the physician and patients with skin of color, special care must be taken when creating a treatment plan. Treatment options include photoprotection, topical skin lightening agents, cosmeceuticals, chemical peels, nonablative laser therapy, or a combination of these modalities[37,38,39,40,41,42,43,44,45,46] (▶ Table 5.2).

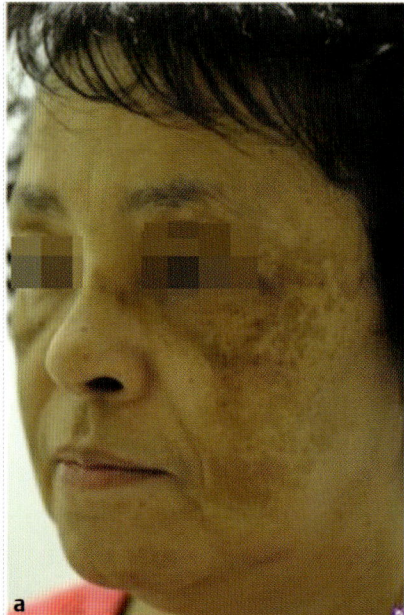
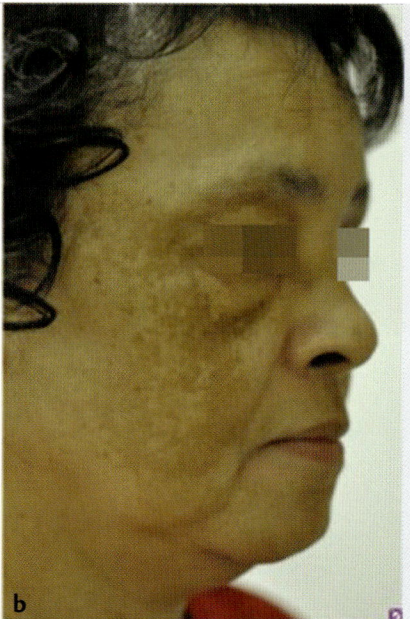

Fig. 5.5 (a,b) Melasma.

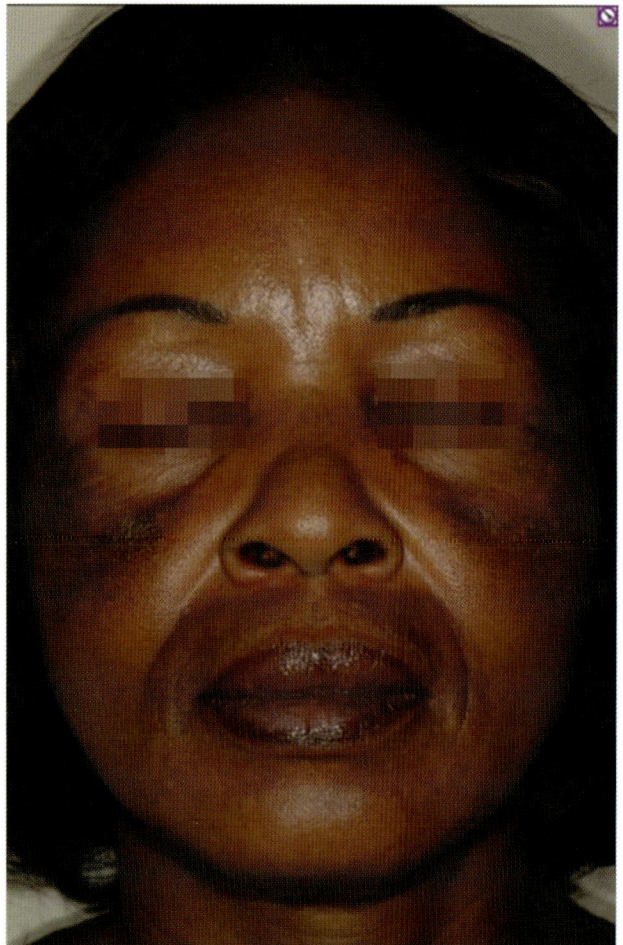

Fig. 5.6 Exogenous ochronosis.

Protection from ultraviolet and visible light is the foundation for all treatment regimens for melasma.[47] Education on the importance of the application of daily broad-spectrum sunscreen is essential in the patient with skin of color who may not use sunscreen on a regular basis.[40,41,42,43,44,45,46,47,48,49] Beyond sun protection, there are numerous topical skin-lightening agents that are considered first-line treatment for melasma.

Topical skin-lightening agents include hydroquinone (HQ), tretinoin, azelaic acid, mequinol, kojic acid, corticosteroids, and an array of cosmeceuticals such as Vitamin C, and are used as monotherapy or in combination to treat melasma. Of these available treatment options, HQ remains the gold standard of therapy and it is usually included in the initial therapy of melasma in patients with skin of color.[47] Although effective in epidermal melasma, especially when used long term and in combination with additional topical agents, HQ has the potential to produce exogenous ochronosis (▶ Fig. 5.7). Exogenous ochronosis, which is also associated with high concentrations of HQ, occurs as a result of homogentisic acid accumulation in the dermis, and presents with facial hyperpigmentation in the affected area.[50]

The most common topical regimen for melasma is a combination of HQ 4%, tretinoin (0.05% to 0.1%), and a corticosteroid.[40] A modification of this triple combination with lower concentrations of the individual components may be beneficial in patients with skin of color due to a lower irritation profile and the reduced risk for PIH.

Chemical peels are considered resurfacing procedures that produce a controlled injury to the skin, which results in exfoliation. The treatment of melasma with chemical peels is a standard treatment, although adverse events, particularly PIH, may occur. Patients with FST IV-VI typically undergo superficial to medium-depth chemical peels after a test area is performed (▶ Table 5.3). Deep chemical peels, such as the Baker phenol peel and higher concentrations of TCA, can result in PIH, scarring, and permanent hypopigmentation in patients with skin of color and should be avoided (▶ Fig. 5.8).

Table 5.2 Treatment Combinations for Melasma

Treatment Combination	Fitzpatrick Skin Type	Comments and Outcomes	Adverse Effects
Hydroquinone (2–4%), Tretinoin (0.05–0.1%), Fluocinolone 0.01% qhs[40]	All skin types (may decrease strength of hydroquinone and tretinoin in darker skin types)	-Most effective first-line treatment	-Mild local irritation, erythema, and skin peeling
Glycolic Acid Peels q 2 weeks + Azelaic Acid 20% cream qhs[38]	IV-VI	-Azelaic acid must be stopped 2 days before and after peel	-Irritation, dryness, photosensitivity
Microneedling followed by application of depigmenting serum[41,42]	III-V	-Depigmenting agents used have been tranexamic acid or serum containing rucinol and sophora-alpha	-No reported adverse effects
Erbium:YAG laser + biweekly glycolic acid peels and daily use of sunscreen and topical azelaic acid cream[43]	II-V	-Glycolic acid peels should be performed 3–6 weeks after laser treatment	-PIH
Microdermabrasion immediately followed by low-fluence Nd:YAG + a daily skin care regimen of hydroquinone with tretinoin or Vitamin C[44]	II-V	-Treatments repeated at 4-week intervals	-Posttreatment erythema, irritation from skin care regimen
Triple-combination topical therapy (azelaic acid + corticosteroid cream or pimecrolimus 1% cream + hydroquinone 4–6% cream) daily and 1064 nm QS Nd:YAG[45]	III-V	-Laser treatments at 4 to 6-week intervals -Significant improvement in overall facial hyperpigmentation	-One case of hyperpigmentation
2% hydroquinone/ 10% glycolic acid gel twice daily + 0.05% tretinoin cream nightly + glycolic acid peels[46]	IV-VI	-Glycolic acid peels at 3-week intervals -More rapid improvement in hyperpigmentation than topical therapy alone	-Mild cutaneous erythema and superficial desquamation

PIH = postinflammatory hyperpigmentation.

Several studies have shown that priming with a topical skin-lightening agent weeks before a chemical peel procedure may be useful in preventing PIH.[37,47,51] In addition, post-peel complications may be decreased by starting at lower concentrations of the peeling agent and titrating upward with each additional chemical peel, extending the intervals between chemical peeling by 2 to 4 weeks, and discontinuing topical retinoid therapy 5 to 7 days before the chemical peel procedure.[51,52]

Recently, microneedling has been reported as a therapy for melasma to provide a means of transdermal drug delivery. Microneedling is a minimally invasive nonablative procedure that uses fine needles to cause controlled injury to the skin by forming microchannels. The injury causes the body to produce new collagen and elastin within the wounds, in addition to neovascularization. Overall, the outcome is skin rejuvenation and scar reduction. Microneedling can be very effective in treating melasma when followed by the application of depigmenting agents such as tranexamic acid or serum containing rucinol and sophora-alpha.[41,42] In addition, as opposed to laser therapy, the risk of hyperpigmentation and scarring in darker skin types is reduced.

Lasers have also been used to treat melasma successfully in patients with skin of color who have lighter skin (FST III-V). However, caution should be used when considering laser surgery in patients with darker skin (FST V-VI), mainly due to the risk of PIH.

5.4.2 Acne Scarring

Acne is one of the most common dermatologic conditions in the United States for which patients, including those with skin of color, seek dermatologic care. The pathogenesis of acne in white patients and patients with skin of color is believed to be the same. However, there are clinical differences of acne and its sequelae in these populations. For example, a common location for acne in African American women is the anterior hairline, primarily due to the use of hair care products used to smooth and moisturize the hair. These products are comedogenic and can result in a condition called *pomade acne*.[53] Postacne sequelae also differ between patients with lighter and darker skin tones. Inflammatory as well as comedonal lesions frequently lead to PIH in darker-skinned individuals (▶ Fig. 5.7), compared with postinflammatory erythema (PIE), which is a common sequela in lighter-skinned individuals. A study by Halder et al[54] demonstrated that in African American skin, papules as well as comedonal lesions histologically displayed inflammatory infiltrates despite appearing noninflammatory clinically. Hence, visible and significant PIH may be present in individuals with darker skin tone who have only mild to moderate acne. Furthermore, inflammatory infiltrates responsible for PIH may activate matrix metalloproteinases that lead to atrophic and ice-pick scarring.[55]

In the acne of the patient with skin of color, treatment may be threefold and include topical, oral, or procedural therapy for

Diverse Skin Type Considerations and Applications for Nonsurgical Combinations

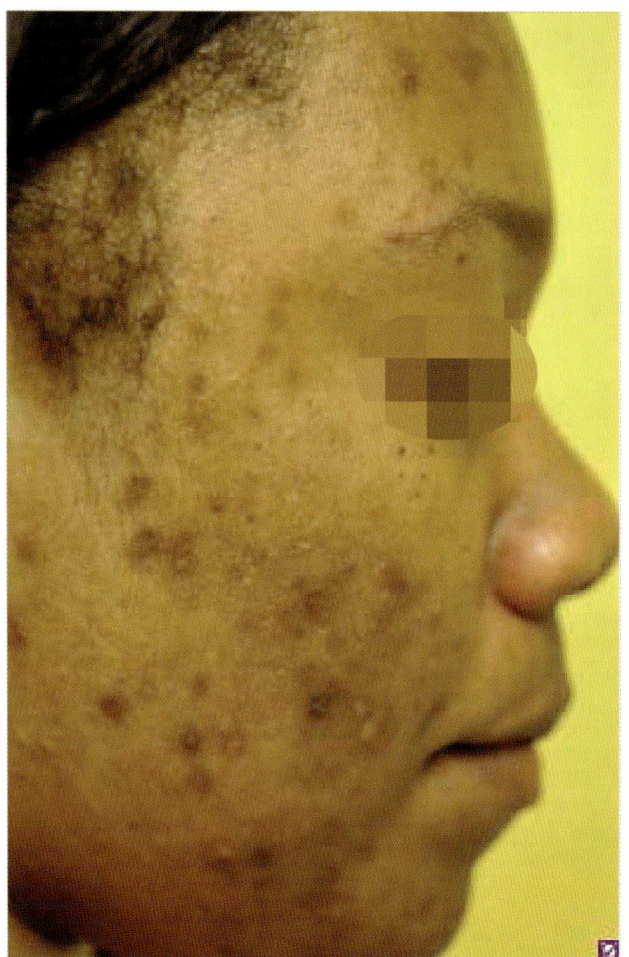

Fig. 5.7 Acne with postinflammatory hyperpigmentation.

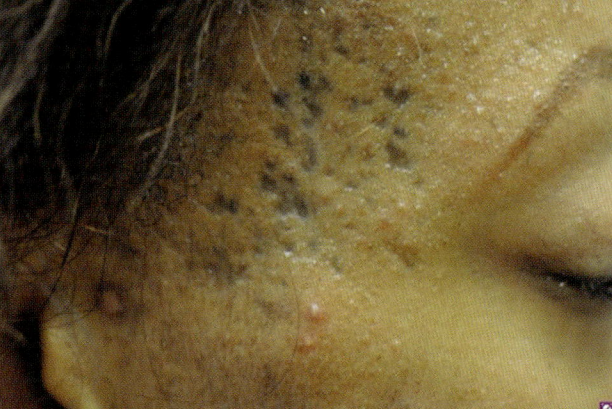

Fig. 5.8 Acne scarring "ice-pick" scars.

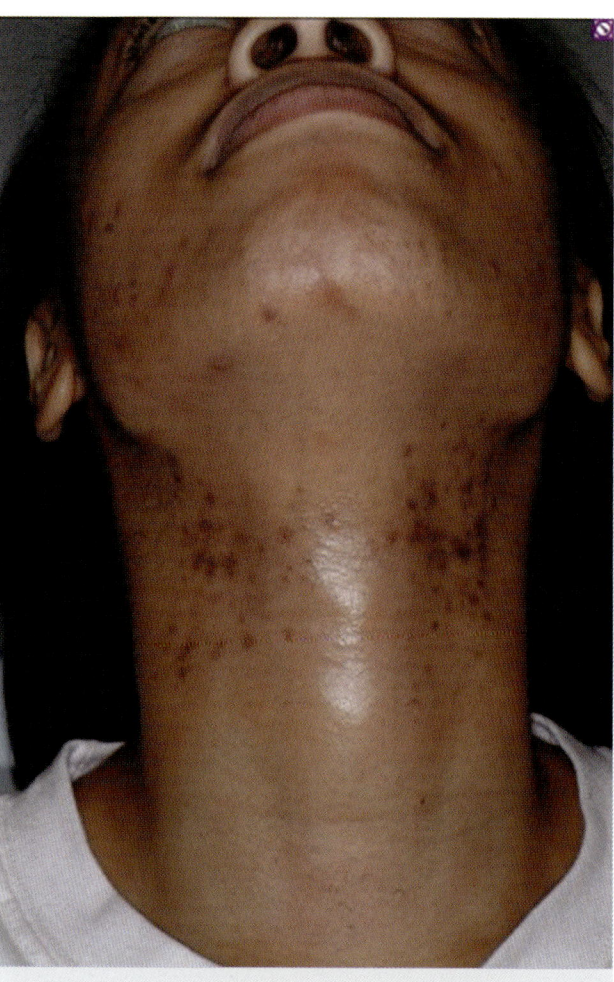

Fig. 5.9 Pseudofolliculitis barbae with postinflammatory hyperpigmentation in a hirsute women of African descent.

Table 5.3 Chemical Peels

Types of Chemical Peels	Depth	Examples
Superficial	Penetrates epidermis only	Glycolic acid, Polyhydroxy acid, Salicylic acid, Trichloroacetic acid, Tretinoin, Jessner's solution
Medium	Penetrates to or through the level of the papillary dermis	TCA 35–40%, Jessner's solution + TCA 35%, GA 70% + TCA 35%
Deep	Penetrates to the reticular dermis	Baker phenol peel

TCA = trichloroacetic acid; GA = glycolic acid.

Table 5.4 Nonsurgical Procedures for Acne Scarring

Treatment	Preferred Fitzpatrick Skin Types	Primary Outcome	Adverse Effects
Priming with hydroquinone 4% and tretinoin 0.025% + CROSS technique of 100% trichloroacetic acid q 2weeks[56]	IV-V	Improvement of ice-pick acne scars	Transient hypopigmentation and transient hyperpigmentation
Nonablative 1064 nm Nd:YAG laser[57]	II-V	Improvement in mild to moderate atrophic acne scars	Transitory erythema, PIH
Nonablative 1550 nm fractional laser at 200 MTZ/cm^2 or 393 MTZ/cm^2, fluence of 40 mJ q 4 weeks[58]	IV-VI	The nonablative 1550 nm fractional laser is safe and efficacious in treating acne scaring in Fitzpatrick skin types IV to VI.	Self-limited PIH
Sublative fractional bipolar radiofrequency + bipolar radio frequency combined with 915 nm diode laser[59]	II-V	Improvement in superficial and deep scarring	Crust formation, erythema, edema, PIH
Microneedling + 35% Glycolic Acid Peels[60]	III-IV	Improvement in grade 1 to 3 acne scarring	Posttreatment erythema and edema, PIH
Subcision + microneedling and 15% TCA peel alternated q 2 weeks[61]	III-V	Improvement in grade 2 to 4 acne scarring	Posttreatment erythema and edema, PIH
PMMA microspheres in collagen[62]	I-VI	Improvement in moderate to severe rolling, atrophic acne scars.	Injection-site pain, injection-site tenderness, swelling, influenza, and nasopharyngitis

PIH = postinflammatory hyperpigmentation; PMMA = polymethylmethacrylate.

acne lesions; topical or procedural therapy for PIH; and procedural therapy for atrophic, rolling or ice-pick scarring.[56,57,58,59,60,61,62] ▶ Table 5.4 lists published data on procedural therapies for acne scarring (▶ Fig. 5.8) in patients with higher FST skin types. When developing a treatment plan for scarring associated with acne in a patient of color, it is important to obtain a history of hypertrophic or keloidal scarring, current topical retinoid therapy, and prior use of isotretinoin.[56,57,58,59,60,61,62] Additionally, these patients are particularly prone to PIH, and it is important to understand that, for some patients, the PIH can be more troubling than the acne itself.[54] Therefore, the propensity to cause PIH should be considered when choosing an appropriate procedural therapy for acnescarring.

5.4.3 Keloids and Hypertrophic Scars

As previously mentioned, hypertrophic scars (HTS) and keloids occur more frequently in patients with skin of color. These benign growths can be aesthetically displeasing to patients and are often symptomatic, causing discomfort, pruritus, or pain. HTS and keloids result from an abnormal scar-healing process that occurs from cutaneous trauma or an inflammatory process. The major difference between these scars is that keloids expand beyond the original wound boundaries, whereas HTS do not.

Histologically, both HTS and keloids are composed of type 1 collagen. Keloids frequently develop in areas of the body with high tension, such as the chest, shoulders, and upper arms, and they can occur after ear piercing and from inflammatory skin in genetically susceptible individuals. Spontaneous keloids are not uncommon.

Keloids are often difficult to treat, and require multiple modalities, surgical and nonsurgical, often used in combination, to produce a therapeutic response. These treatments include pressure therapy, silicone gel sheeting, topical corticosteroids, topical imiquimod, intralesional corticosteroid, 5-fluorouracil or bleomycin injections, cryotherapy, excision, radiation, and laser surgery. Recurrences with any of these approaches are common. ▶ Table 5.5 summarizes several nonsurgical combinations used to address HTS and keloids.[63,64,65,66,67,68,69,70,71] Interestingly, combination therapy utilizing intralesional corticosteroid injections (10 to 40 mg/mL) with treatment sessions performed 4 to 6 weeks apart, produced the most successful outcome in these studies. Other nonsurgical treatment modalities, such as cryotherapy and intralesional corticosteroid injections, must be used with caution in patients with skin of color due to the potential risk of hypopigmentation after the procedure. This complication must be clearly discussed with the patient prior to the procedure, and in the authors' experience, limiting the injecting dose of triamcinolone acetonide to 20 mg/mL or lower may decrease this risk.

5.4.4 Hirsutism

Hirsutism is a very common disorder in female patients with skin of color. This condition can be genetic in nature or associated with polycystic ovarian syndrome (PCOS). A common sequela from a hair removal procedure in male and female patients with curly hair is pseudofolliculitis barbae (PFB) along with subsequent PIH. Combination therapy for hirsutism/PFB/PIH utilizing topical and oral antibiotics, topical corticosteroids, HQ, eflornithine hydrochloride, and laser hair removal can result in significant improvement of the follicular papules, pustules, and hyperpigmentation.

When considering which laser to use for effective hair removal in patients with skin of color, one must consider three factors: the wavelength of the laser, the pulse duration, and the patient's FST. Lasers with shorter wavelengths, such as the 694

Table 5.5 Nonsurgical Treatment Combinations for Keloids and Hypertrophic Scars

Treatment Combination	Scar Type	Comments and Outcomes	Adverse Effects
Silicone gel sheeting and monthly intralesional corticosteroid injections[63]	Hypertrophic scars and keloids	• First-line therapy	• Atrophy • Hypopigmentation
Cryotherapy and intralesional corticosteroid injections monthly[64]	Hypertrophic scars and keloids	• Decreased pain • Decreased itch vs. corticosteroid alone	• Atrophy • Hypopigmentation
Intralesional cryotherapy and silicone gel sheeting[65]	Refractory keloids	• Volume reduction • Decreased pain and discomfort	• Blistering and tissue necrosis in postoperative phase
5-fluorouracil (0.9 mL of 50 mg/mL) and triamcinolone (0.1 mL of 40 mg/mL); 0.1 mL of solution per cm of lesion q 4 weeks[66]	Hypertrophic scars and keloids	• Volume reduction • Reduction of pruritus • Pain resolved	• Telangiectasias
Bleomycin and triamcinolone acetonide; 4–5 mg/cm^2 of solution q 3 months[67]	Hypertrophic scars and keloids	• Flattening • Scar height reduction • Softening	• Erythema • Telangiectasias • Atrophy • Ulceration • Reoccurrence
578 nm copper bromide laser combined with intralesional corticosteroid injections q 4 weeks[68]	Hypertrophic scars and keloids	• Reduced vascular components of scars • Decreased erythema • Improved pruritus • Improve telangiectasia	• Moderate pain during treatment • Transient erythema and edema • Mild hyperpigmentation
CO2 fractional laser (10,600 nm), Pulsed dye laser (585 nm), triamcinolone acetonide injection monthly[69]	Keloids	• Minimal flatness • Minimal effect on size • Pruritus diminished • Lighter pigmentation	• Moderate pain during treatment • Transient erythema and edema • Mild hyperpigmentation
5-fluorouracil (0.9 mL of 50 mg/mL) + triamcinolone (0.1 mL of 40 mg/mL) weekly and 585 nm pulsed dye laser q 4 weeks[70]	Keloids and hypertrophic scars	• Improved flattening • Increased pliability • Decreased pruritus • Decreased erythema	• Moderate pain during treatment • Transient purpura after laser therapy
Radiofrequency followed by triamcinolone (10 mg/mL) injections for 3 to 4 sessions q 8 weeks.[71]	Keloids	• Volume reduction • Increased pliability • Decreased height • Decreased erythema	• Minor bleeding from injection penetration points

ruby laser and the 755 nm alexandrite laser, have a higher affinity for melanin and do not penetrate deeply into the skin.[72] Thus, in darker skin types, thermal epidermal damage may occur due to the increased amount of the target chromophore in not only the hair follicle but also the surrounding epidermis. This results in inflammation and subsequent hyperpigmentation. In contrast, the 810 nm diode laser and the 1064 Nd:YAG laser have less of an affinity for melanin but penetrate deeper into the skin. These lasers are more effective in hair removal for darker skin types, given the lack of epidermal damage that results, compared with the shorter-wavelength lasers and their ability to reach deeply placed hair follicles. ▶ Table 5.6 lists options for hair removal lasers for patients with skin of color.[72,73,74,75,76]

5.4.5 Skin Tightening

Skin-tightening and skin-rejuvenation procedures are becoming more popular. This is due to the public demand for aesthetic procedures that address facial aging and skin laxity, while

Table 5.6 Nonsurgical Procedures for Hirsutism

Laser	Preferred in Fitzpatrick Skin Type	Comments	Adverse Effects
Long Pulsed 1064 nm Nd:YAG laser[72,73]	IV-VI	Proven to be the safest option for hair removal in skin types IV-VI in numerous studies	Short-term hyperpigmentation
755 nm Alexandrite Laser[74,75]	I-IV	Few studies have shown that hyperpigmentation can be reduced in skin types IV and V with the use of topical corticosteroids and epidermal cooling	Blistering, hyperpigmentation, and hypopigmentation (mainly in type VI skin)
800 and 810 nm Diode Laser[76]	I-IV	Longer pulse durations (> 400 msec) should be used in addition to aggressive adjunctive skin cooling in darker skin types	Dyspigmentation in skin types V and VI

Diverse Skin Type Considerations and Applications for Nonsurgical Combinations

Table 5.7 Skin Tightening Devices in Skin of Color

Device	FST	Treatment # (interval)	Primary Outcome	Adverse Effects
Dermaroller (192 needles in eight rows, needle diameter at penetration point of 0.25 mm, roller head, 20 mm)[78]	III-IV	6 (2 wks)	Noticeable clinical improvement of photoaged skin. Significant increase in collagen types I, III, and VII, newly synthesized collagen, and tropoelastin. Significant decrease in mean level of total elastin.	Temporary slight pain, erythema, and facial edema (100%)
Ulthera MFU-V system, lower face and submental regions were treated with 4.4 MHz and 7 MHz transducers with focal depths of 4.5 and 3.0 mm, respectively. Each participant treated with 370 lines of MFU-V with a maximum length of 25 mm and microcoagulation zones spaced 2 to 3 mm apart.[79]	III-VI	1 (n/a)	This trial demonstrated a favorable safety profile for MFU-V in individuals with Fitzpatrick skin types III to VI. Extra care is warranted when using superficial transducers because of the more reactive nature of superficial skin.	Temporary erythema and welting (6%)
EndyMed PRO, 33-W output, facial tightening mode, treatment area: cheeks, heating depth: 3, 12 passes of 30 seconds per area[80]	III-V	3 (1 wk)	Significant improvement in skin laxity. The elastin density was significantly increased compared with controls in all 5 Japanese patients	No adverse events reported
5 Noninsulated microneedle electrode pairs per 10 mm², depth: 0.5–3 mm[81]	II-IV	3 (4 wks)	Addition of the stem cell medium produced a significant benefit in skin roughness and a moderate benefit in overall appearance, compared with FRFM alone	Mild erythema (100%)
Titan infrared nonablative heating device, 32 to 40 J/cm2 over the soft tissue of cheeks and submental area and reduced fluence of 28 to 32 J/cm2 over bony areas and forehead[82]	IV-V	3 (4 wks)	86% of patients with observable lifting of sagging skin folds	Superficial blistering in 11% of the treatments performed

Manufacturers: Fraxel Re:Store 1550 nm; Solta Medical; DERMAROLLER Deutschland S.a.r.l. Lindener Strasse15; Ulthera System, Ulthera, Inc.; EndyMed PRO, EndyMed Medical Ltd.; Titan, Cutera, Inc.
FRFM, Fractional radiofrequency microneedling; FST, Fitzpatrick skin type; MFU-V, microfocused ultrasound with visualization; MPCRF, multisource phase controlled radiofrequency device; MTZ, microthermal zones of injury.
(see Product Index (p.176))

producing little downtime and minimal side effects. Current technologies for skin tightening include noninvasive devices, such as ultrasound and radiofrequency (RF), and minimally invasive devices and techniques, such as microneedling, ablative nonfractional carbon dioxide lasers, and ablative nonfractional carbon dioxide lasers.[77] There is limited data on the use of these devices and procedures for skin tightening in darker skin types. ▶ Table 5.7 summarizes several of the currently available technologies for skin tightening in patients with skin of color and provides some insight on potential adverse events.[78,79,80,81,82] Interestingly, dyschromia with these devices is uncommon and is primarily due to the deep penetration of the tools with a subsequent lack of epidermal damage.

5.4.6 Combining Botulinum Toxin-A with Fillers

The noninvasive injectable market has grown tremendously since 2005.[1] These procedures are well suited for meeting the needs of the aging skin of the face in patients with skin of color.[47] Skin aging differs significantly in dark-skinned patients (FST IV-VI) compared to patients with lighter skin (FST I-III). Signs of aging occur 10 to 20 years later in patients with darker skin because of the photoprotective effects of melanin, which offers a natural sun protection factor of 13.4.[83] Hence, extrinsic aging or photodamage predominates in patients with skin with less pigment, whereas midfacial aging (i.e., infraorbital hollowing, prominent nasolabial fold) predominates in those with pigmented skin.[84]

Nevertheless, botulinum toxin-A (BTX-A) and soft tissue fillers are frequently used in combination to treat superficial lines, folds, and volume loss is patient with all skin types. Safety and efficacy have been assessed for these agents. ▶ Table 5.8 and ▶ Table 5.9 summarize the published literature on the efficacy and safety of BTX-A injections and commonly used fillers in skin of color.[85,86,87,88,89,90,91,92,93,94]

To our knowledge, there have been no reports in the published literature of the development of HTS or keloids in

Table 5.8 FDA Approved BTX-A and the Incidence of Pigmentary Changes in Skin of Color

BTX-A	Variation in Dose	PIH
Onabotulinum toxin A (Botox)[85]	None	0%
Abobotulinum toxin A (Dysport)[86]	Not studied	0%
Incobotulinum toxin A (Xeomin)	Not studied	0%

(see Product Index (p.167))
PIH = postinflammatory hyperpigmentation.

Table 5.9 FDA-approved Fillers and the Incidences of Adverse Events in Skin of Color

Filler	Pigmentary Change	HTS/Keloid	Injection Plane
Hyaluronic acid:			
Juvéderm[87,88]	7.5%	0%	Intradermal
Hylaform[88]	2.5%	0%	Intradermal
Restylane[89,90]	9%	0%	Intradermal
	6%	0%	Intradermal
Belotero[91]	1.1% hypopigmentation	0%	Intradermal
Perlane[89]	2.2% PIH		
Voluma[92]	0%	0%	Subcutaneous or supraperiosteal
Calcium hydroxylapatite (Radiesse)[93]	0%	0%	Subcutaneous
Poly-L-lactic acid (Sculptra Aesthetic)	No data	No data	N/A
Polymethylmethacrylate (Bellafill)[94]	No data	No data	Deep dermal, dermal-subcutaneous junction

(see Product Index (p. 167))
HTS = hypertrophic scarring; PIH = postinflammatory hyperpigmentation.

patients with darker skin types with the injection of either BTX-A or fillers. However, pigmentary changes in patients with skin of color have been reported in several clinical studies involving fillers. The incidences of pigmentary changes, such as PIH from filler injections in patients with darker skin, ranges from 0 to 9%[87,88,89,90,91,95] (see ▶ Table 5.9).

Proper injection technique should be used to decrease the frequency of PIH and to improve the aesthetic outcome in patients with darker skin types. Several authors have recommended minimizing the number of entry points, injecting deeper into the dermis to avoid the dermal-epidermal junction, utilizing the fanning technique (versus multiple serial punctures), and using a slow rate of injection.[84,96] In addition, the application of a mid-potency to high-potency topical corticosteroid immediately after injection, particularly if erythema is present, may help to decrease inflammation and avoid postinflammatory changes.

5.5 Conclusion

Nonsurgical combination therapies are safely and effectively used for rejuvenation of the facial skin of patients with skin of color. Cosmetic concerns for this population include pigmentary disorders, scarring from the inflammatory process of acne, facial hair growth, keloidal scarring, and loss of volume of the midface with sagging and facial frown lines. Combination therapies used to address dyschromias include topical skin-lightening agents combined with microdermabrasion, chemical peels, microneedling, or laser therapy. Factors to consider when selecting an aesthetic procedure in patients with skin of color include the patient's skin type, their ethnic background, the indication for the procedure, and the realistic treatment goals. The combination of neuromodulators and fillers as well as skin-tightening technology addresses volume loss, sagging, and prominent frown lines and nasolabial folds in aging ethnic skin (**see Video 1.1**). Caution must be exercised to avoid PIH with all aesthetic nonsurgical procedures in patients with skin of color.

(The following is an excerpt from Few, J. Facial Aesthetic Surgery in Skin of Color, in Nahai F. The Art of Aesthetics, 2e, 2010, Thieme Publishing Group.)

5.6 Commentary

Julius W. Few Jr.

Based on content elegantly presented, the practitioner needs to avoid trauma to the basal dermal layer, where the greatest concentration of pro-keloid fibroblasts exist. One is left to conclude that treatment of the epidermis and subcutaneous layers are well tolerated, but any treatment that threatens the dermal–epidermal interface or basal dermal layers runs the risk of severe adverse events.

Cosmetic surgical and nonsurgical procedures are becoming ever more popular in our society. According to ASAPS, there was a 94% increase in cosmetic surgery procedures between 1997 and 2015 and a 605% increase in nonsurgical procedures, whereas racial and ethnic minorities accounted for 25% of all procedures, which was a 3% increase from 2014.[1] Because these numbers will only continue to increase, every cosmetic surgeon will need a basic understanding of treating various racial and ethnic groups, which are a growing proportion of our patient population.

First and foremost, the surgeon must understand cultural and ethnic perceptions and focus in on their goals and objectives for cosmetic surgery. Most patients want to look refreshed or improved but do not want to lose their ethnic identity. In 2006, Odunze et al[97] found that regarding blepharoplasty, 40% of African American women were concerned about losing their ethnic identity.[97] Additionally, overcorrection is of great concern, in that ethnic groups seek significant improvement but fear overcorrection much more than their Caucasian counterparts.

Racial and ethnic patients present with dynamic considerations and needs, and although this subset is at risk for pigmentation and scar concerns, the natural resistance to actinic damage often makes rejuvenation efforts very rewarding for racial and ethnic patients. As this chapter alludes to in conjunction with published works, various ethnic and racial groups possess differing skin characteristics, which affect the skin's barrier function, sebum production, sun protection, chemical sensitivity, and effects of aging. In 2001, Hillebrand et al[98] evaluated 3,000 patients of every ethnic and racial background and

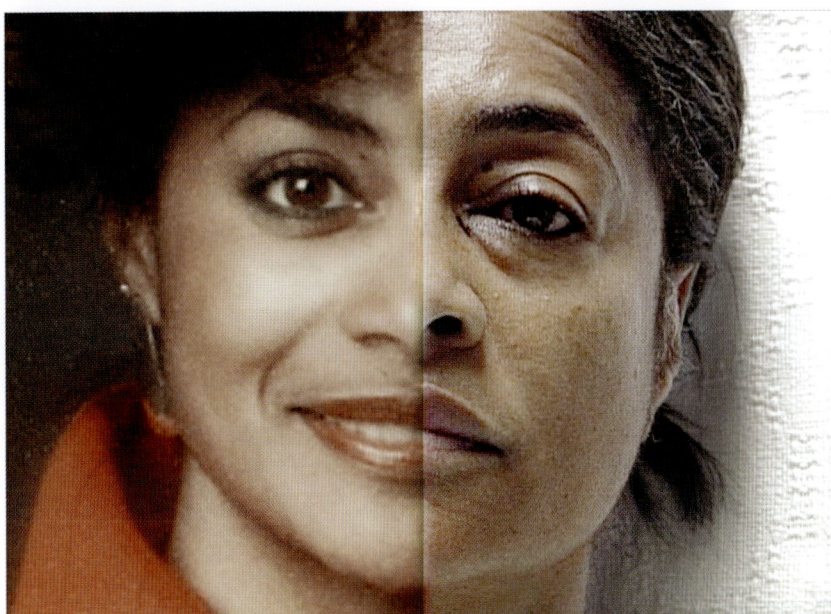

Fig. 5.10 This split image illustrates composite facial aging in an African American woman over a 17-year period. Periorbital aging begins with forehead redundancy and flattening of the brow apex. Crowding of the lateral and central upper eyelid occurs as the brow migrates inferiorly. The upper lid loses septal support, leading to brow prolapse and exacerbation of upper eyelid fullness and congestion. The lateral canthal complex migrates inferiorly, loosening the lower eyelid sling. (Reproduced with permission from Few, J: Facial Aesthetic Surgery in Skin of Color in Nahai, F. The Art of Aesthetics: Principles and Techniques, ed 2, Thieme Publishing, 2010)

differing age groups, and revealed certain age-dependent changes in the skin. The mean facial surface area covered with wrinkles is significantly less in African Americans compared to Caucasians, and the authors suggest that racial differences in other genetic factors besides skin pigmentation, such as DNA repair, are important in determining the development of skin wrinkles.[99,100] However, it behooves the surgeon to be very careful when treating patients of color, in that while darker skin has the tendency to not show wrinkles over time, it must be remembered that darker skin is much more likely to show a scar after an incision.

Although the chapter eloquently discusses applications of nonsurgical modalities in diverse skin types, we will now highlight various aspects of surgical facial rejuvenation and discuss important points as related to treating skin of color. This is particularly important when we look to stack surgical and nonsurgical procedures together in the ethnic patient.

5.6.1 Periorbital Rejuvenation

In our research, we found that African American and Asian eyes, at least subjectively, share a strong association of features, particularly the lateral cant of the eye.[97] A significant number of African American patients when asked, felt their youthful eye had a positive canthal tilt, which is a feature shared among many Asian patients.

From our computer analysis of high-resolution photographs from 500 subjects, we found that canthal ptosis with aging occurs at a faster rate in African Americans than in Caucasians.[101] Hence, although the lateral canthus typically starts higher than the medial canthus in the youthful eye, the drop over time is relatively dramatic and the operating surgeon may be deceived to find the equal canthal points, mistakenly leaving the malposition untreated.

Whereas the lateral canthus may descend drastically in ethnic patients, brow ptosis tends to happen at a lesser extent and at a later age[101,102] (▶ Fig. 5.10). Hence, the surgeon should focus on balancing the brow position while providing support for the planned eyelid repositioning, which in our practice is best performed with an internal browpexy, to help limit the scar burden[103] (▶ Fig. 5.11).

Finally, nonsurgical options such as fillers or neuromodulators provide an excellent option for patients who are uncertain about undergoing surgery, those who want to see potential results before committing to a surgical procedure, or those who wish to avoid surgery altogether, thereby providing a great deal of forgiveness and user-friendliness for the surgeon. Nonsurgical options will be discussed in further detail below.

5.6.2 Rhinoplasty

Nasal aesthetic surgery in people with skin of color is very culturally specific, and although defining points such as alar width, tip fullness, and radix height have been well described for Caucasians, these points are inherently distinct in differing racial and ethnic groups.[103,104] Hence, the goal of the rhinoplasty surgeon should not be to "correct" the nose but rather to enhance the appearance of the nose and bring it closer to a given ethnic/familial definition. To this end, just like with body dysmorphic disorder patients, the treating surgeon must be careful of a small subset of patients who wish to alter their ethnic identity completely, because they have proven to be extremely difficult to satisfy.

From a technical perspective, one should look to avoid visible scar placement such as Weir alar excisions. We developed the internal alarplasty as a viable alternative to externally based alar excisional procedures, avoiding visible scarring issues. If an open approach is undertaken, we suggest placing the incision in the natural recess in the hyperpigmented area of the columella–labial angle, where the scar has proven to be quite forgiving. Common maneuvers for most African, Asian, and Latino rhinoplasty patients include an open tip with the use of a septal strut, lower lateral cephalic trim, and removal of the fibrofat pad collection at the crural dome. Typically, the dorsum is left

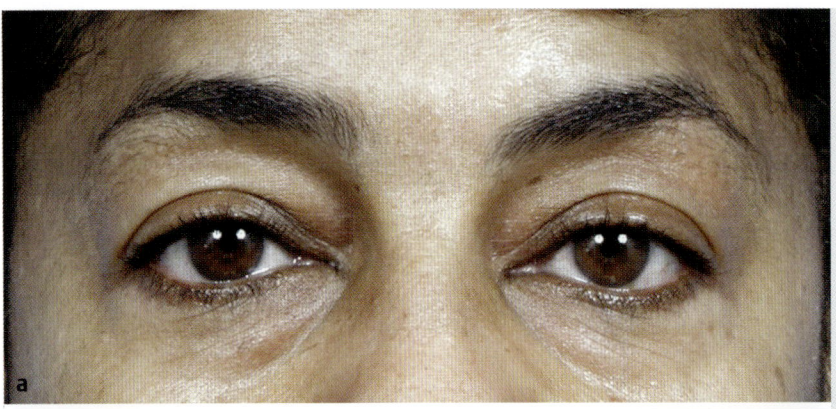

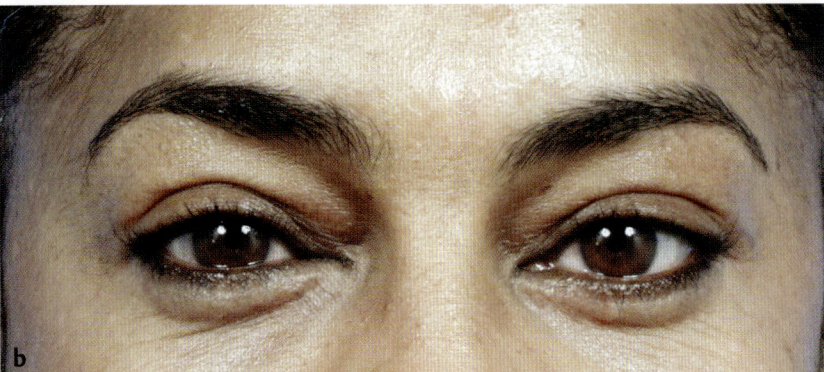

Fig. 5.11 This 50-year old African American woman is shown (**a**) preoperatively and (**b**) 1 year postoperatively after having four-lid blepharoplasty, lateral canthopexy, internal browpexy, and transpalpebral midface lift. (Reproduced with permission from Few, J: Facial Aesthetic Surgery in Skin of Color in Nahai, F. The Art of Aesthetics: Principles and Techniques, ed 2, Thieme Publishing, 2010)

at its original height or augmented with an onlay graft[102] (▶ Fig. 5.12). Although autogenous graft material is often ideal for augmentation rhinoplasty, there can be issues related to donor site scarring, warping, and reabsorption over time. To this end, we have advocated to stack surgical and nonsurgical concepts in some of our patients using hyaluronic acid filler injection to augment the dorsum, at the periosteal and perichondrial level, while surgically enhancing the nasal tip (▶ Fig. 5.13).

It has been our experience that patients with skin of color tend to prefer an undercorrected result rather than having it appear overdone; hence, in patients who are hesitant about surgical intervention, dermal fillers in rhinoplasty have proven to be a useful alternative just like in other areas of rejuvenation (**Video 5.1**).

5.6.3 Facelift

Darker-skinned individuals tend to age prematurely in some areas and late in others because of adipose tissue atrophy, bone remodeling, and gravitational soft tissue changes. African Americans tend to manifest signs of aging in the deeper muscular layers of the face, with sagging of the malar fat pads toward the nasolabial folds. The folds become prominent and cheek ptosis is noted. Given the thicker dermis and subcutaneous tissue of some darker racial ethnic groups combined with infraorbital hypoplasia, midface aging can occur at an earlier age. Although formal rhytidectomy in patients with skin of color can be often be deferred, there continues to be appropriate indications for soft tissue repositioning and the correction of facial rhytids in darker skin.

The primary challenge is that the very nature of a rhytidectomy may cause an increased risk of adverse events, given that hypertrophic and/or keloid scar formation may be exacerbated by increased skin closure tension, foreign body reactions/inflammation, and genetics. Hence, a simple skin-tightening procedure can lead to disastrous results[102] (▶ Fig. 5.14).

The preferred facial rejuvenation procedure is the SMAS plication, allowing for composite preservation and repositioning of soft tissue along with the use of progressive-tension sutures and significantly under-removing redundant skin, to help reduce the resting tension on the periauricular skin closure. The use of a nonabsorbable suture of the mid to superficial dermal closure, removed in 7 to 10 days, greatly reduces the inflammatory response and risk of keloid development[102] (▶ Fig. 5.15).

5.6.4 Nonsurgical Techniques

Lasers

Skin resurfacing in people with skin of color can be quite challenging. While skin of color offers inherent protection from actinic damage, dense sebaceous support to lubricate the skin, and relative thickness, making it very nice to work with, it is also much more prone to PIH and adverse scar formation with resurfacing.

Although traditional ablative technologies, such as CO_2 resurfacing, pose challenges to the treatment of darker-skinned patients, fractional laser technology and nonablative capabilities are very attractive, given the tendency for energy to favor melanin. With the gridlike effect seen with fractional lasers, there is less absolute injury, and areas that are spared aid in dermal recovery.

The primary indications for laser therapy consist of hair reduction, dyschromia, texture irregularities, and scars. Prior to

Diverse Skin Type Considerations and Applications for Nonsurgical Combinations

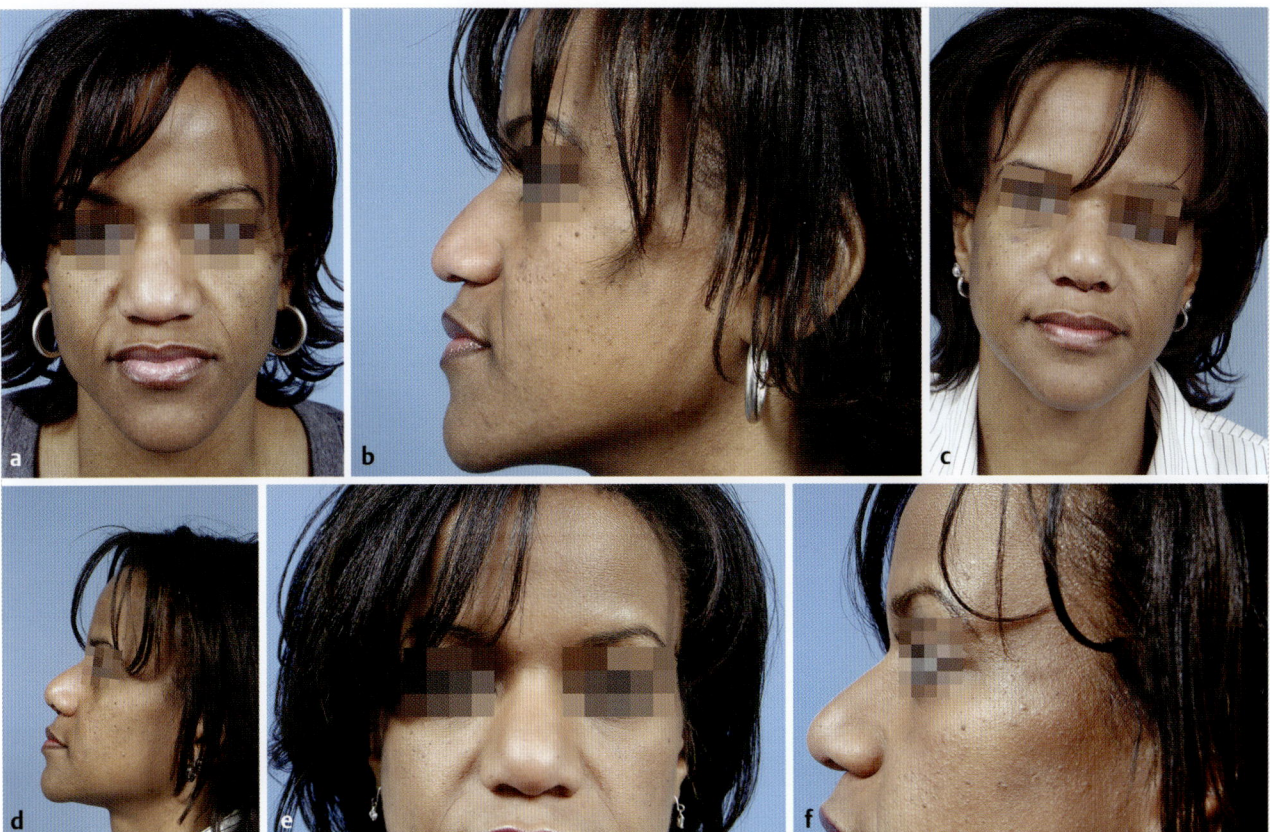

Fig. 5.12 An African American woman with a lack of tip support. Preoperative and postoperative progression after open rhinoplasty, cephalic trim, internal alarplasty, dorsal hump reduction, formal septoplasty, columellar strut, domal sutures, and low-to-low nasal bone in-fracture.
(a,b) Preoperative. (c,d) 1 week postoperatively. (e,f) 2 years postoperatively. (Reproduced with permission from Few, J: Facial Aesthetic Surgery in Skin of Color in Nahai, F. The Art of Aesthetics: Principles and Techniques, ed 2, Thieme Publishing, 2010)

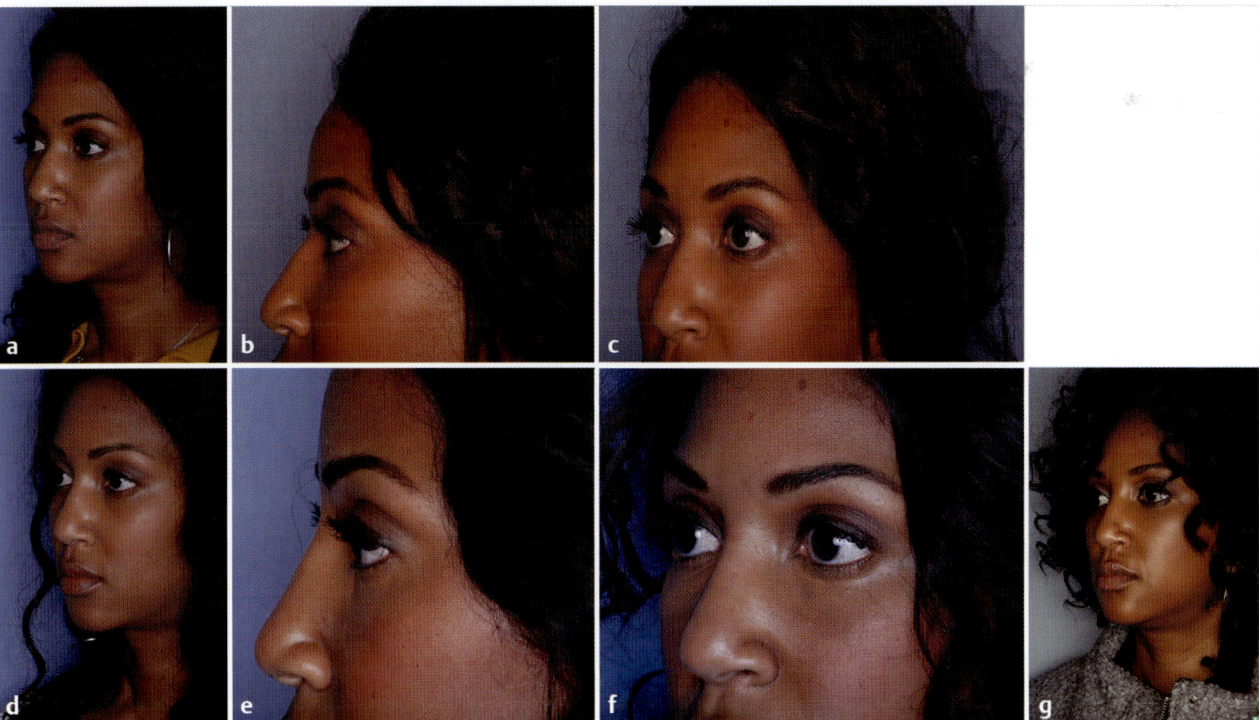

Fig. 5.13 This African American woman sought improvement of her dorsal hump and nasal tip. (a-c) Preprocedure, (d-f) 1-month follow-up after having 0.4 cc of Restylane placed at the preperiosteal level of the proximal dorsum through closed tip rhinoplasty. (g) 22 months after additional dorsal hump rasp reduction.

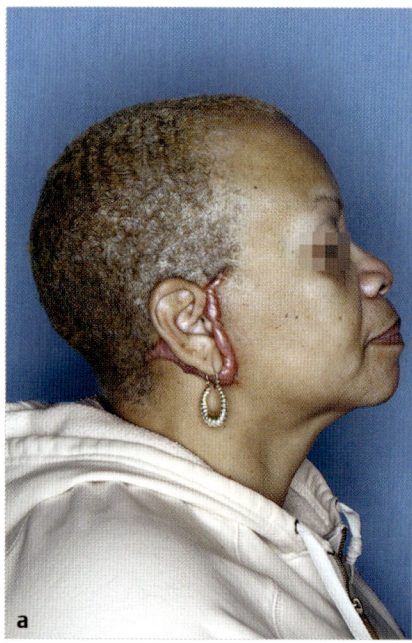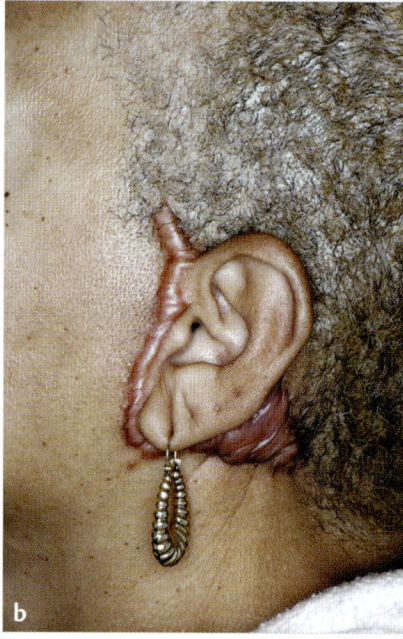

Fig. 5.14 (a,b) This African American woman is shown 1 month after having a skin-only facelift with significant tension-related keloid formation. (Reproduced with permission from Few, J: Facial Aesthetic Surgery in Skin of Color in Nahai, F. The Art of Aesthetics: Principles and Techniques, ed 2, Thieme Publishing, 2010)

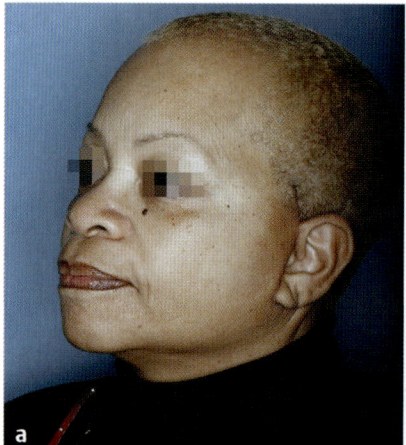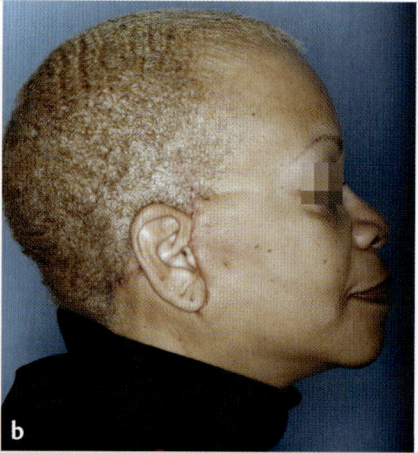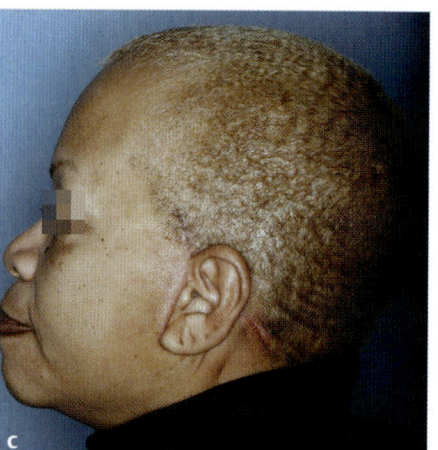

Fig. 5.15 (a-c) Same patient in ▶ Fig. 5.14 is shown 6 months after having a secondary facelift using SMAS plication with conservative skin excision and internal progressive-tension sutures. (Reproduced with permission from Few, J: Facial Aesthetic Surgery in Skin of Color in Nahai, F. The Art of Aesthetics: Principles and Techniques, ed 2, Thieme Publishing, 2010)

any resurfacing, it is vital for patients to use sunscreen, at least an SPF of 20, for 2 to 4 weeks prior to the treatment. HQ and retinoic acid use are beneficial for both preparation of the skin and for control of pigmentation after the treatment, which should typically be held for 1 week before and after. Prior to full treatment, a test patch is often beneficial for understanding how the skin will react. Additionally, dermabrasion, considered the gold standard for skin resurfacing in skin of color, is a relatively low technology that offers precise depth control and accuracy. It can frequently be used as a pretreatment, prior to laser resurfacing or hair removal[102] (▶ Fig. 5.16). Of note, patients must be given a realistic expectation, because understanding the treatment process will likely require a full year or more to achieve the greatest level of correction/enhancement.

Fillers

The use of fillers, particularly hyaluronic acid fillers, in skin of color has many advantages and enjoys the same safety/efficacy profile as seen in Caucasian patients.[90] Due to the increased thickness of skin and the darker pigment, the injection of product into the dermis tends to blend very well.

Based upon our research, there are several general points to consider with injectable fillers.[105] In particular, the primary goal of any injection in skin of color is to minimize the number of needle perforations to the epidermis, thereby reducing the risk of PIH. Additionally, it is important to inject the material into the deeper dermis to minimize the risk of dermal/epidermal separation, which can lead to epidermolysis and PIH.

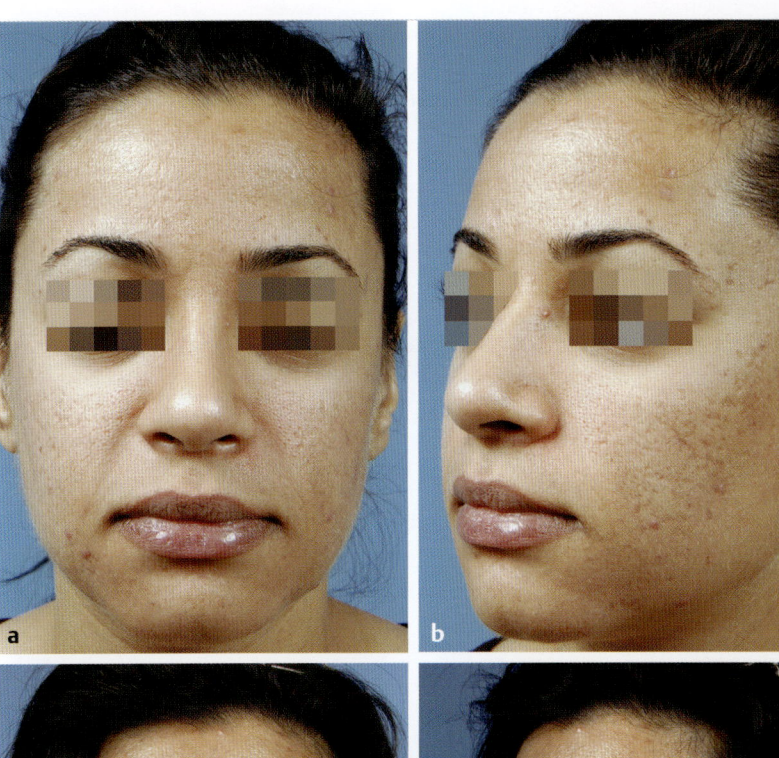
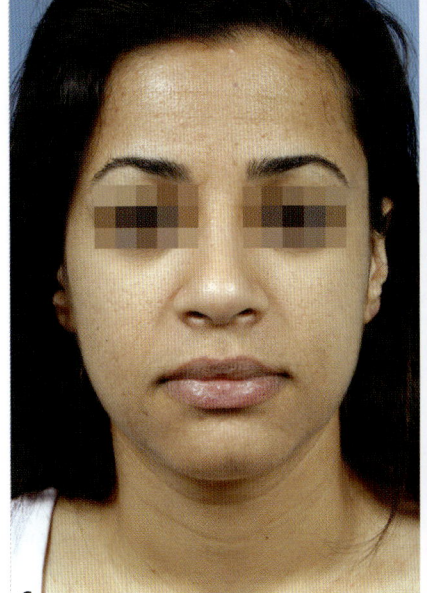
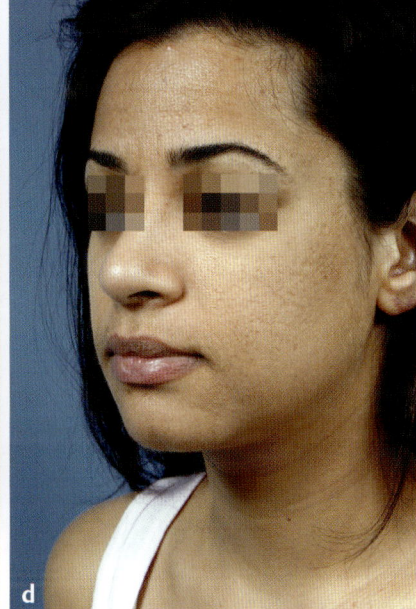

Fig. 5.16 Fitzpatrick skin type IV with active acne and scarring. After acne control and three rounds of dermabrasion, nonablative (wavelength 1540 nm) and ablative (wavelength 2940 nm) were performed. **(a,b)** Preprocedure, **(c,d)** 6-month follow-up. (Reproduced with permission from Few, J: Facial Aesthetic Surgery in Skin of Color in Nahai, F. The Art of Aesthetics: Principles and Techniques, ed 2, Thieme Publishing, 2010)

5.6.5 Conclusion

Racial and ethnic minorities are a growing proportion of patients receiving cosmetic surgery, and a basic understanding of skin of color is mandatory for all cosmetic surgeons. The salient points and techniques discussed in this chapter can lead to safe and predictable outcomes in patients with skin of color.

References

[1] American Society for Aesthetic Plastic Surgery. 2015 data. www.surgery.org. Accessed 30 April, 16
[2] English RS, Shenefelt PD. Keloids and hypertrophic scars. Dermatol Surg. 1999; 25(8):631–638
[3] Weigand DA, Haygood C, Gaylor JR. Cell layers and density of Negro and Caucasian stratum corneum. J Invest Dermatol. 1974; 62(6):563–568
[4] Freeman RG, Cockerell EG, Armstrong J, Knox JM. Sunlight as a factor influencing the thickness of epidermis. J Invest Dermatol. 1962; 39:295–298
[5] Thomson ML. Relative efficiency of pigment and horny layer thickness in protecting the skin of Europeans and Africans against solar ultraviolet radiation. J Physiol. 1955; 127(2):236–246
[6] Reed JT, Ghadially R, Elias PM. Effect of race, gender, and skin type on epidermal permeability barrier function. J Invest Dermatol. 1994; 102:537
[7] McKnight A, Momoh AO, Bullocks JM. Variations of structural components: specific intercultural differences in facial morphology, skin type, and structures. Semin Plast Surg. 2009; 23(3):163–167
[8] La Ruche G, Cesarini JP. [Histology and physiology of black skin]. Ann Dermatol Venereol. 1992; 119(8):567–574
[9] Kompaore F, Marty JP, Dupont C. In vivo evaluation of the stratum corneum barrier function in blacks, Caucasians and Asians with two noninvasive methods. Skin Pharmacol. 1993; 6(3):200–207
[10] Hicks SP, Swindells KJ, Middelkamp-Hup MA, Sifakis MA, González E, González S. Confocal histopathology of irritant contact dermatitis in vivo and the impact of skin color (black vs white). J Am Acad Dermatol. 2003; 48 (5):727–734

[11] Szabo G. Mitochondria and other cytoplasmic inclusions. In: Gordon M, ed. Pigment Cell Biology. New York: Academic Press; 1959

[12] Staricco RJ, Pinkus H. Quantitative and qualitative data on the pigment cells of adult human epidermis. J Invest Dermatol. 1957; 28(1):33–45

[13] Toda K, Pathak MA, Parrish JA, Fitzpatrick TB, Quevedo WC, Jr. Alteration of racial differences in melanosome distribution in human epidermis after exposure to ultraviolet light. Nat New Biol. 1972; 236(66):143–145

[14] Bolognia JL, Orlow SJ. Melanocyte biology. In: Bolognia JL, Jorizzo JL, Rapini RP, eds. Dermatology. St Louis, MO: Mosby; 2003:935

[15] Masson P. Pigment cells in man. In: Miner RW, Gordon M, eds. The Biology of Melanosomes, Vol IV. New York: New York Academy of Sciences; 1948:10–17

[16] Szabó G, Gerald AB, Pathak MA, Fitzpatrick TB. Racial differences in the fate of melanosomes in human epidermis. Nature. 1969; 222(5198):1081–1082

[17] Yoshida-Amano Y, Hachiya A, Ohuchi A, et al. Essential role of RAB27A in determining constitutive human skin color. PLoS One. 2012; 7(7):e41160

[18] Montagna W, Carlisle K. The architecture of black and white facial skin. J Am Acad Dermatol. 1991; 24(6 Pt 1):929–937

[19] Herzberg AJ, Dinehart SM. Chronologic aging in black skin. Am J Dermatopathol. 1989; 11(4):319–328

[20] Kotrajaras R, Kligman AM. The effect of topical tretinoin on photodamaged facial skin: the Thai experience. Br J Dermatol. 1993; 129(3):302–309

[21] Colby SL, Ortman JM. Projections of the Size and Composition of the US Population: 2014 to 2060. US Census Bureau, ed.; 2015 Mar:25–1143

[22] Fitzpatrick TB. The validity and practicality of sun-reactive skin types I through VI. Arch Dermatol. 1988; 124(6):869–871

[23] Kawada A. UVB-induced erythema, delayed tanning, and UVA-induced immediate tanning in Japanese skin. Photodermatol. 1986; 3(6):327–333

[24] Glogau RG. Chemical peeling and aging skin. J Geriatric Dermatol. 1994; 2: 31

[25] Lancer HA. Lancer Ethnicity Scale (LES). [letter]. Lasers Surg Med. 1998; 22 (1):9

[26] Goldman M. Universal classification of skin type. J Cosmet Dermatol. 2002; 15:53–54, 57

[27] Fanous N. A new patient classification for laser resurfacing and peels: predicting responses, risks, and results. Aesthetic Plast Surg. 2002; 26(2): 99–104

[28] Willis I, Earles MR. A new classification system relevant to people of African descent. J Cosmet Dermatol. 2005; 18(3):209–216

[29] Taylor S, Westerhof W, Im S, Lim J. Noninvasive techniques for the evaluation of skin color. J Am Acad Dermatol. 2006; 54(5) Suppl 2:S282–S290

[30] Roberts WE. The Roberts skin classification system. J Drugs Dermatol. 2008; 7(5):452–456

[31] Halder RM, Grimes PE, McLaurin CI, Kress MA, Kenney JA, Jr. Incidence of common dermatoses in a predominantly black dermatologic practice. Cutis. 1983; 32(4):388–390, 390

[32] Alexis AF, Sergay AB, Taylor SC. Common dermatologic disorders in skin of color: a comparative practice survey. Cutis. 2007; 80(5):387–394

[33] Sanchez MR. Cutaneous diseases in Latinos. Dermatol Clin. 2003; 21(4):689–697

[34] Kang SJ, Davis SA, Feldman SR, McMichael AJ. Dyschromia in skin of color. J Drugs Dermatol. 2014; 13(4):401–406

[35] Chua-Ty G, Goh CL, Koh SL. Pattern of skin diseases at the National Skin Centre (Singapore) from 1989–1990. Int J Dermatol. 1992; 31(8):555–559

[36] Pu LLQ. Aesthetic Plastic Surgery in Asians: Principles and Techniques. Thieme Publishing Group; 2015

[37] Sarkar R, Bansal S, Garg VK. Chemical peels for melasma in dark-skinned patients. J Cutan Aesthet Surg. 2012; 5(4):247–253

[38] Mahajan R, Kanwar AJ, Parsad D, Kumaran MS, Sharma R. Glycolic Acid peels/azelaic Acid 20% cream combination and low potency triple combination lead to similar reduction in melasma severity in ethnic skin: results of a randomized controlled study. Indian J Dermatol. 2015; 60(2): 147–152

[39] Sarkar R, Arora P, Garg KV. Cosmeceuticals for Hyperpigmentation: What is Available? J Cutan Aesthet Surg. 2013; 6(1):4–11

[40] Guevara IL, Pandya AG. Melasma treated with hydroquinone, tretinoin, and a fluorinated steroid. Int J Dermatol. 2001; 40(3):212–215

[41] Fabbrocini G, De Vita V, Fardella N, et al. Skin needling to enhance depigmenting serum penetration in the treatment of melasma. Plast Surg Int. 2011; 2011:158241

[42] Budamakuntla L, Loganathan E, Suresh DH, et al. A randomized, open-label, comparative study of tranexamic acid microinjections and tranexamic acid with microneedling in patients with melasma. J Cutan Aesthet Surg. 2013; 6 (3):139–143

[43] Manaloto RM, Alster T. Erbium:YAG laser resurfacing for refractory melasma. Dermatol Surg. 1999; 25(2):121–123

[44] Cohen BE, Elbuluk N. Microneedling in skin of color: A review of uses and efficacy. J Am Acad Dermatol. 2016; 74(2):348–355

[45] Ho SG, Yeung CK, Chan NP, Shek SY, Kono T, Chan HH. A retrospective analysis of the management of acne post-inflammatory hyperpigmentation using topical treatment, laser treatment, or combination topical and laser treatments in oriental patients. Lasers Surg Med. 2011; 43(1):1–7

[46] Burns RL, Prevost-Blank PL, Lawry MA, Lawry TB, Faria DT, Fivenson DP. Glycolic acid peels for postinflammatory hyperpigmentation in black patients. A comparative study. Dermatol Surg. 1997; 23(3):171–174, discussion 175

[47] Davis EC, Callender VD. Aesthetic dermatology for aging ethnic skin. Dermatol Surg. 2011; 37(7):901–917

[48] Hall HI, Rogers JD. Sun protection behaviors among African Americans. Ethn Dis. 1999; 9(1):126–131

[49] Briley JJ, Jr, Lynfield YL, Chavda K. Sunscreen use and usefulness in African-Americans. J Drugs Dermatol. 2007; 6(1):19–22

[50] Levin CY, Maibach H. Exogenous ochronosis. An update on clinical features, causative agents and treatment options. Am J Clin Dermatol. 2001; 2(4): 213–217

[51] Davis EC, Callender VD. A review of acne in ethnic skin: pathogenesis, clinical manifestations, and management strategies. J Clin Aesthet Dermatol. 2010; 3(4):24–38

[52] Draelos ZD, Carter E, Maloney JM, et al. United States/Canada Dapsone Gel Study Group. Two randomized studies demonstrate the efficacy and safety of dapsone gel, 5% for the treatment of acne vulgaris. J Am Acad Dermatol. 2007; 56(3):439.e1–439.e10

[53] Plewig G, Fulton JE, Kligman AM. Pomade acne. Arch Dermatol. 1970; 101 (5):580–584

[54] Halder RM, Holmes YC, Bridgeman-Shah S, Kligman AM. A clinicohistopathologic study of acne vulgaris in black females. (abstract). J Invest Dermatol. 1996; 106:888

[55] Fabbrocini G, Annunziata MC, D'Arco V, et al. Acne scars: pathogenesis, classification and treatment. Dermatol Res Pract. 2010; 2010:893080

[56] Khunger N, Bhardwaj D, Khunger M. Evaluation of CROSS technique with 100% TCA in the management of ice pick acne scars in darker skin types. J Cosmet Dermatol. 2011; 10(1):51–57

[57] Keller R, Belda Júnior W, Valente NY, Rodrigues CJ. Nonablative 1,064-nm Nd:YAG laser for treating atrophic facial acne scars: histologic and clinical analysis. Dermatol Surg. 2007; 33(12):1470–1476

[58] Alexis AF, Coley MK, Nijhawan RI, et al. Nonablative Fractional Laser Resurfacing for Acne Scarring in Patients With Fitzpatrick Skin Phototypes IV-VI. Dermatol Surg. 2016; 42(3):392–402

[59] Taub AF, Garretson CB. Treatment of Acne Scars of Skin Types II to V by Sublative Fractional Bipolar Radiofrequency and Bipolar Radiofrequency Combined with Diode Laser. J Clin Aesthet Dermatol. 2011; 4(10):18–27

[60] Sharad J. Combination of microneedling and glycolic acid peels for the treatment of acne scars in dark skin. J Cosmet Dermatol. 2011; 10(4):317–323

[61] Garg S, Baveja S. Combination therapy in the management of atrophic acne scars. J Cutan Aesthet Surg. 2014; 7(1):18–23

[62] Karnik J, Baumann L, Bruce S, et al. A double-blind, randomized, multicenter, controlled trial of suspended polymethylmethacrylate microspheres for the correction of atrophic facial acne scars. J Am Acad Dermatol. 2014; 71(1): 77–83

[63] Gold MH, McGuire M, Mustoe TA, et al. International Advisory Panel on Scar Management. Updated international clinical recommendations on scar management: part 2–algorithms for scar prevention and treatment. Dermatol Surg. 2014; 40(8):825–831

[64] Yosipovitch G, Widijanti Sugeng M, Goon A, Chan YH, Goh CL. A comparison of the combined effect of cryotherapy and corticosteroid injections versus corticosteroids and cryotherapy alone on keloids: a controlled study. J Dermatolog Treat. 2001; 12(2):87–90

[65] Stromps JP, Dunda S, Eppstein RJ, Babic D, Har-Shai Y, Pallua N. Intralesional cryosurgery combined with topical silicone gel sheeting for the treatment of refractory keloids. Dermatol Surg. 2014; 40(9):996–1003

[66] Davison SP, Dayan JH, Clemens MW, Sonni S, Wang A, Crane A. Efficacy of intralesional 5-fluorouracil and triamcinolone in the treatment of keloids. Aesthet Surg J. 2009; 29(1):40–46

[67] Camacho-Martínez FM, Rey ER, Serrano FC, Wagner A. Results of a combination of bleomycin and triamcinolone acetonide in the treatment of keloids and hypertrophic scars. An Bras Dermatol. 2013; 88(3):387–394

[68] Son IP, Park KY, Kim B, Kim MN. Pilot study of the efficacy of 578 nm copper bromide laser combined with intralesional corticosteroid injection for treatment of keloids and hypertrophic scars. Ann Dermatol. 2014; 26(2):156–161

[69] Martin MS, Collawn SS. Combination treatment of CO2 fractional laser, pulsed dye laser, and triamcinolone acetonide injection for refractory keloid scars on the upper back. J Cosmet Laser Ther. 2013; 15(3):166–170

[70] Asilian A, Darougheh A, Shariati F. New combination of triamcinolone, 5-Fluorouracil, and pulsed-dye laser for treatment of keloid and hypertrophic scars. Dermatol Surg. 2006; 32(7):907–915

[71] Weshay AH, Abdel Hay RM, Sayed K, El Hawary MS, Nour-Edin F. Combination of radiofrequency and intralesional steroids in the treatment of keloids: a pilot study. Dermatol Surg. 2015; 41(6):731–735

[72] Uddhav A. Patil and Lakshyajit D. Dhami. Overview of Lasers. Indian J Plast Surg. 2008 Oct; 41(Suppl): S101–S113, Patients with skin types IV–VI: efficacy, safety, and the role of topical corticosteroids in preventing side effects. J Drugs Dermatol. 2007; 6(1):60–66

[73] Ismail SA. Long-pulsed Nd:YAG laser vs. intense pulsed light for hair removal in dark skin: a randomized controlled trial. Br J Dermatol. 2012; 166(2):317–321

[74] Aldraibi MS, Touma DJ, Khachemoune A. Hair removal with the 3-msec alexandrite laser in patients with skin types IV-VI: efficacy, safety, and the role of topical corticosteroids in preventing side effects. J Drugs Dermatol. 2007; 6(1):60–66

[75] Breadon JY, Barnes CA. Comparison of adverse events of laser and light-assisted hair removal systems in skin types IV-VI. J Drugs Dermatol. 2007; 6(1):40–46

[76] Battle EF, Jr, Hobbs LM. Laser-assisted hair removal for darker skin types. Dermatol Ther (Heidelb). 2004; 17(2):177–183

[77] Morton LM, Dover JS. Foreseeing the future of skin tightening. Dermatol Surg. 2014; 40 Suppl 12:S199–S202

[78] El-Domyati M, Barakat M, Awad S, Medhat W, El-Fakahany H, Farag H. Multiple microneedling sessions for minimally invasive facial rejuvenation: an objective assessment. Int J Dermatol. 2015; 54(12):1361–1369

[79] Harris MO, Sundaram HA. Safety of Microfocused Ultrasound With Visualization in Patients With Fitzpatrick Skin Phototypes III to VI. JAMA Facial Plast Surg. 2015; 17(5):355–357

[80] Tanaka Y, Tsunemi Y, Kawashima M, Tatewaki N, Nishida H. Treatment of skin laxity using multisource, phase-controlled radiofrequency in Asians: visualized 3-dimensional skin tightening results and increase in elastin density shown through histologic investigation. Dermatol Surg. 2014; 40(7):756–762

[81] Seo KY, Kim DH, Lee SE, Yoon MS, Lee HJ. Skin rejuvenation by microneedle fractional radiofrequency and a human stem cell conditioned medium in Asian skin: a randomized controlled investigator blinded split-face study. J Cosmet Laser Ther. 2013; 15(1):25–33

[82] Chua SH, Ang P, Khoo LS, Goh CL. Nonablative infrared skin tightening in Type IV to V Asian skin: a prospective clinical study. Dermatol Surg. 2007; 33(2):146–151

[83] Kaidbey KH, Agin PP, Sayre RM, Kligman AM. Photoprotection by melanin–a comparison of black and Caucasian skin. J Am Acad Dermatol. 1979; 1(3):249–260

[84] Harris MO. The aging face in patients of color: minimally invasive surgical facial rejuvenation-a targeted approach. Dermatol Ther (Heidelb). 2004; 17(2):206–211

[85] Grimes PE, Shabazz D. A four-month randomized, double-blind evaluation of the efficacy of botulinum toxin type A for the treatment of glabellar lines in women with skin types V and VI. Dermatol Surg 2009;35:429-36

[86] Taylor SC, Callender VD, Albright CD, Coleman J, Axford-Gatley RA, Lin X. AbobotulinumtoxinA for reduction of glabellar lines in patients with skin of color: post hoc analysis of pooled clinical trial data. Dermatol Surg. 2012; 38(11):1804–1811

[87] Heath CR, Taylor SC. Fillers in the skin of color population. J Drugs Dermatol. 2011; 10(5):494–498

[88] Grimes PE, Thomas JA, Murphy DK. Safety and effectiveness of hyaluronic acid fillers in skin of color. J Cosmet Dermatol. 2009; 8(3):162–168

[89] Taylor SC, Burgess CM, Callender VD. Safety of nonanimal stabilized hyaluronic acid dermal fillers in patients with skin of color: a randomized, evaluator-blinded comparative trial. Dermatol Surg. 2009; 35 Suppl 2:1653–1660

[90] Odunze M, Cohn A, Few JW. Restylane and people of color. Plast Reconstr Surg. 2007; 120(7):2011–2016

[91] Downie JB, Grimes PE, Callender VD. A multicenter study of the safety and effectiveness of hyaluronic acid with a cohesive polydensified matrix for treatment of nasolabial folds in subjects with Fitzpatrick skin types IV, V, and VI. Plast Reconstr Surg. 2013; 132(4) Suppl 2:41S–47S

[92] Jones D, Murphy DK. Volumizing hyaluronic acid filler for midface volume deficit: 2-year results from a pivotal single-blind randomized controlled study. Dermatol Surg. 2013; 39(11):1602–1612

[93] Marmur ES, Taylor SC, Grimes PE, Boyd CM, Porter JP, Yoo JY. Six-month safety results of calcium hydroxylapatite for treatment of nasolabial folds in Fitzpatrick skin types IV to VI. Dermatol Surg. 2009; 35 Suppl 2:1641–1645

[94] Cohen S, Dover J, Monheit G, et al. Five-year safety and satisfaction study of PMMA-collagen in the correction of nasolabial folds. Dermatol Surg. 2015; 41 Suppl 1:S302–S313

[95] Alexis AF, Alam M. Racial and ethnic differences in skin aging: implications for treatment with soft tissue fillers. J Drugs Dermatol. 2012; 11(8):s30–s32, discussion s32

[96] Glogau RG, Kane MA. Effect of injection techniques on the rate of local adverse events in patients implanted with nonanimal hyaluronic acid gel dermal fillers. Dermatol Surg. 2008; 34 Suppl 1:S105–S109

[97] Odunze M, Reid RR, Yu M, Few JW. Periorbital rejuvenation and the African American patient: a survey approach. Plast Reconstr Surg. 2006; 118(4):1011–1018

[98] Hillebrand GG, Levine MJ, Miyamoto K. The age-dependent changes in skin conditions in African American, Asian Indians, caucasians, East Asians and Latinos. IFSCC Magazine. 2001; 4:259–266

[99] Grimes P, Edison BL, Green BA, Wildnauer RH. Evaluation of inherent differences in ethnic skin types and response to topical polyhydroxy acid (PHA) use. Washington DC: American Acadamy of Dermatology Poster Exhibit; March 2001

[100] Grimes PE, Hunt SG. Considerations for cosmetic surgery in the black population. Clin Plast Surg. 1993; 20(1):27–34

[101] Odunze M, Rosenberg DS, Few JW. Periorbital aging and ethnic considerations: a focus on the lateral canthal complex. Plast Reconstr Surg. 2008; 121(3):1002–1008

[102] Few J. Facial Aesthetic Surgery in Skin of Color in Nahai, F. The Art of Aesthetics: Principles and Techniques. ed 2. Thieme Publishing; 2010

[103] Hoefflin SM. Ethnic Rhinoplasty. New York: Springer-Verlag; 1997

[104] Matory EW. Ethnic Considerations in Facial Aesthetic Surgery. Philadelphia: Lippincott Williams & Wilkins; 1998

[105] Grimes PE, Few JW. Injectable Fillers in Skin of Color. In: Carruthers J, Carruthers A, eds. Procedures in Cosmetic Dermatology; Soft Tissue Augmentation. 2nd ed. Amsterdam: Sanders Elsevier; 2008:143–151

6 Noninvasive Devices Used in Combination with Volumizing

Rachel N. Pritzker, Shraddha Desai, and Brian S. Biesman

Summary

Noninvasive and minimally invasive devices have become very attractive because of their lower risk, less downtime, and more gradual approach to aging. A new trend in combining or offering sequential noninvasive treatments, such as using fillers and lasers together, is gaining in popularity due to the short downtime. A review of the literature is necessary, because the amount of information regarding the use of fillers and other treatments, and the safety of such combinations, should be extensive. However, the information is sparse. This chapter provides some guidelines for patient selection and tips when performing multiple treatments.

Keywords: Botulinum toxin type A, combination treatments, devices, fillers, lasers, noninvasive, resurfacing

> **Key Points**
> - The patient population is seeking more nonsurgical treatment options with less downtime, resulting in high demand for concomitant procedures.
> - The scientific literature is starting to demonstrate safety and efficacy of the concurrent use of various treatments.
> - Proper patient selection and consultation is imperative when determining the best combination and sequence of noninvasive or minimally invasive procedures.

6.1 Introduction

Facial aging is the result of a complex combination of multiple factors, and our professional understanding of this process continues to expand. The visible signs of aging are a combination of, among other factors, fat loss and redistribution, bony resorption, and collagen/elastic tissue denaturation. If all of these elements are not dealt with in proper combination, patients may be deprived of their optimal potential outcomes.

Although the field of both invasive and noninvasive cosmetic procedures is growing exponentially, the most notable and recent advancements lie within the noninvasive and minimally invasive categories, which is reflective of patient demand. In fact, the American Society of Plastic Surgeons' (ASPS) statistics for 2014[1] demonstrated the greatest rise since the prior year within the cosmetic minimally invasive procedures category. Within this category, botulinum toxin type A (Botox) and soft tissues fillers remain in the top two, but lasers such as those for resurfacing (both ablative and nonablative) continue to rise, increasing 6% from 2013 (see product Index and **Video 2.3**).[1] Patients are seeking procedures with lower risk profiles, less downtime, and a more gradual approach to enhancing the aging process. Patients are also undergoing procedures at an earlier age, leading to the demand for noninvasive procedures that produce more subtle, yet preventative results. If a procedure requires downtime, the emphasis is to minimize the duration, thus there is increased importance on completing multiple procedures in the same session. This new trend is changing the way many physicians address facial aging.

There are several hesitancies that prevent a practitioner from performing sequential treatments, such as the possibility of changing the properties of the filler, leading to diminished effectiveness or potentiating the risk of both short- and long-term side effects. The package inserts approved by the U.S. Food and Drug Administration (FDA) for both filler substances and devices include warnings against using other procedures in conjunction with their products. For example, injectable poly-L-lactic acid (injectable PLLA, Sculptra Aesthetic) warns against the use of any laser or procedure based on "active dermal response" due to "possible risk of eliciting an inflammatory reaction at the implant site."[2] The insert of the microfocused ultrasound (MFUS) device Ulthera states that there has not been an evaluation of use over materials, therefore "treatment is not recommended directly over those areas with any of the following: mechanical implants, dermal fillers, implanted electrical devices" (see Product Index (p. 185) and **Videos 2.1 and 2.2**).[3] There is no mention of a suggested time frame for using procedures in combination, except for recommendations to allow for complete healing and waiting until the effects are completely realized before proceeding with other procedures. Clinically, complete healing can take up to 6 months for certain treatments, making this timeline unrealistic and undesirable for patients with several cosmetic concerns to address. The question facing the practitioner is not if one can combine noninvasive treatments, but if and when it is safe to do so. As one can see, the combination of treatments is not black and white, and safety concerns from the FDA approvals have not been corroborated to date within the literature. Fortunately, investigations are slowly being published to help answer some of these questions, which may help guide the clinician.

6.1.1 Literature Review of Combination Noninvasive Treatments

The scientific literature is beginning to explore the effectiveness and safety of sequential treatments, but concrete conclusions remain sparse. Our goal is to evaluate the existing evidence for these combinations and to create practical methods based on these scientific principles. When trying to conceive the ideal plan for combining noninvasive treatments, it is paramount to review the literature pertinent to these combinations.

One of the earliest investigations of combining noninvasive treatments was conducted in 2005 by England et al[4] to determine the effects of monopolar radiofrequency (RF) treatment over soft tissue filler in an animal model. Monopolar RF is known to have a depth of heating dependent on the geometry of the electrode, with the 1.5 cm² hand piece penetrating up to

8 mm, making it one of the deepest modalities. At this depth, it is especially important to investigate its use over dermal fillers, because it would contact the filler substance placed more superficially. Using monopolar RF, they [England et al.] investigated, through histology, the effects on various filler substances when used either at the same time as the RF treatment or 1 month after treatment within a juvenile pig model.[4] The five filler substances used were

1. Cross-linked human collagen.
2. Hyaluronic acid (HA).
3. Calcium hydroxylapatite (caHA).
4. Poly-L-lactic acid (PLLA).
5. Liquid silicone.

The filler substance was injected from the middle to deep dermal layer down to the subcutaneous tissue, depending on the substance and placement typically employed during cosmetic applications. The monopolar RF treatment was performed at relatively high settings (1.5 cm^2 treatment tip, 130 and 162 J, 3 passes). Histologic evaluations done sequentially up to 4 months after treatment did not demonstrate any decrease in filler persistence. Moreover, there were no increased adverse events seen clinically due to bulk heating. Therefore, in this animal model, the various filler substances did not change the conductivity of the RF treatment and cause unwanted thermal effects. Over the 4-month follow-up, histology demonstrated trends, although not statistically significant, toward an increased collagen response with HA, PLLA, and caHA when combined with the RF procedure. In a follow-up study, Shumaker et al[5] found significant increases in the foreign body, inflammatory, and fibrotic responses associated with these fillers when treated sequentially with monopolar RF over those treated with RF alone at the 1-month follow-up. It is possible that these changes led to the trend toward increased collagen response seen in their previous study, but this is unable to be confirmed.[4,5] Further, Kim et al[6] found a greater change in the wrinkle severity score and an increase in procollagen production when RF was applied prior to HA filler placement in both a human model and an animal model, respectively.

In human tissue, Alam et al[7] injected HA and caHA filler to the upper arm and performed monopolar RF treatment (1.5 cm^2 treatment tip, 63.5 setting, 2 passes) to the same area 2 weeks later. A control subject did not receive the RF treatment over the injected filler. Within punch biopsy specimens obtained 3 days after the RF treatment, there were no differences seen with light microscopy and digital photomicrographs of the filler substance between areas treated with RF and those areas not treated with RF. There were no differences in signs or symptoms between the control and experimental groups, except a slight transitory pain reported when RF was delivered over the filler.[7]

Beyond RF treatments, Farkas et al[8] examined the histologic effects of several light and laser-based technologies on filler substances in an animal model. HA filler was placed within the dermis of a pig model, and then 2 weeks later, the same area was given one of seven different lasers/light devices. These devices included (see Product Index (p. 176))

- Intense pulsed light (IPL) 560 nm filter (Sciton, Inc.).
- Nd:YAG 1,064 nm (Sciton, Inc.).
- Er:glass 1,540 nm (Lux1540, Palomar Medical Technologies, Inc.).
- erbium 2,940 nm (ProFractional, Sciton, Inc.).
- Er:YAG 2,940 nm (Palomar Medical Technologies, Inc.).
- CO2 10,600 nm (ActiveFX and DeepFX, Lumenis).

Within the 8 mm punch biopsies performed immediately after the laser treatment, there were no signs of interaction of the filler and laser when using the superficially reaching devices, but there was clear interaction when treating with the deep ablative systems (Er:YAG 2,940 nm and CO_2). On histology, the microablative columns created by the laser were interspersed in the pool of filler. Some of the HA filler was seen to migrate into the ablated microchannels or was trapped within collapsed ablated columns in the reticular dermis. The filler substance itself did not show any denaturation or significant morphologic changes, even at higher energy settings.[8]

A similar study was performed on human skin by Goldman et al,[9] who investigated the effects of HA filler followed by a laser or light device in a split-face study, randomized trial. Thirty-six patients received HA filler to the nasolabial folds and postauricular area, followed by either 1,320 nm Nd:YAG, 1,450 nm diode, monopolar RF, or IPL with a 560 nm cutoff filter on one side over the filler. After sequential biopsies over 28 days, there were no significant differences in histology demonstrating damage to the filler, although sampling was an issue within this study, because several biopsies did not demonstrate any filler on histology in either the group treated with an energy device or the group not treated with an energy device. There were no reported adverse events related to overlapping any of the devices over the filler on the same day.[9]

Another deeply penetrating device is the MFUS, which is frequently used for tissue tightening on the face, neck, and chest. MFUS is able to penetrate up to 4.5 mm while employing a commonly used treatment hand piece. Friedmann et al[10] reported the efficacy and safety of using sequential IPL, then MFUS, followed by PLLA injection, in one treatment session on the face. The sequence of procedures, as noted, was chosen specifically to avoid potential increased energy absorption secondary to erythema from MFUS, if IPL was performed afterward. The authors did mention that if MFUS and IPL were not performed on the same day, they would wait 2 weeks before performing MFUS following any PLLA injection to allow for the swelling to subside. A case review by Hart et al[11] demonstrated similar findings in which MFUS and PLLA were used in different areas (face, chest, and back) on the same day. They performed the MFUS procedure first to avoid the water from the PLLA displacing the tissue depth being targeted and to prevent blood contamination of the transducer. There were no increased adverse events from the combination treatment, even when treating the neck and chest. A larger dilution of PLLA, 16 cc in these cases, was used when treating the chest.[10,11]

In another study of the combination of device and filler treatment on human skin, Casabona and Michalany[12] injected both HA and caHA into the inner thigh and studied the histologic effects of MFUS performed over the site. With a control area of filler without MFUS treatment, biopsies were compared at days 0, 15, 30, and 180. There were no significant differences in the inflammatory process or product migration. In comparing qualitative neocollagenesis and neoelastinogenesis, the retroauricular area of the same patient was injected and treated with MFUS, and a control area was left untreated with the device.

Histologic samples stained with Masson's trichrome stain and Verhoff von Giesen stain at day 60 showed an increase in density of the collagen fibers in the areas treated with both fillers and the device simultaneously as compared to the control area in this patient. There were no adverse events noted in the study, and there was no difference in the clinical appearances between the experimental and control areas.[12]

Park et al[13] performed a split-face study of the use of HA filler (Teosyal, Teoxane Laboratories) alone to the nasolabial fold versus concomitant HA filler with a nonablative infrared (IR) device (Titan, Cutera, Inc.). Each of these modalities alone had been shown to improve the clinical appearance of these studied areas. The histologic findings on each side were similar, and there was preservation of filler at the deep dermal–subcutaneous junction. There were no increased adverse events among the 12 patients receiving combination treatment, yet there were also no significant clinical improvements using combination treatment over HA filler alone.[13]

Finally, more well-known, widely used, and important to acknowledge is the combination of botulinum toxin and laser. Treatment with the toxin in the same area treated by a laser has been shown to decrease the degradation of filler, which resulted in a higher volume remaining at the end of muscle paralysis in an animal model.[14]

With treatment on the hand, injecting toxin 1 week prior to resurfacing improved healing of the skin after resurfacing.[15,16] A small study of 10 female patients showed that botulinum toxin injection to the glabella, forehead, and crow's-feet to one side of the face 1 week prior to full-face laser resurfacing resulted in greater improvement on the combination-treatment side.[16] Additional studies with botulinum toxin injection 1 day to 2 weeks prior to fractional resurfacing demonstrated similar results.[17,18,19] Treatment with botulinum toxin injection immediately prior to IPL, nonablative lasers, and radiofrequency devices, in contrast, did not reveal any adverse events.[19,20] On the other hand, the diffusion of botulinum toxin to the neighboring zygomatic muscle when treating periorbital rhytides with neuromodulator and CO_2 ablative resurfacing same day has also been reported.[21]

We can see from the review of the literature that heat generated during a procedure does not change the basic morphology of the filler substance. Further, we know that collagen denaturation occurs at approximately 55 to 70 °C and that temperatures reached within the targeted tissue for devices are estimated to be 50 to 65 °C for neocollagenesis and the tissue-tightening effect.[4] The HA fillers are sterilized during manufacturing at 120 °C, therefore enduring much higher temperatures without changes to its stability.[9]

It is equally important to note that the energy from the device and filler most often do not significantly interact. Theoretically, midface volumizers properly placed at the preperiosteal plane would be below the depth of penetration of the noninvasive devices, as would fillers placed in the deep reticular dermis (▶ Fig. 6.1). Further, what may be important to consider is the type of device, because the longevity of HA and caHA placed from the subcutaneous plane to the superficial dermis did not demonstrate decreased longevity over 6 months when used in combination with the MFUS device, yet dissolution of a caHA nodule inadvertently placed superficially in the dermis was witnessed with the CO_2 device. Reddy et al[22] described a case successfully employing a CO_2 laser to dissolve a misplaced nodule of caHA. The patient experienced a visible nodule of caHA immediately after injection of this filler to the tear trough area, a location typically not injected with this filler substance. After one session of CO_2 fractionated ablative resurfacing, performed 6 months after the initial injection, complete clinical

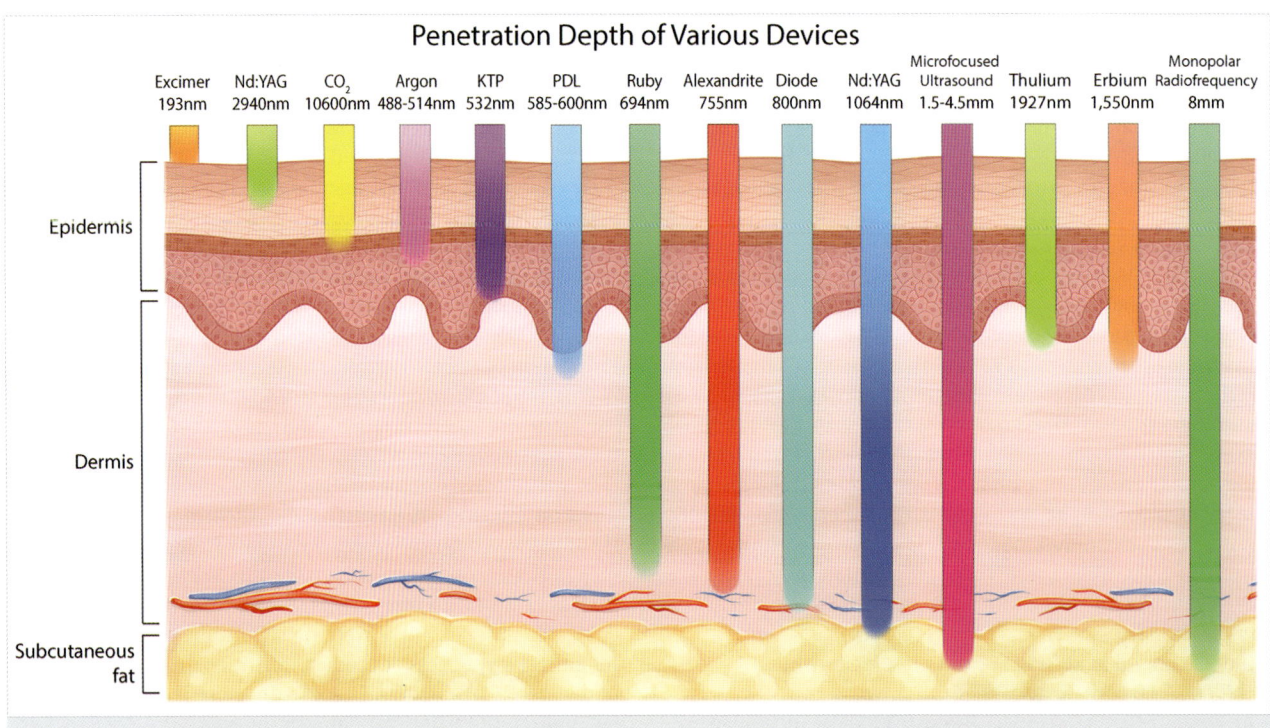

Fig. 6.1 Layers of the face with the depths of commonly used lasers.

resolution at the 2-week follow-up was seen.[22] The depth of penetration for the CO_2 device is more superficial than the MFUS device, and therefore greater interaction was noted in these examples. The extent to which placement depth impacts longevity of the product after a particular combination treatment requires further evaluation; however, safety does not seem to be affected.

There are several concerns regarding using filler and laser treatments sequentially, ranging from the effect of the heat from the laser on the filler to the risk of adverse events from the combination of treatments. The theoretical risks have not thus far been supported by research, but the synergistic effects are documented. Moreover, many physicians are performing such treatments within the same day, but most have yet to publish their findings.

6.2 Patient Selection and Preoperative Considerations

Choosing the appropriate procedure(s) for the patient's aging concerns is always paramount. Incorporating clinical goals for the patient as well as selecting procedures based on social and occupational downtime is also important to consider. When choosing a plan that requires more downtime, the ideal approach would be to perform all of the procedures safely within the same treatment day or as close together as possible. Management of patient expectations is essential with any procedure, but especially when discussing noninvasive procedures. Preprocedural photography and a detailed review of the potential changes based specifically on the individual's cosmetic complaints, rather than broad outcomes, are necessary. Also, the number of treatments and frequency of treatments should be emphasized.

In choosing the type of filler substance to be used, one must consider the amount of volume loss, where the volume loss is most located, and the age/preference of the patient. If moderate to severe midface volume correction is needed for series of PLLA, an HA filler with a combination of low and high molecular weight, or caHA placed preperiosteally, is recommended. Frequently, this clinical volume loss is accompanied by laxity of the lower face, so a skin-tightening procedure, such as RF or MFUS, is often recommended. Alternatively, another common combination of cosmetic complaints is etched perioral or periocular rhytides along with pigment and textural concerns of the skin. In this scenario, one would ultimately combine low-molecular-weight HA fillers placed in the superficial dermis and ablative or nonablative resurfacing. Ideal candidates do not have excessive tissue laxity or severe rhytides, which may require the use of an unreasonable number of filler syringes or aggressive laser resurfacing settings. Treatment response and meeting expectations is typically higher for those with mild to moderate findings. Although fine lines do well with resurfacing and deeper folds respond better to volume replacement with soft tissue fillers, combination therapy is necessary to treat patients with both concerns. Therefore, a physician must explain each component during a consultation.

The most preoperative attention is paid to ablative resurfacing. A patient must be prepared for pretreatment (prophylactic medications, if necessary), postoperative care, and frequent follow-up. Patients who are unable or unwilling to do so should not be treated. All patients, regardless of whether they have a history of cold sores or not, are treated prophylactically with famciclovir, valacyclovir, or acyclovir. Those with concern for acne flares are started on doxycycline to avoid complications. Some clinicians will pretreat all of their patients with oral antibiotics for prophylaxis, and other clinicians even treat the nares with mupirocin to cover for methicillin-resistant *Staphylococcus aureus* (MRSA) colonization.[23] The use of prophylactic, oral antibiotic treatment is controversial, and some clinicians do not use it at all.[24]

Contraindication to laser resurfacing and soft tissue fillers include active skin infection and conditions that koebnerize or inhibit wound healing.[23] Although there is no literature on the effect of anticoagulants on laser resurfacing or soft tissue fillers, ideally the patient should be at a therapeutic level and be cautioned about the possibility of extensive bruising, increased pinpoint bleeding, and prolonged healing. A baseline international normalized ratio (INR) taken a few days prior to treatment is helpful for those on warfarin. If the level is outside the therapeutic range, it may be better to delay the procedure until it is within range. Caution should also be taken in patients who have undergone recent radiation therapy in the field of intended treatment; their skin may be more sensitive, so the settings may have to be modified.[23] Recent isotretinoin therapy, which is an ongoing debate, appears to be safe, yet the standard of care currently is to wait 6 months after completion of therapy.[25] Fractional ablative resurfacing of acne scars in Asian patients, who received isotretinoin within 1–3 months prior to treatment, had no significant side effects even after 6 months of follow-up. There was no evidence of hypertrophic scars or keloids.[25]

6.3 Technical Steps and Tips

Within this new space of combining multiple cosmetic treatments, there is no clear consensus regarding either the ideal timeline for multiple procedures or the necessary order of same-day treatments. We can address recommendations for obtaining the best results and learning points aimed toward creating an efficient plan based on the literature and experience thus far. In general, it is always imperative to use the same caution one would use with a single procedure and apply it to each sequential procedure. The skin is prepped with the same aseptic, clean technique prior to each injection and again repeated prior to any laser device that is used, or vice versa.

When considering performing laser and filler on the same day, there are two considerations to determine which procedure is completed first.

1. Consideration is the swelling or other immediate barriers that may occur that presen a technical issue for your second procedure. Several dermatologic and plastic surgeons perform filler injections prior to laser treatment to ensure that landmarks are clearly seen, so that the filler can be placed in the appropriate area. This is especially true if performing full-face ablative or nonablative resurfacing, because the swelling is immediate and intense, altering the contours of the face. In addition, if a patient is premedicated for pain relief, placing the patient in an upright position to

visualize the target areas may be difficult, requiring placement of filler substance prior to completing the preoperative protocols. Furthermore, if topical anesthetic is used over the entire face for a laser procedure, it may be difficult to visualize any early signs of vascular compromise such as blanching; therefore, one may consider placing filler prior to a topical anesthetic. Topical anesthesia can also provide excessive hydration of the area to be treated and render treatment outcomes more difficult to judge. This is especially true when treating the lips.

2. When planning sequential treatments, it is the target chromophore one must consider. For example, CO_2 and Er:YAG ablative lasers target intracellular water as a chromophore. The depth of penetration could potentially be limited if contacting a hydrophilic HA filler substance. When studied, the overall morphology of the HA filler was not changed immediately on histopathology, but filler was observed within microablative channels in spite of it being placed in the deep dermis.[8] Furthermore, Reddy et al[22] described a case report in which a CO_2 laser was successfully employed to dissolve a misplaced nodule of caHA in the tear trough. Therefore, these changes can demonstrate the importance of injection depth and the type of device used when combining treatments. Several lower-concentration HA fillers are placed higher within the papillary or superficial reticular layers, especially for etched perioral lines, an area that is frequently also treated with more aggressive ablative lasers. In this scenario, it is best to treat separately, laser first followed by HA filler after re-epithelialization or after visualization of results from the laser resurfacing.

Many patients also have vascular and pigmentary concerns along with textural issues. In these cases, it is suggested that treatment with IPL, pulsed dye laser (PDL), or potassium titanium phosphate (KTP) laser for vascular lesions, and q-switched alexandrite or cryotherapy for pigmented lesions, be performed prior to resurfacing. This order allows the vessels and/or lentigines to be targeted directly. If performed afterward, the erythema from the resurfacing makes the underlying lesions more difficult to appreciate, and the chromophore for the vascularity is obscured. If treating larger lentigines or thin seborrheic keratoses prior to resurfacing, one would decrease the fluence of the initial device, so as to not ultimately create bulk heating of the lesion when combining treatments on the same day.

If planning on using tissue-tightening procedures in conjunction with laser and filler treatments, there are various recommendations about the order of the procedures. There have not been issues with excessive heating when RF was performed over dermal filler, yet there may be an issue if the filler substance is reconstituted with another fluid.[7,12] In a report of several cases of same-day IPL, MFUS, and PLLA, the IPL is performed first, followed by the MFUS, and then the PLLA. By performing the semipermanent filler last, one can avoid blood contamination of the laser and ultrasound tips. Further, since the PLLA is reconstituted with water and lidocaine, there is at least a theoretical concern that the excess water may result in a deeper target and more adverse effects from thermal injury.[10,11] Interestingly, when traditional ablative resurfacing is performed under local anesthesia with extensive infiltration of tissues versus general anesthesia where no supplemental local anesthetic is provided, there are no apparent clinical differences in efficacy, safety, or recovery despite keeping the laser setting constant. Of note, if layering several procedures at once (i.e., tissue tightening, fillers, and several lasers), it is prudent to adjust settings for the latter treatments as heat continues to build up in the skin. Also when performing tissue-tightening devices and injectables together, it may be worthwhile to wait to visualize the effects of the tightening procedure prior to injection, because early-onset tightening may result in a lower filler requirement than originally expected. However, each case is handled on an individual basis. If tissue tightening is primarily targeting the jowls, perioral injections, then injections of the temples and periorbital region, or other injections, can be administered simultaneously.

The synergy of combining neuromodulator and filler or laser resurfacing is well documented.[14,16,17,18,19,24] The main concern of performing botulinum toxin on the same visit as another procedure is swelling and the potential for subsequent diffusion of the toxin to unwanted neighboring muscles. The risk is highest in the periorbital area. Although there have been no reports of inactivation or clinical changes with botulinum toxin injection immediately prior to IPL, nonablative lasers, and RF devices, there have been reports of zygomatic muscle weakness after botulinum toxin and CO_2 periorbital resurfacing simultaneously.[19,20] For any procedure that creates swelling, it is best to treat the swelling during a separate visit either before or after a surgical or resurfacing procedure. It has been suggested that neuromodulator administration prior to ablative resurfacing procedures will enhance the clinical results with respect to wrinkle reduction (**see Video 1.1**).[16,17,24]

6.4 Results

We routinely perform soft tissue filler injection and noninvasive skin tightening during the same treatment session. Although it has been clearly demonstrated that soft tissue fillers are not degraded by the thermal effects produced with most noninvasive skin-tightening techniques, we prefer to perform skin tightening in advance of soft tissue volume augmentation. The swelling induced by noninvasive skin tightening of the head and neck is modest enough that soft tissue volume augmentation can generally be performed with outstanding results (**see Video 2.11**).

6.4.1 Case 1

(▶ Fig. 6.2)

6.4.2 Case 2

(▶ Fig. 6.3)

6.4.3 Case 3

(▶ Fig. 6.4)

6.4.4 Case 4

(▶ Fig. 6.5)

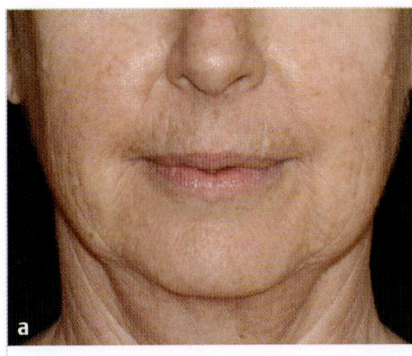
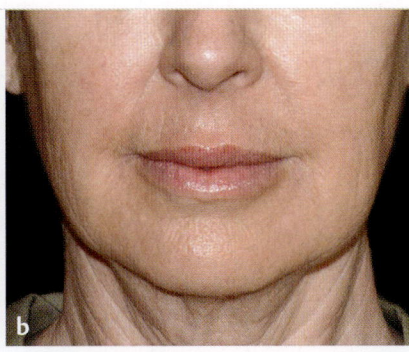

Fig. 6.2 This 59-year-old woman is shown (a) before and (b) 3 months after final treatment with a combination regimen. First, a neuromodulator was administered to lips, Depressor Anguli Oris (DAO), and mentalis muscles followed 2 weeks later by nonablative fractional resurfacing to the face, neck, and chest. Then, 2 weeks later, noninvasive skin tightening was performed over the full face. Finally, 2 weeks later, ablative fractional resurfacing and hyaluronic acid injection to the perioral region was performed. (Courtesy of Dr. Suzanne Kilmer.)

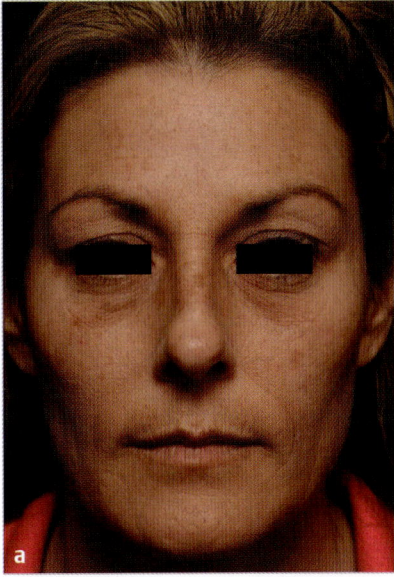
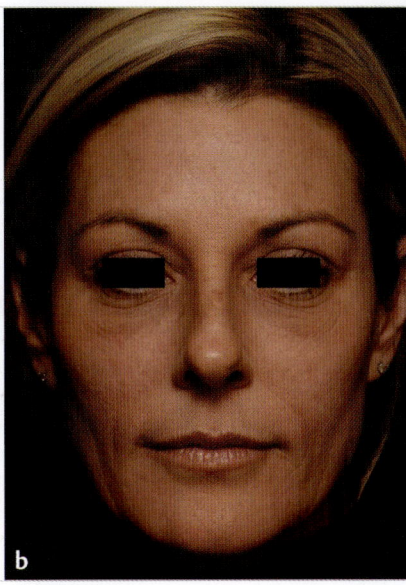

Fig. 6.3 This 45-year-old woman is shown (a) before and (b) 3 months after having upper blepharoplasty and full-face ablative fractional laser skin resurfacing, and 2 months after having a neuromodulator to the upper face, HA filler to the midface and perioral region, and PLLA to the lateral cheeks. (Courtesy of Dr. Brian Biesman.)

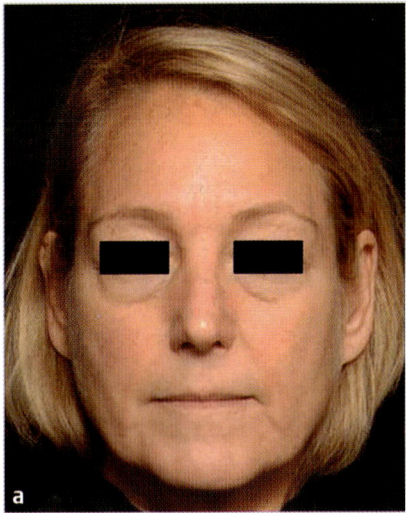
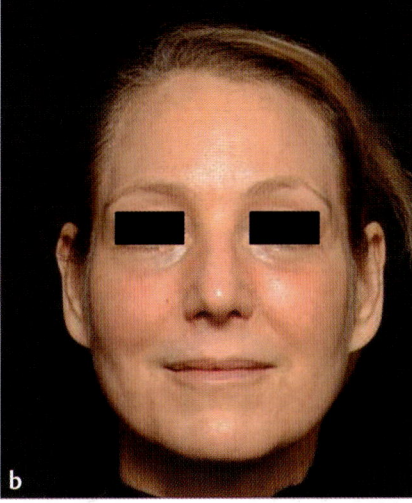

Fig. 6.4 This 58-year-old woman is shown (a) before and (b) 3 months after having bilateral upper lid blepharoplasty and full-face ablative fractional resurfacing, and 2 months after having a hyaluronic acid filler to her midface, temples, and perioral region.

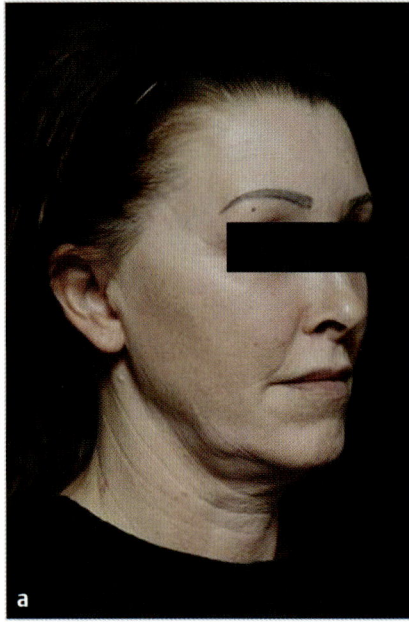 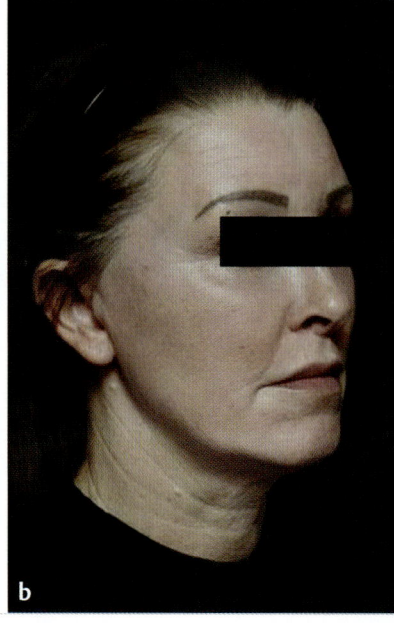

Fig. 6.5 This 53-year-old woman is shown (a) before and (b) 1 week after having lower face/neck MFUS (4.5/3.0) and full-face ablative fractional laser skin resurfacing performed on the same treatment day. No injectables were administered despite a plan to do so at follow-up due to the substantial improvement she achieved. (Courtesy Dr. Brian Biesman.)

6.5 Postoperative Care

For the most part, there is no difference between postoperative care for laser resurfacing alone versus resurfacing with concomitant filler injection. Prevention of infection and bacterial colonization is crucial during the postoperative period. For that reason, patients are often required to perform daily vinegar soaks. The exact proportion of vinegar to water may vary, but typically 1 teaspoon of white vinegar is diluted in 1 cup of cool water.[23] A cloth is dampened with the solution and gently applied to the treated area. This not only helps protect against infection, but also decreases redness and swelling. To avoid crusting and poor wound healing, bland ointments such as petrolatum or Aquaphor (Beiersdorf Inc.) are applied to keep the skin moist. Patients should refrain from the use of other topicals at this time. After re-epithelialization (3 to 5 days), a light moisturizer and sunscreen can be applied instead. Patients should be educated on the expected duration of redness and potential side effects. A written handout with these points and the contact information for the office and/or physician should be provided.

6.6 Avoiding and Treating Complications

Given the evolution and years of experience with different types of injectables and treatment techniques, we have good data on the most common complications. Complications with filler injection alone range from mild to severe in consequence, most of which resolve quickly within the postoperative phase. These side effects and complications include
- Swelling.
- Bruising.
- Intravascular injection leading to necrosis or vision impairment.
- Acute or late-onset nodules resulting from possible biofilm, hypersensitivity, and foreign body reaction.

Methods of avoiding and treating these complications are well documented.[26] Frequently, when combining treatments, the additive swelling becomes the most difficult side effect for a patient to endure within the immediate postprocedural period. When considering how to minimize posttreatment swelling with filler alone, Glogau and Kane[27] determined that rapid-injection, rapid-flow rates (over 0.3 mL/min), and higher volumes lead to more local reactions. A common fear of practitioners when witnessing excessive swelling is filler migration and diffusion. To our knowledge, except for botulinum toxin with ablative laser resurfacing as previously discussed, there are no studies or reports of adverse events from a particular combination of treatments in this regard.[21]

Recently, Jordan and Stoica[28] published a review on filler migration. Causes for migration fell into several categories including
- Injection technique (poor technique, high volume injected, filler injected under pressure).
- Massage.
- Muscle activity.
- Gravity.
- Antigravity.
- Pressure-induced.
- Lymphatic spread.
- Intravascular injection.

Although some of the cases in this review noted the possibility of employing multiple fillers over time as a potential causative agent, none reviewed the potential for the combination of filler substance and devices in this context.[28]

When performing sequential laser or device-based procedures on the same visit, the acute phases of healing are as expected, but they are often more intense for the patient. For example, when treating with both MFUS and ablative fractionated resurfacing (AFR) during the same treatment session, there was more significant swelling within the first postoperative days, but no other complications were attributed to this combination. Re-epithelialization from the AFR was not delayed, making the length of the postoperative period the same as doing either procedure alone.[29] If the postprocedural period is expected to be more intense when combining procedures, it is important to counsel the patients about clinical signs signaling a complication. For example, evidence of a postinjection vascular compromise may be difficult to appreciate if performing laser resurfacing or another device on the same day, because the erythema from the device can mask the color changes or other clinical signs of impending necrosis. Similarly, signs of infection may be masked by the epidermal slough from the laser or edema.

After ablative laser treatment, patients are cautioned to be strict with wound care, which often includes performing vinegar soaks and taking oral antibiotics and antivirals to help reduce the risk of superficial infection. Herpes simplex infection after fractional resurfacing is the most common infection.[30,31] Bacterial infection after fractional resurfacing has an incidence of 0.1%.[30,31] Other potential pathogens that can occur after ablative laser resurfacing include *Candida albicans* and atypical mycobacterium, therefore culture is necessary at the first signs of infection.[32] Although rare, cases of bacterial infection after nonablative 1,550 nm/1927 nm resurfacing have now been reported. These cases did not endure any sequelae, but they required antibiotics and a visit to the hospital for one patient.[33] As a result, it would be particularly important for the physician to educate patients on other clinical signs of infection such as pain, crusting, pustular eruption, or prolonged healing time, to notify their physician immediately. Further, all procedures regardless of whether they are done simultaneously or separately, should be managed with appropriate postprocedural care to minimize the potential for complications. With any ablative or nonablative resurfacing treatment, it is of the utmost importance to review in detail which products patients may or may not use and when. Frequently, patients layer on topical products that "promote healing" or "anti-aging" found outside of the performing physician's office, which can lead to irritation dermatitis, postinflammatory hyperpigmentation (PIH), and a delay in re-epithelialization. Finally, some filler substances require massaging the area after placement to help avoid nodule formation, such as PLLA. It may be tougher and more painful if an ablative laser is done at the same time, but it still should be emphasized for a patient to perform the massages in the areas.

One author (B.B.) has anecdotally witnessed the disappearance of previously placed Hylacross filler in the midfacial region following treatment with microfocused ultrasound. The patient had been treated many months ago with filler and was stable from that perspective. Within 48 hours after undergoing microfocused ultrasound treatment, substantial indentation was noted in the treatment area overlying the previously placed soft tissue filler. Following replacement of the filler, the patient regained his pretreatment appearance. Since then, we have treated many patients with previously placed HA fillers who have not experienced degradation of product. We do recommend discussing potential changes created by microfocused ultrasound on HA fillers with patients, but we do not view previously placed HA fillers as a contraindication to microfocused ultrasound treatment.

6.7 Conclusion

Overall, the growing demand for the combination of noninvasive or minimally invasive procedures is evident to any practitioner. It is essential to determine which combination of treatments is appropriate for a particular patient based on the patient's unique signs of aging, downtime constraints, budgetary restrictions, and overall expectations. The literature is quickly beginning to reveal the benefits, safety, and possible pitfalls of combining treatments.

6.8 Commentary

Julius W. Few Jr.

I applaud the authors for highlighting how so many manufacturers have been limited in their ability to evaluate combination approaches to nonsurgical rejuvenation for both commercial and regulatory reasons. First, the commercial concern that is linked to the idea that suggesting that more than a given proprietary application is needed suggests inadequacy, making no real incentive to look at combination approaches. Second, the U.S. FDA gives approval for a given technology within specific parameters of investigation, making marketing of combination approaches illegal and punishable. One can find the warnings in the package inserts, as the warnings relate to using microfocused ultrasound after filler injection. With all of these incentives against innovation in combination approaches, the needs of our patients are a strong incentive in favor of delivering more nonsurgically.

I agree with the authors regarding antibiotic prophylaxis and laser use; the science does not support routine use. The most crucial component to prevent posttreatment infection is good, consistent wound care after laser ablation. We routinely instruct patients to cleanse the resurfaced area 2 to 3 times per day and then to apply a nonirritating occlusive while using routine herpetic prophylaxis. Ultimately, one of the more valuable principles shared is the idea that caution should rule over convenience. As the authors highlight, stacking skin tightening, fillers, and laser (stackable treatment) often requires a reduction in energy delivery to make the given treatment safe and effective. We recommend that a 25% reduction in energy to achieve the same or better result safely will combine multimodality treatment. The synergistic effects can often lessen the volume needed for filler, compared to the same case with filler alone.

References

[1] American Society of Plastic Surgeons. (2015) 2014 Plastic surgery statistics report. Retrieved form http://www.plasticsurgery.org/Documents/news-resources/statistics/2014-statistics/plastic-surgery-statsitics-full-report.pdf

[2] Galderma Laboratories L.P. Sculptra® Aesthetic (injectable poly-L-lactic acid) [package insert]. Fort Worth, TX

[3] Ulthera, Inc. Ulthera (microfocused ultrasound with visualization) [package insert]. Meza, AZ

[4] England LJ, Tan MH, Shumaker PR, et al. Effects of monopolar radiofrequency treatment over soft-tissue fillers in an animal model. Lasers Surg Med. 2005; 37(5):356–365

[5] Shumaker PR, England LJ, Dover JS, et al. Effect of monopolar radiofrequency treatment over soft-tissue fillers in an animal model: part 2. Lasers Surg Med. 2006; 38(3):211–217

[6] Kim H, Park KY, Choi SY, et al. The efficacy, longevity, and safety of combined radiofrequency treatment and hyaluronic Acid filler for skin rejuvenation. Ann Dermatol. 2014; 26(4):447–456

[7] Alam M, Levy R, Pajvani U, et al. Safety of radiofrequency treatment over human skin previously injected with medium-term injectable soft-tissue augmentation materials: a controlled pilot trial. Lasers Surg Med. 2006; 38(3):205–210

[8] Farkas JP, Richardson JA, Brown S, Hoopman JE, Kenkel JM. Effects of common laser treatments on hyaluronic acid fillers in a porcine model. Aesthet Surg J. 2008; 28(5):503–511

[9] Goldman MP, Alster TS, Weiss R. A randomized trial to determine the influence of laser therapy, monopolar radiofrequency treatment, and intense pulsed light therapy administered immediately after hyaluronic acid gel implantation. Dermatol Surg. 2007; 33(5):535–542

[10] Friedmann DP, Fabi SG, Goldman MP. Combination of intense pulsed light, Sculptra, and Ultherapy for treatment of the aging face. J Cosmet Dermatol. 2014; 13(2):109–118

[11] Hart DR, Fabi SG, White WM, Fitzgerald R, Goldman MP. Current Concepts in the Use of PLLA: Clinical Synergy Noted with Combined Use of Microfocused Ultrasound and Poly-L-Lactic Acid on the Face, Neck, and Décolletage. Plast Reconstr Surg. 2015; 136(5) Suppl:180S–187S

[12] Casabona G, Michalany N. Microfocused ultrasound with visualization and fillers for increased neocollagenesis: clinical and histological evaluation. Dermatol Surg. 2014; 40 Suppl 12:S194–S198

[13] Park KY, Park MK, Li K, Seo SJ, Hong CK. Combined treatment with a nonablative infrared device and hyaluronic acid filler does not have enhanced efficacy in treating nasolabial fold wrinkles. Dermatol Surg. 2011; 37(12):1770–1775

[14] Küçüker İ, Aksakal IA, Polat AV, Engin MS, Yosma E, Demir A. The effect of chemodenervation by botulinum neurotoxin on the degradation of hyaluronic acid fillers: an experimental study. Plast Reconstr Surg. 2016; 137(1):109–113

[15] Alter TS, Lupton JR. Laser resurfacing and fillers. Head and Neck Aesthetics. 327–32. http://www.skinlaser.com/wp-content/uploads/2011/06/Laser-Skin-Resurfacing-and-Fillers.pdf

[16] Zimbler MS, Holds JB, Kokoska MS, et al. Effect of botulinum toxin pretreatment on laser resurfacing results: a prospective, randomized, blinded trial. Arch Facial Plast Surg. 2001; 3(3):165–169

[17] Zimbler M, Undavia S. Update on the effect of botulinum toxin pretreatment on laser resurfacing results. Arch Facial Plast Surg. 2012; 14(3):156–158

[18] Yamauchi PS, Lask G, Lowe NJ. Botulinum toxin type A gives adjunctive benefit to periorbital laser resurfacing. J Cosmet Laser Ther. 2004; 6(3):145–148

[19] Beer K, Waibel J. Botulinum toxin type A enhances the outcome of fractional resurfacing of the cheek. J Drugs Dermatol. 2007; 6(11):1151–1152

[20] Semchyshyn NL, Kilmer SL. Does laser inactivate botulinum toxin? Dermatol Surg. 2005; 31(4):399–404

[21] Chacur R, Chacur N, Alves D, et al. Complications associated with the use of CO2 fractional laser for the treatment of skin renewal (resurfacing). Lasers Surg Med. 2015; 47(S26):22

[22] Reddy KK, Brauer JA, Anolik R, et al. Calcium hydroxylapatite nodule resolution after fractional carbon dioxide laser therapy. Arch Dermatol. 2012; 148(5):634–636

[23] Ramsdell WM. Fractional carbon dioxide laser resurfacing. Semin Plast Surg. 2012; 26(3):125–130

[24] Alster TS. Against antibiotic prophylaxis for cutaneous laser resurfacing. Dermatol Surg. 2000; 26(7):697–698

[25] Kim HW, Chang SE, Kim JE, Ko JY, Ro YS. The safe delivery of fractional ablative carbon dioxide laser treatment for acne scars in Asian patients receiving oral isotretinoin. Dermatol Surg. 2014; 40(12):1361–1366

[26] Vanaman M, Fabi SG, Carruthers J. Complications in the Cosmetic Dermatology Patient: A Review and Our Experience (Part 1). Dermatol Surg. 2016; 42(1):1–11

[27] Glogau RG, Kane MA. Effect of injection techniques on the rate of local adverse events in patients implanted with nonanimal hyaluronic acid gel dermal fillers. Dermatol Surg. 2008; 34 Suppl 1:S105–S109

[28] Jordan DR, Stoica B. Filler migration: a Number of mechanisms to Consider. Ophthal Plast Reconstr Surg. 2015; 31(4):257–262

[29] Woodward JA, Fabi SG, Alster T, Colón-Acevedo B. Safety and efficacy of combining microfocused ultrasound with fractional CO2 laser resurfacing for lifting and tightening the face and neck. Dermatol Surg. 2014; 40 Suppl 12: S190–S193

[30] Shah S, Alam M. Laser resurfacing pearls. Semin Plast Surg. 2012; 26(3):131–136

[31] Metelitsa AI, Alster TS. Fractionated laser skin resurfacing treatment complications: a review. Dermatol Surg. 2010; 36(3):299–306

[32] Palm MD, Butterwick KJ, Goldman MP. Mycobacterium chelonae infection after fractionated carbon dioxide facial resurfacing (presenting as an atypical acneiform eruption): case report and literature review. Dermatol Surg. 2010; 36(9):1473–1481

[33] Xu LY, Kilmer SL, Ross EV, Avram MM. Bacterial infections following non-ablative fractional laser treatment: a case series and discussion. Lasers Surg Med. 2015; 47(2):128–132

7 Microneedling and Platelet-Rich Plasma

Johnson C. Lee and Z. Paul Lorenc

Summary

Platelet-rich plasma (PRP) contains concentrated platelet-derived growth factor (PDGF), transforming growth factor-beta (TGF-β), vascular endothelial growth factor (VEGF), epidermal growth factor (EGF), and insulin-like growth factor (IGF), all of which promote local tissue repair. PRP is created by centrifuging autologous whole blood collected from a peripheral vein. PRP is applied as a topical or injectable adjunct to microneedling for synergistic augmentation of collagen production, angiogenesis, and tissue regeneration. PRP by itself has shown beneficial effects in the literature across various fields including orthopedic, cardiac, plastic, and oral and maxillofacial surgery. The process of microneedling creates microchannels into the dermis while stimulating collagen production and remodeling through the PDGF release. Microneedling is a successful treatment modality for several skin conditions including postacne atrophic scars, androgenic alopecia, and alopecia areata.

Keywords: platelet-rich plasma (PRP), microneedling, platelet-derived growth factor (PDGF), transforming growth factor-beta (TGF-β), vascular endothelial growth factor (VEGF), epidermal growth factor (EGF), insulin-like growth factor (IGF), percutaneous collagen induction (PCI), collagen induction therapy, fibroblast growth factor (FGF), microchannels, alopecia

Key Points

- Platelet-rich plasma (PRP) is concentrated by centrifuging autologous whole blood collected from a peripheral vein.
- PRP contains highly concentrated platelet-derived growth factor (PDGF), transforming growth factor-beta (TGF-β), vascular endothelial growth factor (VEGF), epidermal growth factor (EGF), and insulin-like growth factor (IGF), all of which promote local tissue repair.
- Microneedling creates microchannels into the dermis while stimulating collagen production and remodeling through PDGF release.
- PRP is applied as a topical or injectable adjunct to microneedling for synergistic augmentation of collagen production, angiogenesis, and tissue regeneration beyond either modality alone.

7.1 Introduction

Microneedling, also known as percutaneous collagen induction (PCI) or collagen induction therapy, was first described in the 1990s as a novel method of skin resurfacing.[1,2,3] Microneedling utilizes direct mechanical trauma to modify tissues and requires very little downtime and a shorter healing phase when compared to ablative modalities such as laser or dermabrasion.

Microneedle devices create controlled microchannels within the skin that close within minutes. Skin penetration stimulates platelets to release chemotactic factors causing invasion of other platelets, neutrophils, and fibroblasts. These cells release numerous growth factors including PDGF, fibroblast growth factor (FGF), TGF-α and TGF-β, all of which stimulate the migration and proliferation of fibroblasts, promote collagen production, and promote regeneration of a normal collagen lattice structure.[4,5] Microneedling has also been reported as a successful treatment modality for several skin conditions including postacne atrophic scars, androgenic alopecia, and alopecia areata.[6,7,8]

More recently, microneedling technology has been augmented with additional modalities. One promising adjunct takes advantage of the temporary microchannels to directly introduce growth factors and cytokines in the form of PRP into the dermis. PRP is defined as the portion of the plasma fraction of autologous blood with higher-than-baseline platelet concentrations. This is achieved by centrifugation of whole blood drawn from a peripheral vein. High-speed centrifugation concentrates platelet levels fivefold to eightfold per volume of plasma.[9] The most common and important growth factors found in PRP include

- PDGF
- TGF-β
- VEGF
- EGF
- IGF

These factors are chemotactic and mitogenic, promoting angiogenesis and subsequence migration of macrophages. Macrophages supplement the healing environment with additional growth factors and cytokines producing local tissue repair and continuous regeneration. Other affected cells include fibroblasts, stem cells, endothelial cells, osteoblasts, smooth muscle cells, and keratinocytes, which contribute to collagen production and angiogenesis.[10,11] Given these effects, the addition of PRP to a treatment modality is sometimes advertised with the descriptive term *vampire* in reference to the creature of ancient folklore who sustains its immortality by drinking the blood of the living.

PRP by itself has shown beneficial effects in the literature across various fields including orthopedic, cardiac, plastic, and oral and maxillofacial surgery.[12] Multiple in vitro studies of PRP since 2007 have demonstrated increase in endothelial cell, stem cell, procollagen, fibroblasts, growth factor, and Type 1 collagen proliferation. Animal studies of PRP have also shown clinical benefit including increased wound healing, enhanced neurotrophic effects, increased fat grafting survival in rabbits and rats, reduction in wrinkling with increased fibroblasts, and increased bone formation in skull defects. Conversely, some studies have shown equivocal or deleterious effects of PRP including increased inflammation, diminished bony repair, and no effect on free fat graft survival in mice. In human trials, studies have been more consistently positive, with decreased edema and ecchymosis after facelifts, increased wound-healing rates, more rapid epithelialization of skin graft donor sites, decreased erythema after laser treatments, increased skin elasticity and collagen promotion, increased hair count in alopecia, improved diabetic wounds, and improved appearance of acne scars.[13,14,15,16,17] In a review by

Sommeling et al,[18] 36 out of 40 studies consisted of randomized controlled trials and case-control studies that demonstrated favorable outcomes with PRP use in plastic surgery.

Because both microneedling and PRP are relatively new technologies in aesthetic medicine, the currently available literature evaluating the efficacy of the combined modalities is sparse but consistently positive. Akcal et al[19] reported increased skin flap survival ($p < 0.01$) when PRP was combined with microneedling of ischemic skin flaps in a rat model. The increase in flap survival when compared to the control and microneedling-only groups suggests a benefit from PRP growth factors beyond microneedling alone.[19] Similarly, in a split-face comparative study of microneedling with PRP versus microneedling with Vitamin C, Chawla[20] found the PRP group to have significantly higher patient satisfaction after rolling and boxcar acne scar treatment, although Vitamin C provided more benefit for post-inflammatory hyperpigmentation.

Given the known and similar benefits of microneedling and PRP, it is reasonable to expect that the combination of these two regenerative modalities can provide a synergistic effect on the regeneration and rejuvenation of skin (**see Video 1.1**).

7.2 Patient Selection

The patient selection criteria for microneedling with PRP are similar to those of microneedling alone. Beyond skin rejuvenation, patients who can benefit from microneedling with PRP include patients with surgical or postacne scarring, aging or sun-damaged skin, and hair disorders. Extra caution should be taken in patients with excess superficial vascularity, active skin inflammation or disease, sensitive or eczematous skin, diminished healing, or anticoagulant history, because recovery may be extended or complicated.

7.3 Technical Steps and Treatment Plan

Prior to treatment, patients should avoid prolonged sun exposure or sunburns for at least 24 hours to avoid excessive inflammation and injury. Topical products are discontinued 12 hours prior to treatment, and the skin must be clean and free from cosmetic products. Any patient with active or resolving infection should have treatment delayed until resolution.

7.3.1 Patient Preparation

1. All makeup and jewelry is removed, and standardized patient photos are taken.
2. The skin is degreased with alcohol prep, and a topical anesthetic cream composed of 20% benzocaine, 6% lidocaine, and 4% tetracaine is applied to the planned treatment areas. This cream is allowed to penetrate the skin for 30 to 45 minutes.

7.3.2 Platelet-Rich Plasma Preparation

1. Using sterile technique, 10 mL of autologous whole blood is drawn from a peripheral vein into tubes containing the anticoagulant, acid citrate dextrose (ACD).
2. Tubes are gently and manually inverted and turned 5 to 10 times prior to placement into a centrifuge.
3. Tubes are centrifuged 3,500 rpm for 15 minutes at a room temperature of 22 °C to obtain a platelet count at least 4.5 times higher than baseline.
    a) Using an 18-gauge needle, serum is extracted and placed into separate 3-mL syringe vials for use.
4. The supernatant platelet-poor plasma (PPP) can be partly removed and partly used to resuspend the platelets or, preferably, the entire serum volume can be used to resuspend and minimize the loss of platelets.
5. Although calcium gluconate can be added as an activator 1:0 (i.e., 1 mL of calcium gluconate in 9 mL of PRP), platelets will become activated upon contact with dermis or blood during microneedling.[10] Early activation of PRP with calcium may create clumping or gelling and could prevent penetration into the dermal microchannels.

7.3.3 Treatment

1. After 45 minutes or when the patient is sufficiently numb, the face is wiped clean and cleansed with a gentle cleanser and sterilized with alcohol. Sterile saline is used to wipe the skin, and the skin is pat dry.
2. The face is divided into sections (cheeks, perioral, periocular, and forehead).
3. The forehead and upper lip are the most sensitive areas and are therefore treated first while they are still numb. PRP is applied to the skin with the needleless syringe and spread evenly in the section to be treated. Appropriate needle depth selection should allow sufficient penetration of the PRP. Alternatively, intradermal injection of PRP can be performed.
4. Needle depth is chosen according to the section to be treated:
    a) Forehead: 1.0 to 1.25 mm.
    b) Periocular: 1.0 to 1.25 mm.
    c) Perioral: 1.5–2.0 + mm × 3 to 5 passes in each direction AND 0.5–1.0 mm × 2 passes in each direction.
5. Cheeks: 1.5–2.0 mm + × 3 to 5 passes in each direction AND 0.5–1.0 mm × 2 passes in each direction.
6. Three horizontal passes and 3 vertical passes (more if tolerated) are made per section, while additional PRP is added throughout the process to keep the skin from drying and to allow penetration into the skin. Needle depth is decreased if purpura is observed. Extra, superficial passes on the cheeks and mouth are used to maximize textural change by targeting different depths.
7. Once the microneedling is complete and all of the serum is used, the skin is gently wiped with a wet, nonwoven gauze pad and a biocellulose mask composed of aloe vera, Argireline (acetyl hexapeptide-3, Lipotec SA), glycerin, and hyaluronic acid is applied and left on for 15 minutes. The mask decreases erythema and recovery time, and it provides a cooling effect. An ice roller can be used alternatively or concurrently on the mask for added patient comfort.
8. After removing the mask, hyaluronic acid serum can be applied if desired, and a thin layer of occlusive moisturizer can be placed for skin protection.

7.4 Results
7.4.1 Case 1
(▶ Fig. 7.1)

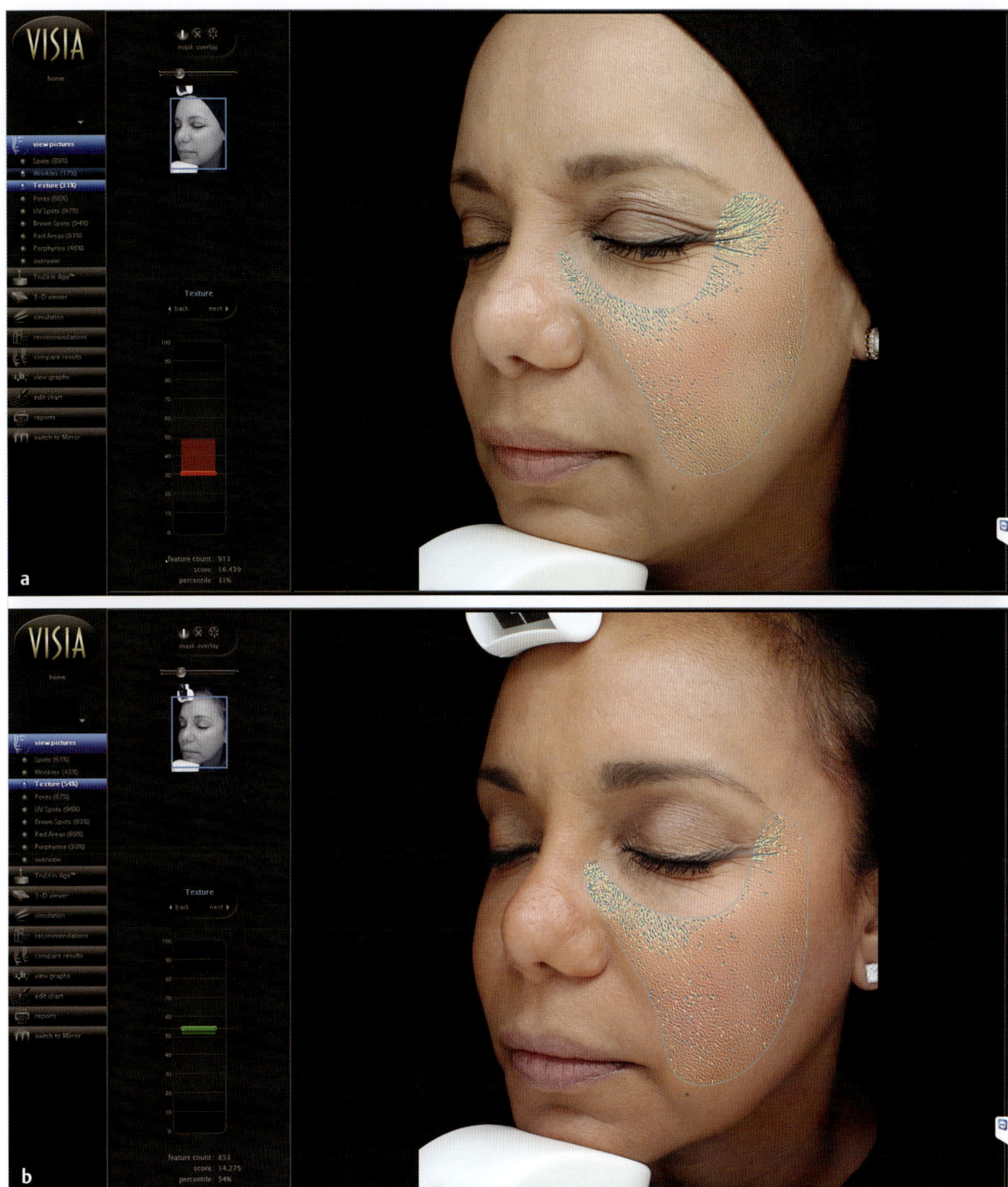

Fig. 7.1 This 52-year-old woman is shown **(a)** before and **(b)** after two treatments with microneedling and platelet-rich plasma. These images, taken 6 weeks apart, show a 23% improvement in skin texture as measured using VISIA.

7.5 Postprocedural Care

Immediately after treatment, there may be slight burning or discomfort that can be treated with over-the-counter analgesics. Sunscreen and cosmetic products are to be avoided for at least 24 hours. The patient can return to work the next day, although swelling may persist into the second or third day. Erythema and mild desquamation may occur for 3 to 5 days, after which regular skin care, including the use of tretinoin, can be restarted. By 1 week, patients can expect to be free of postprocedural side effects although they should avoid any alcohol, acid-based toners, and direct sun exposure for 2 weeks. Antiviral medication is indicated to prevent a herpes simplex outbreak.[21]

7.6 Complications and Shortcomings

There are a few reports of complications in the literature about microneedling, given its minimally invasive, superficial mechanism of action and no reports of complications directly attributable to PRP administration.[22,23] Increasing needle depth is associated with improved results but with longer downtime and greater swelling, bruising, and bleeding.[24] Thorough skin preparation is vital to avoid introducing immunogenic particles that may initiate local or systemic hypersensitivity reactions within the dermis.[25] Perhaps the most concerning potential complication is "tram track" scars, in which multiple lines of pigmented punctate hypertrophic scars form in the direction of the microneedle application. These occur more commonly over the bony prominences of the zygoma, forehead, and temporal area, and they may be improved with silicone gel therapy.[26] Patients with a history of keloidal or hypertrophic scar formation should be carefully treated with more superficial settings if treatment is planned over bony prominences. Using circular movements and avoiding repetitive passes over the same areas can additionally reduce scarring trauma.

7.7 Commentary

Julius W. Few Jr. and Alec Semersky

Microneedling Depth Penetration, Presence of Pigment Particles, And Fluorescein-Stained Platelets: Clinical Usage for Aesthetic Concerns [Reused with permission from Few JW, Semersky A. Commentary on Micro-Needling Depth Penetration, Presence of Pigment Particles, and Fluorescein-Stained Platelets: Clinical Usage for Aesthetic Concerns. Aesthet Surg J (2016) 37 (1): 84–85.)]

Microneedling is a relatively novel technique that uses needles ranging from 0.5 mm to 2.5 mm to create microwounds or channels in the skin. The microneedles are designed to penetrate the stratum corneum without traveling into the nerve fibers of the skin. In doing so, microneedling can create micro channels in the skin relatively painlessly. The channels allow for the delivery of macromolecules through the skin, and, while healing, promote collagen production in the skin. As a result, microneedling is an effective tool for treating aesthetic skin concerns such as wrinkling, as well as delivering transdermal medications and vaccines.

The authors of this chapter aimed to determine the average depth penetration of microneedles, as well as the optimal time of topical application to achieve maximum depth of macromolecule dissemination through the skin after microneedling treatment. In studies I, II, and III, low sample sizes of only facial skin excised from Caucasian patients aged 72, 73, and 62, respectively, were utilized. The use of only these preauricular skin strips from a narrow ethnic background limits the broader applications of these studies. It would be advantageous to examine needle penetration depth and time-dependent dissemination of macromolecules after microneedling on skin excised from different areas of the body, and on skin of different ages and ethnicities. The authors of this chapter do increase the sample size by examining five sections within each $1 \times 1\,cm^2$ section of excised skin, although a larger selection of skin samples is still required for complete study. Size indeed may not matter for microneedling.

Despite a small sample size, the varying penetration depths of different needle lengths provide meaningful information. The authors of this chapter found that the level of needle penetration was consistent between 0.5 and 1.5 mm, as validated by histology and tissue marking. When the investigators in this chapter used needle lengths of 1.5-, 2-, and 2.5-mm lengths, the results were less consistent and the level of penetration was greater for the 2-mm length than the 2.5-mm length. They appropriately indicate that there is a need for additional research for longer-length applications, and we concluded that the outcomes were impressive across varying lengths of penetration, making 1- to 1.5-mm needles an optimal choice for the described indication.

The findings in this chapter related to the time-dependent dissemination of macromolecules through the skin are particularly important. With an increased sample size, the massage times of topical products into the skin posttreatment indicated in the study could serve as a guideline for doctors who employ these topical products after treatment.[28,29] The study results suggest that the optimal time of skin penetration is at 5 minutes and that the window of tissue access starts to close drastically after 30 minutes, making a truly essential contribution to the literature.

The authors of this chapter achieved excellent results in treating aged skin, wrinkling, laxity, alopecia, atrophic acne scars, and striae through microneedling. Both patients and observers unanimously reported aesthetic improvements 12 months after completing microneedling treatment for each of the previously mentioned categories. The minimally invasive nature of microneedling is enticing for both patients and healthcare professionals because of its efficacy, low complication rate, and relative simplicity. For patients, the minimal pain of the microneedles is also an alluring benefit over more invasive alternatives.[30]

At The Few Institute, microneedling is used to treat aesthetic concerns ranging from static wrinkles, to atrophic acne scars, to a wide range of other scars. Occasionally, microneedling will also be utilized for repigmenting skin. Patients opt for microneedling to treat these aesthetic concerns because of its positive results as well as its relative painlessness. Our results from 100 microneedling patients sampled were overwhelmingly positive. Like the study, we encountered few complications other than prolonged erythema and occasional swelling. Aesthetically, our patients also experienced consistent improvement, and the demand for retreatment has been high. To improve results, the authors of the study employed topical PRP after microneedling. Although the results are significant, we would like to have seen a head-to-head, blinded comparison between the use of PRP and a placebo. Given that using microneedles releases a variety of growth factors, including PCGF, PRP may not add a statistically significant benefit.[4,5,6,7,31,32,33,34]

We congratulate the authors of this chapter for presenting a very elegant, well-controlled study on microneedling, which is a powerful tool in cosmetic medicine. We believe that this study validates the importance of adjunct cosmetic procedures in the plastic surgery patient, because the results shown could not be achieved by surgery alone. Microneedling shows promise as an effective, minimally invasive tool for long-lasting improvements in skin appearance. The data found on microneedling depth penetration and the time-dependent dissemination of macromolecules are an important step in the advancement of microneedling for use in other applications such as vaccines and the delivery of medication impermeable to the skin.

7.8 Acknowledgements

The authors thank Carissa McCormack, medical esthetician, for her technical support and contribution to this chapter.

References

[1] Fernandes D. Percutaneous collagen induction: an alternative to laser resurfacing. Aesthet Surg J. 2002; 22(3):307–309

[2] Camirand A, Doucet J. Needle dermabrasion. Aesthetic Plast Surg. 1997; 21(1):48–51

[3] Fernandes D. Skin needling as an alternative to laser. Presented at the International Confederation for Plastic, Reconstructive, and Aesthetic Surgery Conference, San Francisco, Calif., June 26–30, 1999

[4] Ferguson MW, O'Kane S. Scar-free healing: from embryonic mechanisms to adult therapeutic intervention. Philos Trans R Soc Lond B Biol Sci. 2004; 359(1445):839–850

[5] Bandyopadhyay B, Fan J, Guan S, et al. A "traffic control" role for TGFbeta3: orchestrating dermal and epidermal cell motility during wound healing. J Cell Biol. 2006; 172(7):1093–1105

[6] El-Domyati M, Barakat M, Awad S, Medhat W, El-Fakahany H, Farag H. Microneedling therapy for atrophic acne scars: an objective evaluation. J Clin Aesthet Dermatol. 2015; 8(7):36–42

[7] Dhurat R, Mathapati S. Response to microneedling treatment in men with androgenetic alopecia who failed to respond to conventional therapy. Indian J Dermatol. 2015; 60(3):260–263

[8] Chandrashekar B, Yepuri V, Mysore V. Alopecia areata-successful outcome with microneedling and triamcinolone acetonide. J Cutan Aesthet Surg. 2014; 7(1):63–64

[9] Marx RE, Carlson ER, Eichstaedt RM, Schimmele SR, Strauss JE, Georgeff KR. Platelet-rich plasma: growth factor enhancement for bone grafts. Oral Surg Oral Med Oral Pathol Oral Radiol Endod. 1998; 85(6):638–646

[10] Eppley BL, Pietrzak WS, Blanton M. Platelet-rich plasma: a review of biology and applications in plastic surgery. Plast Reconstr Surg. 2006; 118(6):147e–159e

[11] Sclafani AP, Romo T, III, Ukrainsky G, et al. Modulation of wound response and soft tissue ingrowth in synthetic and allogeneic implants with platelet concentrate. Arch Facial Plast Surg. 2005; 7(3):163–169

[12] Redler LH, Thompson SA, Hsu SH, Ahmad CS, Levine WN. Platelet-rich plasma therapy: a systematic literature review and evidence for clinical use. Phys Sportsmed. 2011; 39(1):42–51

[13] Sclafani AP, Azzi J. Platelet preparations for use in facial rejuvenation and wound healing: a critical review of current literature. Aesthetic Plast Surg. 2015; 39(4):495–505

[14] Tobita M, Tajima S, Mizuno H. Adipose tissue-derived mesenchymal stem cells and platelet-rich plasma: stem cell transplantation methods that enhance stemness. Stem Cell Res Ther. 2015; 6:215

[15] Picard F, Hersant B, Bosc R, Meningaud JP. The growing evidence for the use of platelet-rich plasma on diabetic chronic wounds: a review and a proposal for a new standard care. Wound Repair Regen. 2015; 23(5):638–643

[16] Singh B, Goldberg LJ. Autologous platelet-rich plasma for the treatment of pattern hair loss. Am J Clin Dermatol. 2016; 17(4):359–367

[17] Serra-Mestre JM, Serra-Renom JM, Martinez L, Almadori A, D'Andrea F. Platelet-rich plasma mixed-fat grafting: a reasonable prosurvival strategy for fat grafts? Aesthetic Plast Surg. 2014; 38(5):1041–1049

[18] Sommeling CE, Heyneman A, Hoeksema H, Verbelen J, Stillaert FB, Monstrey S. The use of platelet-rich plasma in plastic surgery: a systematic review. J Plast Reconstr Aesthet Surg. 2013; 66(3):301–311

[19] Akcal A, Savas SA, Gorgulu T, et al. The effect of platelete rich plasma combined with microneedling on full venous outflow compromise in a rat skin flap model. Plast Reconstr Surg. 2015; 136(4) Suppl:71–72

[20] Chawla S. Split face comparative study of microneedling with PRP versus microneedling with vitamin C in treating atrophic post acne scars. J Cutan Aesthet Surg. 2014; 7(4):209–212

[21] Lee JC, Daniels MA, Roth MZ. Mesotherapy, microneedling, and chemical peels. Clin Plast Surg. 2016; 43(3):583–595

[22] Schwarz M, Laaff H. A prospective controlled assessment of microneedling with the Dermaroller device. Plast Reconstr Surg. 2011; 127(6):146e–148e

[23] Hartmann D, Ruzicka T, Gauglitz GG. Complications associated with cutaneous aesthetic procedures. J Dtsch Dermatol Ges. 2015; 13(8):778–786

[24] Fernandes D, Signorini M. Combating photoaging with percutaneous collagen induction. Clin Dermatol. 2008; 26(2):192–199

[25] Soltani-Arabshahi R, Wong JW, Duffy KL, Powell DL. Facial allergic granulomatous reaction and systemic hypersensitivity associated with microneedle therapy for skin rejuvenation. JAMA Dermatol. 2014; 150(1):68–72

[26] Pahwa M, Pahwa P, Zaheer A. "Tram track effect" after treatment of acne scars using a microneedling device. Dermatol Surg. 2012; 38(7 Pt 1):1107–1108

[27] Few JW, Semersky A. Commentary on: Micro-needling depth penetration, presence of pigment particles, and fluorescein-stained platelets: clinical usage for aesthetic concerns. Aesthet Surg J. 2017; 37(1):84–85

[28] Microneedle applicator designs for transdermal drug delivery applications." Donnelly/Microneedle-Mediated Transdermal and Intradermal Drug Delivery (2012): 57–78. Web. 1 July 2016

[29] Koutsonanos DG, del Pilar Martin M, Zarnitsyn VG, et al. Transdermal influenza immunization with vaccine-coated microneedle arrays. PLoS One. 2009; 4(3):e4773

[30] Gill HS, Denson DD, Burris BA, Prausnitz MR. Effect of microneedle design on pain in human volunteers. Clin J Pain. 2008; 24(7):585–594

[31] Faler BJ, Macsata RA, Plummer D, Mishra L, Sidawy AN. Transforming growth factor-beta and wound healing. Perspect Vasc Surg Endovasc Ther. 2006; 18(1):55–62

[32] Fitzpatrick RE, Rostan EF. Reversal of photodamage with topical growth factors: a pilot study. J Cosmet Laser Ther. 2003; 5(1):25–34

[33] Fisher GJ, Varani J, Voorhees JJ. Looking older: fibroblast collapse and therapeutic implications. Arch Dermatol. 2008; 144(5):666–672

[34] Quan T, Wang F, Shao Y, et al. Enhancing structural support of the dermal microenvironment activates fibroblasts, endothelial cells, and keratinocytes in aged human skin in vivo. J Invest Dermatol. 2013; 133(3):658–667

8 Use of Light- and Energy-Based Therapies with Cosmetic Surgery

Michael I. Kulick and Natasha Kulick

Summary

Perceived aesthetic appearance is based in part on the amount of redundant skin, the impact of the underlying supporting structures, and the quality of the skin itself. Normal aging changes such as hyperpigmentation and hypopigmentation, hypervascularity, fine wrinkles, skin laxity, and skin pore size and texture can be treated with light- and energy-based therapies (LAEBT) with high patient satisfaction.

Keywords: ablative therapy, aging process, carbon dioxide (CO_2), chromophore, erbium, hyperpigmentation, hypervascularity, hypopigmentation, ionizing radiation, light- and energy-based therapy (LAEBT), nonablative fractional resurfacing, photorejuvenation, radiofrequency (RF), skin damage, supplements

> **Key Points**
>
> - What defines a youthful appearance? How can providing patients ancillary light- and energy-based therapies (LAEBT) result in a more complete aesthetic improvement?
> - Patient selection and skin analysis is critical to obtain good outcomes.
> - Understanding the limitation of one's device is important.
> - Thermal energy and resultant dermal heating is responsible for skin tightening. Which patients are ideal for treatment with these modalities? How can the clinician optimize patient safety and outcomes?
> - When using LAEBT, complications can be minimized by initially using manufacturers, device settings, and staying up-to-date by attending certified, CME education courses.

8.1 Introduction

One's perceived aesthetic appearance is based in part on the amount of redundant skin, the impact of the underlying supporting structures, and the quality of the skin itself. Although surgeons often focus on the skin envelope and supporting structures, the remaining skin has changed from its original, youthful manifestation. Signs of this change are evident through undesirable hyperpigmentation and hypopigmentation, hypervascularity, fine wrinkles, and items difficult to quantify such as skin pore size and texture (▶ Fig. 8.1). To date, light- and energy-based therapies (LAEBT) have not been shown to provide skin tightening that parallels the results obtained through surgery. However, LAEBT can significantly improve patient satisfaction regarding their appearance after surgery. They also provide nonsurgical options, which would allow the treating clinician to improve the patient's appearance.

The etiology of the signs of skin aging is multifactorial. An acknowledged source of skin damage is the effect of ionizing radiation from the sun. Despite medical advice, many patients still do not wear sunscreen or do not apply them as directed. The cumulative impact of the sun's radiation on unprotected skin can cause dyschromia.[1]

A genetic component also factors into one's aging process. Not all individuals age the same way given parallel environmental exposure. Systemic conditions such as diabetes, scleroderma, or other connective tissue disorders impact the appearance of one's skin and the ability to heal.[2] Cystic acne during adolescence can leave scars that may become more unsightly as one ages.[3,4] Hormonal changes can affect the appearance of an individual's skin.[5]

Even one's lifestyle beyond the harmful effects of the sun's radiation can impact the aging process of the skin. Smoking is harmful to the skin and wound healing.[6] Proper skin hygiene can mitigate the signs of aging by keeping skin pores open and minimizing unwanted melanin in the epidermis. Individuals trying to optimize the appearance of their skin spend millions of dollars using over-the-counter, topical agents that do not have peer review papers substantiating their efficacy.

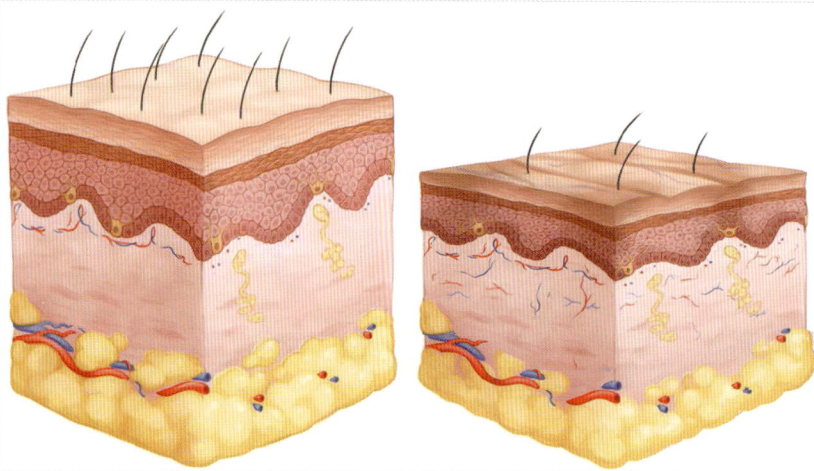

Fig. 8.1 This is a good representation of a graphic example of the difference between younger and older skin.

Once a surgical procedure has been performed, skin laxity and the underlying support structures have been corrected. The ancillary use of LAEBT can enhance the appearance of the remaining facial skin by improving its color and texture. Such therapies can also be used on nonfacial regions. Frequently patients do not want surgery. In this clinical setting, utilizing LAEBT can significantly improve one's appearance.

8.2 Patient Selection

8.2.1 Safety

There are many factors that influence the outcome of nonsurgical LAEBT results. To actualize the patient's expectations requires effective communication between the clinician and patient. Selecting the correct LAEBT to address the patient's concern is predicated upon proper patient selection and understanding the limitations and capabilities of one's device. If a patient has unrealistic expectations, then the final outcome could be compromised regardless of the skin treatment therapy utilized. When providing treatment alternatives, it is better to underpromise than to deal with the perceived promises that may not be fulfilled. A comprehensive informed consent and written pretreatment and posttreatment instructions can mitigate posttreatment misunderstandings.

Many LAEBTs rely on the energy being focused to a chromophore, which can be water, melanin, and/or hemoglobin (▶ Fig. 8.2). When a patient presents with a "tan," they should be given the option to wait until the tan fades before initiating treatment if the energy source efficacy is impacted by skin color. This way, the energy that is intended for undesirable melanin will not be drawn to the skin pigment because of the transient tan. Patients with hypervascularity should be advised to avoid anything that would cause vasodilatation prior to treatment. If a patient has a hypersensitivity to sunlight, using a device that provides light energy as a therapeutic modality should not be recommended.[2]

Patients who have taken recent medications such as isotretinoin or oral antibiotics, which are known to cause hyperpigmentation, should have their aesthetic treatment delayed until the systemic effects of these medications have expired. Even nonprescribed medications such as St. John's Wort can negatively impact the final outcome, because the use of such a nonprescribed medication can contribute to hyperpigmentation. Prescribed medications such as Coumadin (warfarin, Bristol-Myers Squibb Company) or over-the-counter medications that impact the coagulation cascade should be stopped prior to treatment if it would not compromise the patient's health to minimize the potential complication of bruising (▶ Table 8.1 and ▶ Table 8.2). Pregnancy is a "relative" contraindication. Most companies have not performed studies that demonstrate safety in such a clinical setting.

Patients with active autoimmune or connective tissue disorders should not be treated.[7] However, patients with stable lupus may still have unwanted skin redness once their condition becomes stable and they are not receiving treatment for their

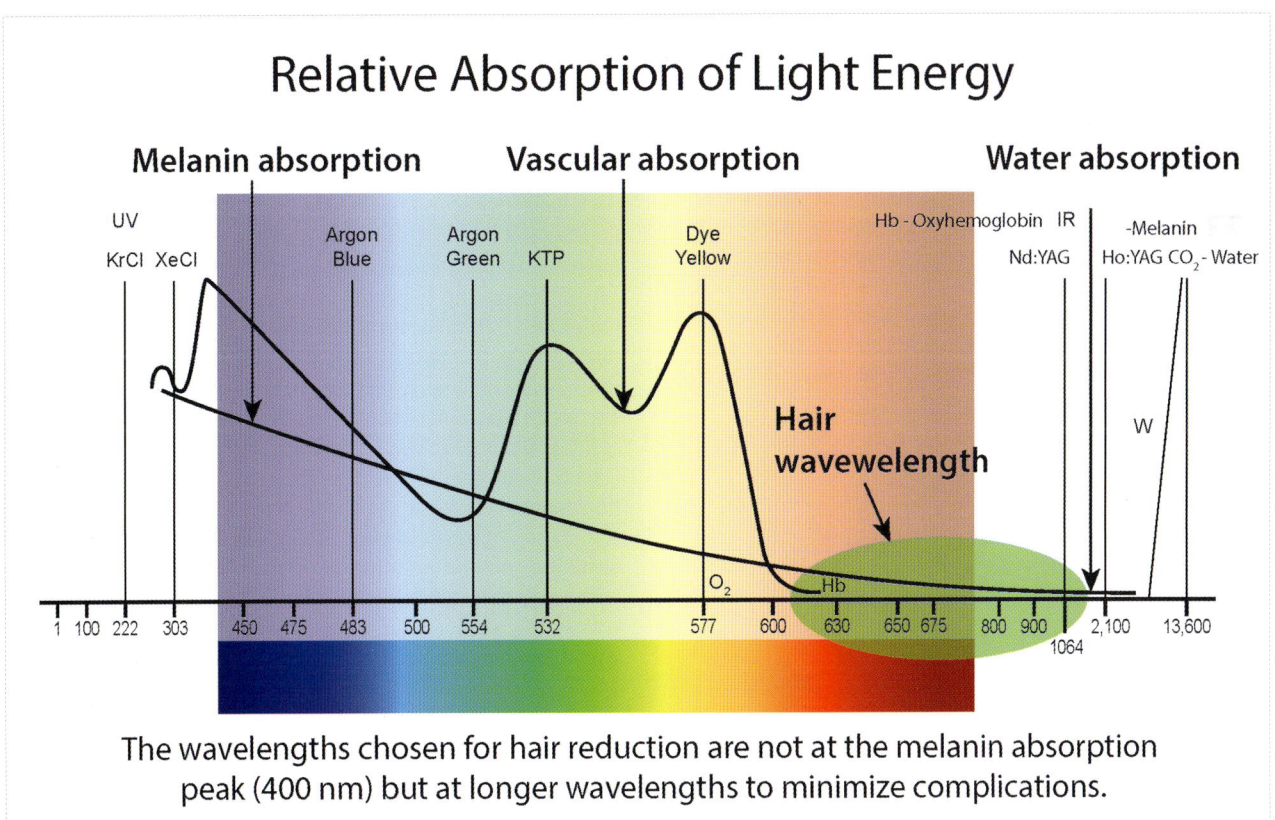

Fig. 8.2 Relative absorption of light energy and the various types of laser energy.

Table 8.1 Medications that may complicate LAEBT*

Acelite	Actifed	Advil
Alka Seltzer	Aleve**	Anacin
Anaprox**	APC Tablets	A.R.M.
Arthritis Pain Tabs**	Ascodeen	Ascriptin**
Asperbuf**	Aspergum**	Aspirin**
Aspirin Suppository	Axotal	Baby Aspirin**
Bayer**	Bismol	Buff A Comp Tabs
Bufferin	Clinoril**	Celebrex**
Congespirin	Contact	Cope
Coricidin D Decongestant	Coricidin Tablets	Cospirin
Coumadin	Darvon With Aspirin	Dolobid
Caspirin	Emprazil	Emperin With Codeine
Equagesic	Excedrin**	4-Way Cold Tablets
Feldene	Fiorinal	Fiorinal With Codeine
Gemnisyn	Hyco Pap	Ibuprofen**
Indocin	Indomethacin	Nurofen**
Medigesic Plus Caps	Medpro Compound Tabs	Midol
Monacet	Motrin**	Naprosyn**
Norgesic	Norgesic Forte	Orudis**
Pabirin	Panalgesic	Pepto Bismol
Percodan	Rhinex	Rufen
Sk-65	Sudafed	Supac
Synalgos	Talwin	Vanquish
Vioxx**		

*When taken 2 weeks before surgery
**Or any type of anti-inflammatory medication

medical condition. Good results can be obtained in terms of improving residual hypervascularity.

The treatment of patients with a history of wound-healing problems, such as keloid and hypertrophic scarring, needs to be evaluated to determine why such conditions occurred. Hypertrophic scarring can occur after burn injuries and can be improved with ablative technology and or pulsed light treatments.[8] Potentially cancerous skin lesions in the treatment area should be biopsied prior to addressing aesthetic concerns. In contrast, benign conditions such as actinic keratosis can be treated with LAEBT, cryotherapy, or other modalities.

As part of patient safety, topics to include in an informed consent for LAEBT are prolonged redness, transient "speckling" (hyperpigmentation), scabbing, edema, hair loss, purpura, hyperpigmentation, hypopigmentation, bruising, activation of a cutaneous herpetic skin eruption, infection, scarring, and dissatisfaction. In general, the more ablative the device, the greater the potential for these adverse side effects.

8.2.2 Analysis of the Skin

It is very important to address the individual's skin color. The gold standard for rating skin color is the Fitzpatrick scale[7] (▶ Fig. 8.3). Patients with a lighter skin color (Fitzpatrick I–III) are easier to treat when dealing with dyschromia, because the adjacent, untreated skin does not have as much innate pigment, allowing for an easier "blending" to the untreated region. Patients with Fitzpatrick skin types IV–VI can be treated successfully with LAEBT. To minimize the chance of posttreatment hyperpigmentation, these patients should be pretreated with a bleaching cream such as hydroquinone or kojic acid.[8] These topical agents should be continued until the patient has obtained his or her optimized, final skin color. Patients with a history of herpetic skin breakouts in the treatment area should be prescribed antiviral medication, which should be continued until the patient has fully recovered.

Determining the basis of the dyschromia is a critical component to providing optimal care. Hyperpigmentation is the most common manifestation of the aging process of the skin; this can consist of isolated spots or an overall yellow or brown discoloration on the skin. When hyperpigmentation manifests as overall yellow or brown skin discoloration, it can hinder identifying the underlying hypervascularity as the redness is camouflaged. Reducing the undesirable brown skin discoloration will reveal this vascular problem. Thus, a thorough evaluation of the skin regarding the desired improvement in hyperpigmentation, hypervascularity, and skin wrinkling is needed prior to selecting the best modality for treatment.

It is important to appreciate the various densities of the undesirable chromophore or skin rhytides, which can vary within the treatment region. Patients with rosacea often have a prominence of hypervascularity in the malar region. Not adjusting device parameters in response to chromophore density may result in a complication or inadequate results. The perioral and orbital regions are often left with skin wrinkles after a successful surgical procedure. Ablative energy may reduce these signs of aging. To optimize ablative therapy in areas with deeper skin wrinkles, a second or third pass is often needed.

The patient's age also can influence the treatment parameters and outcome. Parameters successfully used treating individuals in their thirties may need to be adjusted for those who are 50 to 60 years of age due in part to a thinning of the dermis, wound healing, and concomitant medical conditions.

The location of the treatment is also an important consideration. Although the desired results are similar to those for facial skin, the device settings used for facial skin may need to be adjusted when treating the skin on the neck, chest, or hands. Depending on the technology used, the recovery process can be more difficult when treating nonfacial skin.[9]

Table 8.2 Supplements that may impact LAEBT adversely*

Arnica montana (unless prescribed)	Bilberry
Cayenne	Don quai
Echinacea	Feverfew
Fish oil	Garlic
Ginger	Ginkgo biloba
Ginseng	Hawthorne
Kava kava	Licorice root
Ma huang (ephedra)	Melatonin
Red clover	St. John's wort
Valerian	Vitamin E
Yohimbe	

*When taken 2 weeks before surgery

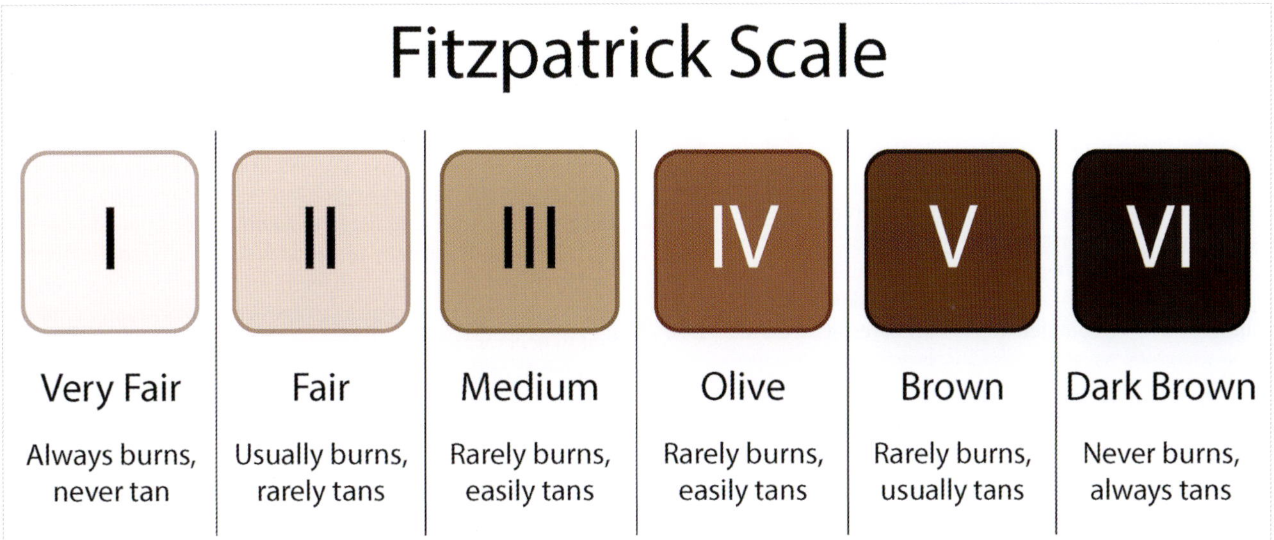

Fitzpatrick Scale

I	II	III	IV	V	VI
Very Fair	Fair	Medium	Olive	Brown	Dark Brown
Always burns, never tan	Usually burns, rarely tans	Rarely burns, easily tans	Rarely burns, easily tans	Rarely burns, usually tans	Never burns, always tans

Fig. 8.3 The Fitzpatrick scale. Assessing skin color is an important factor when treating a patient's skin. The clinician should be aware that certain individuals, such as those from Asian or Mediterranean descent, may present with a skin type II or III but react like a skin type IV person. Thus, establishing their "tanning" history is important. Starting with lower energy settings and doing a "test patch" may be prudent to avoid complications. (Adapted with permission from Fitzpatrick, T. B. "Soleil et peau" [Sun and skin]. Journal de Médecine Esthétique (in French) (2): 33–34) 1975)

8.2.3 Understanding the Technology

There are many LAEBT that can improve the appearance of the skin. Each manufacturer has enabled its device with unique features, which prevents the clinician from transferring specific treatment parameters from one manufacturer's device to another's manufacturer's device despite using the same type of therapeutic energy. Thus, the operator must have a thorough understanding of how the device settings can impact the final result. Variables that impact outcomes include but are not limited to the type of energy, number of treatments, wavelength, fluence, density pattern, overlapping of pulses, and number of "passes." Adequate training is imperative when incorporating LAEBT into one's practice. Using treatment parameters within the manufacturers guidelines is the best way to minimize complications.

8.2.4 Combining Modalities

As clinicians understand LAEBT, their limitations, and how to avoid complications, combining different modalities may enhance outcomes. Photorejuvenation following ablative therapy can be helpful with blending to adjacent skin areas. Providing radiofrequency (RF) treatments to the perioral or periorbital regions can smooth skin wrinkles following the improvement in dyschromia through photorejuvenation.[10,11] During the recovery process after ablative therapy, affording patients photorejuvenation treatments with the fluence reduced and selecting a cutoff filter that delivers energy primarily directed toward red can shorten the recovery time.

8.3 Pretreatment and Posttreatment Protocols

Although the clinician should use his or her judgment as to what protocol to follow, the following guidelines are helpful when using LAEBT regardless of the specific device.

Prior to Treatment

- Avoid medications with anticoagulant effects.
- Avoid medications that are known to create hyperpigmentation.
- Avoid high-dose topical Vitamin C and retinoids 1 week prior to treatment.
- Stress the importance of applying topical sun blocks during therapy.
- Recommend topical pretreatment and posttreatment of bleaching creams for IV skin types.
- Advise patients who receive routine skin treatments from their esthetician to avoid chemical peels or vigorous extractions during the course of LAEBT.
- Stress the importance of the prophylactic use of antiviral medication if the patient has a history of herpetic skin eruptions.
- Ensure that there is enough time for the medication to work prior to LAEBT treatment if a topical anesthetic cream is to be used for pain control.
- Provide protective eyewear during treatment.

8.4 Incorporating Nonsurgical LAEBT

There are many pathways to improve the appearance of the skin using LAEBT. Providing patients these types of opportunities should enhance their overall aesthetic experience. Given the gamut of nonsurgical techniques currently available, it is impossible to demonstrate the efficacy of all therapies. The cases presented reflect some of the possible nonsurgical options in which the appearance of the skin is improved and embraces a more complete rejuvenation result (**see Video 1.1**).

8.4.1 Ablative Therapy

Prior to the early 1990s, chemical peels and dermabrasion were the mainstay of topical, nonincisional treatment for wrinkles and unwanted brown spots. These modalities are still used effectively. The implementation of lasers to treat hyperpigmentation and skin wrinkling became popular in the early 1990s.[8] Usually lasers provide a single, collimated wavelength delivered to the skin. The primary wavelengths used for laser skin resurfacing are CO_2 (10,600 nm) or erbium YAG (2,940 nm). The dynamic ability to control the depth of injury through the device settings during treatment enhanced the use of lasers compared to topical chemical agents. The "target" of the energy is the water content within the skin. The evolution of laser therapy has been focused on minimizing the recovery period by reducing the initial zones of injury. Providing smaller focal injury spots and delivering laser energy in a scattered pattern has helped shorten recovery times and treatment discomfort. This modification may require more than one treatment to provide parallel results, however. Depending on the amount, density, and pattern of the energy delivered, lasting results may be seen after one to three treatments. In general, the greater the energy delivered and the higher the density, the longer the recovery for each treatment (▶ Fig. 8.4). The end point for a fully ablative single treatment is a light tan skin color. When providing less energy to the skin, hyperemia may reflect the desired initial skin reaction.

Initial recovery times can be short, 2–3 days or longer, for 3–8 weeks. Multiple laser treatments may be required when patients opt for shorter recovery periods. Typically, there is some initial skin crusting, because the energy penetrates into the dermis and ablates tissue within the zone of injury. Posttreatment protocols may parallel the protocols provided to individuals with second-degree burns, including topical creams and or bandages. Camouflage makeup can be applied once the skin is healed. Treatment analgesia is customized to the fluence, the density of the energy delivered, and the energy wavelength, and it can range from topical analgesics with oral supplementation to general anesthesia.

In terms of the wavelengths for each laser, it is CO_2 or erbium for the fully ablative image, erbium for the nonablative fractional resurfacing, and CO_2 for the ablative fractional resurfacing. The ideal patient does not have underlying redness but is looking for an improvement in skin wrinkling and hyperpigmentation. Removing the undesirable "brown" skin color may reveal pre-existing redness that was masked by the unwanted melanin in the epidermis. Because of the potential for hypopigmentation posttreatment, treating patients with Fitzpatrick skin type IV–VI requires a modification of one's protocol for treating skin types II–III. Being able to "blend" the treated area to the adjacent skin by altering the energy settings or delivery pattern is important. The need to adjust the pattern and amount of energy delivered also needs to be considered when treating regional areas, such as the perioral and periorbital regions, which are often left with wrinkles following a rhytidectomy or blepharoplasty.

Clinical Results

This woman had a facelift performed by another physician. Her concerns were the residual fine wrinkling and brown spots on her face (▶ Fig. 8.5a). She underwent full-face, CO_2 laser skin resurfacing. The clinical end point of laser treatment on the deep wrinkles was a chamois color of the skin. Other regions without such deep wrinkles had skin erythema as the treatment end point. Two years after this treatment, this woman had smoother skin and a reduction in her hyperpigmentation

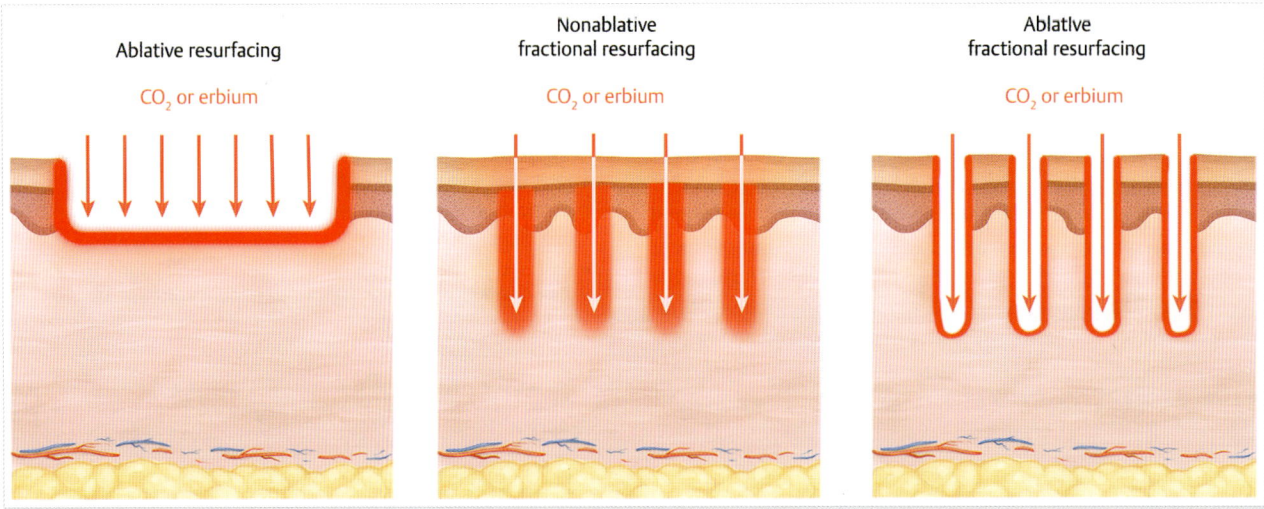

Fig. 8.4 Manufacturers have improved their delivery systems to provide variable epidermal and dermal impact for the same wavelength.

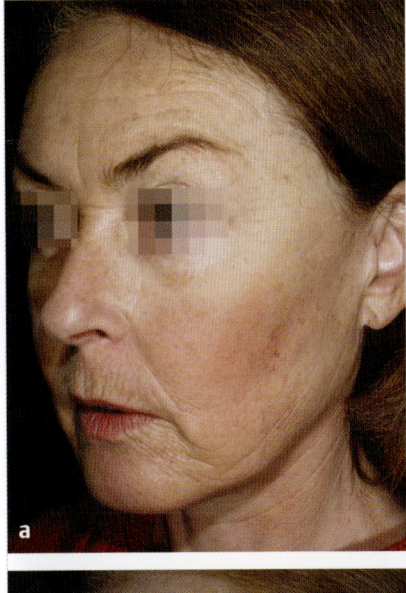
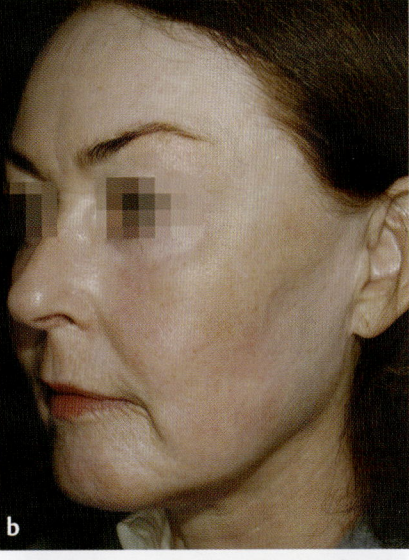
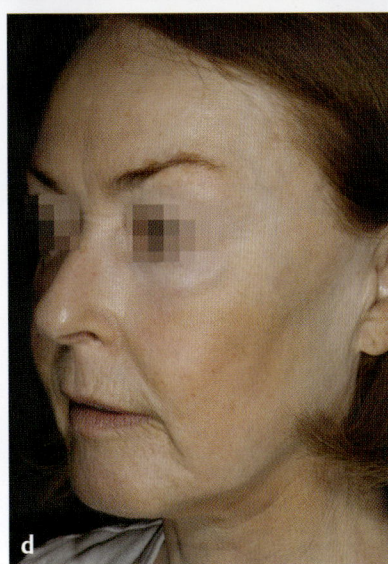

Fig. 8.5 (a) Prior to treatment, this patient did not like the skin wrinkles and hyperpigmentation of her skin. It is important to note that hyperpigmentation can conceal any hypervascularity that is present. Removal of the hyperpigmentation may allow the hypervascularity to become more obvious once the patient is fully recovered. It can also cause hypopigmentation in the treatment zone. To avoid a line of demarcation, the adjacent skin requires an adjustment of treatment parameters. This is often facilitated by reducing the device energy settings as one goes beyond the primary treatment area. Laser skin resurfacing and neurotoxin use were also used on this patient. (b) After treatment, she has a clear, lasting improvement of her unwanted perioral and facial skin wrinkles. She also has areas of hypopigmentation and a light pink tone to her skin, because her preexisting hypervascularity is more obvious. Her jawline served as the area for "blending" to her nontreated neck. (c) Without any intervention other than neurotoxins, once or twice per year, she has maintained her improvement in wrinkles and skin color. (d) She still has an improvement in her fine skin wrinkling. Despite using sun block, she has an increase in her skin hyperpigmentation.

(▶ Fig. 8.5b). As she continued to age, she received periodic neurotoxin injections on her forehead and in the lateral orbital and perioral regions. She has maintained an improvement in her skin color and wrinkle reductions using this protocol, as shown 5 years (▶ Fig. 8.5c) and 10 years (▶ Fig. 8.5d) after her ablative treatment.

This woman would have optimally benefited from a rhytidectomy. She did not have an underlying problem with hypervascularity (▶ Fig. 8.6a). However, she did not want surgery and thus had full-face, CO_2 laser skin resurfacing. Anesthesia was provided by regional nerve blocks and IV conscious sedation. In the areas of skin wrinkling, a chamois skin color indicated the treatment end point. Adjacent skin received less laser energy. Six months after her single treatment, she has a smoother skin surface and no lines of demarcation between the deeper skin lines that received more laser energy than the adjacent skin (▶ Fig. 8.6b).

Ablative LAEBT can be used on darker skin types. Routinely pretreating these patients with a bleaching cream for 2–3 weeks is important. This cream is continued until the final desired skin color is obtained. This young woman had multiple hyperpigmentation spots on her face that she wanted to be removed (▶ Fig. 8.7a). These spots were assessed to be benign nevi of varying depth and size. She requested a single treatment modality. She was pretreated with topical 10% hydroquinone for 3 weeks and then underwent a CO_2 skin surface ablation of the multiple lesions using regional nerve block anesthesia supplemented with IV conscious sedation. Two weeks after her CO_2 ablation of these multiple lesions, she had hyperpigmentation of the treated areas. She restarted her 10% hydroquinone cream applied to her treatment areas twice a day (▶ Fig. 8.7b). Six months after stopping her hydroquinone cream and 1½ years after her treatment, she has an even tone throughout her skin and elimination of her unwanted nevi (▶ Fig. 8.7c).

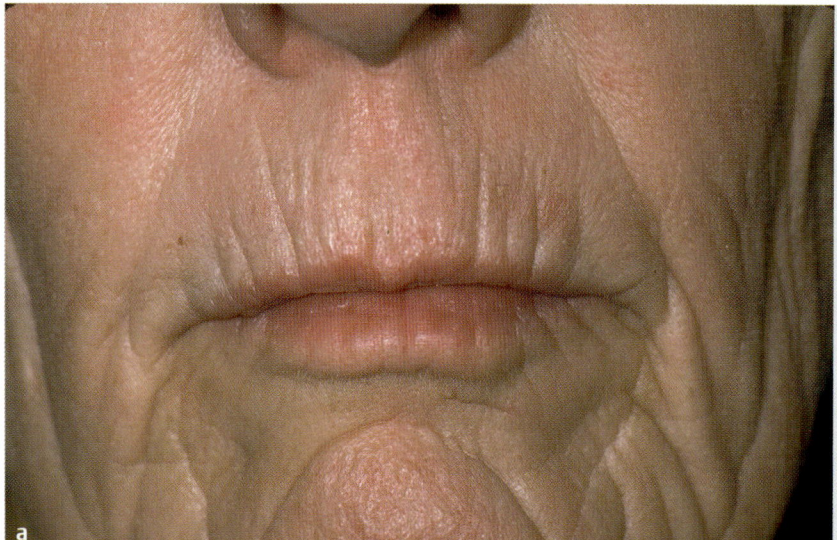
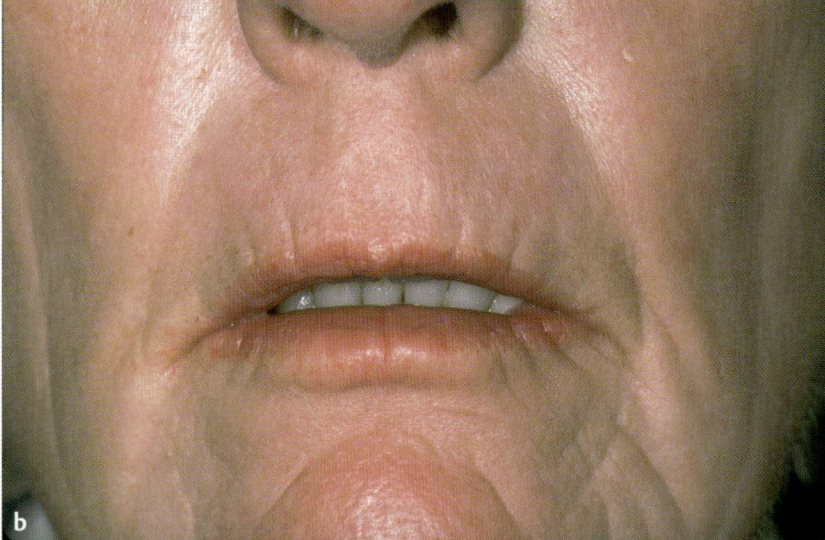

Fig. 8.6 CO_2 laser resurfacing. **(a)** Pretreatment. The deep lines and redundant skin would be hard to correct with skin "fillers." Even if she underwent a facelift, she would have been left with deep perioral lines. **(b)** Six months posttreatment. Adjusting the energy delivered allowed for an improvement in her deep wrinkles without obvious lines of demarcation (hypopigmentation) in terms of perioral skin color. No other modalities were used to obtain this result.

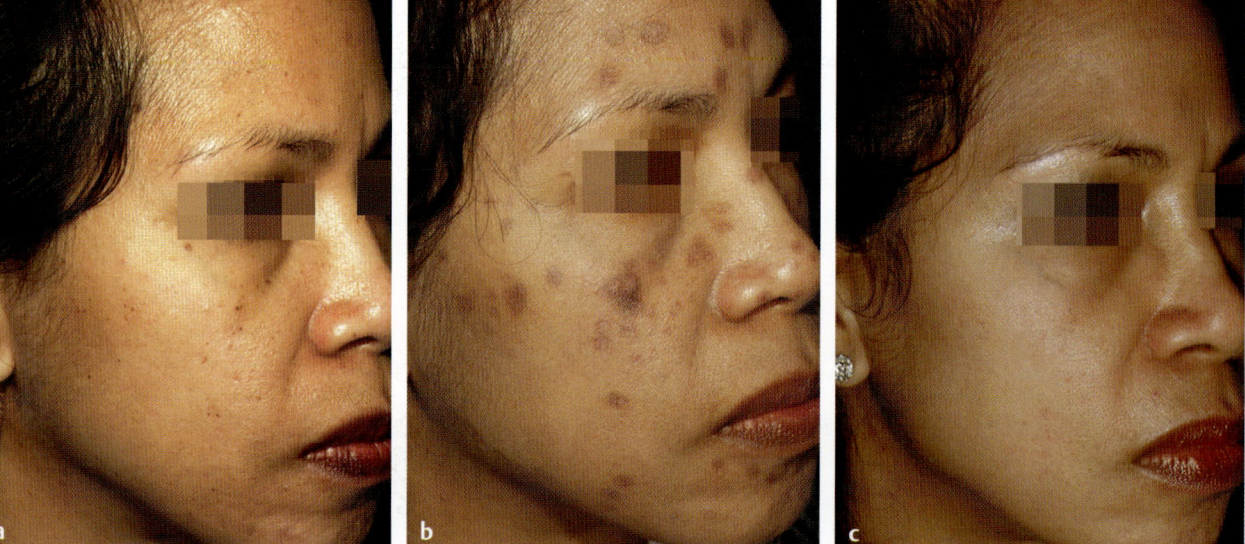

Fig. 8.7 Ablative LAEBT. **(a)** Multiple benign nevi. **(b)** Two weeks posttreatment. Despite pretreatment with hydroquinone and attention to blending the primary areas (location of the nevi) to the adjacent skin, she had hyperpigmentation in the areas that received a higher energy setting required to remove the nevi. During her recovery period, she was able to conceal the hyperpigmentation with topical makeup. **(c)** 18 months posttreatment. She has no areas of skin color demarcation and no return of her unwanted nevi 1½ years after treatment.

8.4.2 Ablative LAEBT in Conjunction With a Surgical Procedure

Ablative therapy can be performed at the same time as a surgical procedure. Patients may request this to reduce the cumulative recovery time if both ablative and LAEBT treatments were performed independently. Performing these procedures together requires the clinician to have a complete understanding of the potential impact of the ablative modality on the blood supply of an elevated skin flap. Altered blood supply due to skin flap elevation requires an adjustment in device settings. In addition, simultaneous ablative regional treatment requires an accurate assessment of adjacent skin color and the skill set to "blend" skin ablation in order to minimize the chance of a line of demarcation after treatment.

This woman had a previous rhytidectomy, and she serves as a good example of how multiple LAEBT can optimize one's aesthetic result (▶ Fig. 8.8). She expressed multiple concerns preoperatively; she wanted a one-treatment improvement of her perioral wrinkles, improvement of her nasolabial folds, improvement of the dyschromia of her face and neck, and a change in the appearance of her nose (▶ Fig. 8.8**a,b**). After a thorough discussion of her treatment options, she decided to have a redo rhytidectomy, lower blepharoplasty, and revision rhinoplasty. In terms of her skin appearance, an ablative treatment of her perioral region at the time of her surgery was a safe option, because the ablative "blending" zone was not undermined and because a fully ablative CO_2 skin resurfacing would improve the wrinkles around her mouth and satisfy her desire for a single treatment to improve these wrinkles. However, skin color "blending" of her perioral region to the adjacent skin dyschromia on her cheek was an issue because of the skin pigment and vascularity adjacent to the perioral region (▶ Fig. 8.8**c**). To address this vascularity adjacent to the perioral region, the patient underwent five photorejuvenation treatments of her face and neck after surgery. This reduced the time of skin redness following a fully ablative laser resurfacing of her perioral region, and it facilitated the skin color blending to the adjacent cheek. Six months after her last photorejuvenation treatment, she has an improvement in her perioral wrinkles and no evidence of a line of demarcation (▶ Fig. 8.8**d-f**).

8.4.3 Photorejuvenation

The use of intense pulsed light (IPL) provides the clinician with a significant tool to improve the appearance of the skin.[12] RF energy has been added by companies to augment the clinical impact of the light energy source.[10] Unlike lasers that deliver one wavelength, IPL devices emit noncoherent light with wavelengths in the range of 515 to 1200 nm but at a much lower

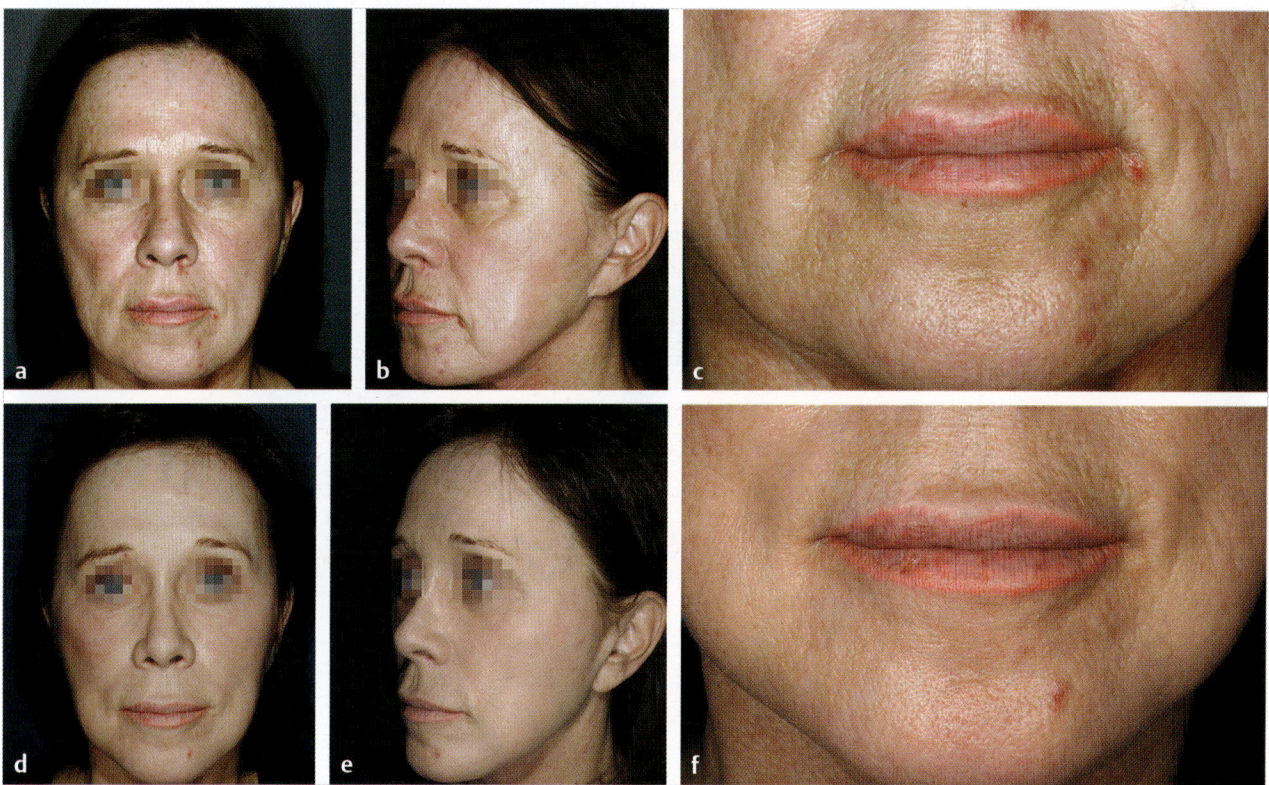

Fig. 8.8 (a–c) Pretreatment. This patient had significant hyperpigmentation of the skin on her face, neck, and chest. She also had deep perioral lines. The majority of her facial skin was smooth. A fully ablative skin resurfacing would provide an improvement of her perioral skin wrinkles. However, this would create a skin color line of demarcation that cannot be prevented even through optimal blending techniques. Thus, another modality, photo rejuvenation (IPL) was added after her surgery to blend her facial skin color to the perioral region that received a full CO_2 ablation to improve the perioral wrinkles. **(d–f)** Six months after a rhytidectomy, lower blepharoplasty, and revision rhinoplasty. After her surgical procedure, which also included a perioral fully ablative skin resurfacing, she received five full-face IPL treatments to blend the skin dyschromia. Combining LAEBT modalities provided the patient with a single surgical procedure, improvement in her perioral lines, and overall improvement in her facial skin color.

energy density for each wavelength than laser devices. Filters are used to limit the spectrum of light and "target" the energy to the primary, undesirable chromophore within the skin. Such filtering technology also limits potentially harmful light radiation. Depending on the device, physicians can select the primary therapeutic wavelength by using a designated handpiece or cutoff filter, which focuses the energy more towards red (vascular) or brown (melanin). The broad-spectrum light energy that is delivered allows this technology to simultaneously reduce unwanted hyperpigmentation and hypervascularity with each treatment. The ideal patient does not have skin laxity as his or her primary concern but rather wants an improvement in dyschromia and or vascular concerns.

The clinical effect and recovery time is primarily based on the chromophore density, energy wavelengths delivered to the skin, fluence (radiant energy), and pre-treatment skin temperature. Typically, the epidermis is protected through the use of a topically applied cool gel or device handpiece, which contains an internal cooling system. Treatment analgesia is usually afforded through a topical cream and/or an oral medication. Compared to lasers, the spot size is larger allowing for treatment of greater surface areas expeditiously. To achieve the optimal results with a minimum recovery time for each treatment, a series of treatments are required, often three to six treatments. The number of treatments is predicated by patient expectations and clinical presentation. Initial treatment device parameters are usually provided by the manufacturer and require the physician to assess the innate skin color, the skin response to sunlight, and the concentration of an undesirable chromophore. After each treatment, settings can be adjusted for subsequent sessions, usually by increasing the fluence, because the preceding treatment should have made improvements. If there is an adverse effect, prolonged recovery (more than 4 to 6 hours of erythema), or an expressed intolerance to treatment, device settings may need to be reduced. While there is a recovery period (initial erythema/edema of the skin), this time is short compared to that of ablative technologies. Patients with hyperpigmentation can expect a darkening of these regions before the epidermal layer slowly sloughs. The resolution of this appearance can take 3 to 10 days. The greater the density of undesirable pigment, the longer it will take to shed the darkened epithelium.

It is important to understand that it may be hard to initially determine the extent of hypervascularity in patients with moderate to severe hyperpigmentation, because the brown/yellow epidermal color can camouflage underlying redness. In such clinical settings, I (M.I.K.) initially select cutoff filters (therapeutic wavelengths) that focus the light energy toward correcting hyperpigmentation and then adjust the light energy filters to focus on the vascular component for subsequent treatments. Reducing the unwanted hyperpigmentation initially provides a better visualization of the remaining redness. This allows subsequent sessions to have the device settings customized to focus on improving the vascular condition.

The ideal patient's primary concern should be unwanted brown spots and redness as opposed to wrinkles. However, in certain clinical situations in which the patient has hypervascularity in the same region as fine skin wrinkling (usually the periorbital region), the heat absorbed within the dermis and subsequent dermal neocollagenesis can improve fine skin wrinkling. In my experience, the greater the degree of undesirable hypervascularity within the area of fine skin wrinkling, the greater the improvement in skin texture and wrinkles after treatment (▶ Fig. 8.9**a,b**).

Patients with darker skin (Fitzpatrick classification IV – VI), can be safely treated by optimizing therapeutic parameters.[6] Depending on one's device, the settings that can be altered to accommodate these skin types include the following; pulse width, pulse duration, inter-pulse delay, wavelength filter, number of pulses per activation, adjusting the RF energy, depth of energy penetration, epidermal cooling, and light fluence.

Once competency is established treating facial skin, most IPL devices allow for the treatment of nonfacial skin. Usually, the settings suggested by the device manufacturer are less aggressive for these locations. Definition of the area that is to be improved must be clearly outlined and the clinician must be able to "blend" the treated area to the adjacent zone to minimize the possibility of a line of demarcation. Reducing fluence is one way of "blending" the primary treatment area as you approach the adjacent sun-damaged areas that will not be treated. The optimal result may require more than the initially prescribed number of sessions.

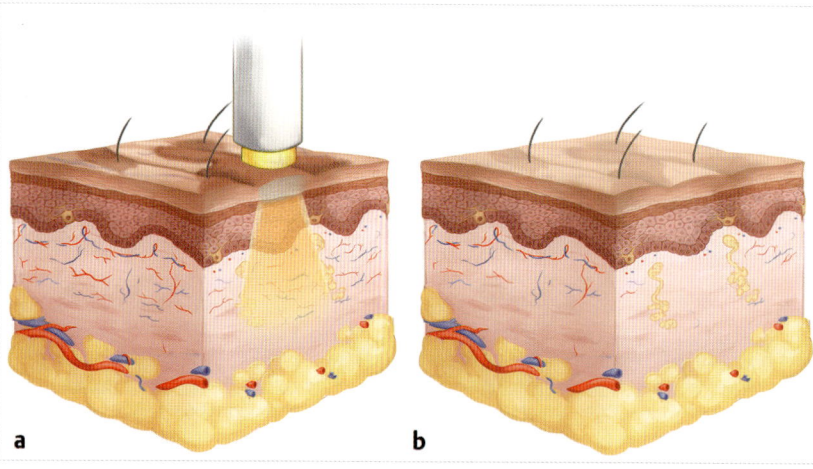

Fig. 8.9 (a) The high density of undesirable vasculature in the dermis attracts the light thermal energy into the dermis. (b) The resultant dermal inflammatory response results in neocollagenesis, which provides skin smoothening.

Clinical Results

This woman did not like the redness and brown spots on her face (▶ Fig. 8.10**a**) She underwent five full-face photorejuvenation treatments. The recovery time did not require her to miss work. Three months after her last treatment, she has an improvement of her skin appearance (▶ Fig. 8.10**b**). Analysis through Canfield's VISIA Complexion Analysis System confirms the improvement in unwanted brown spots (▶ Fig. 8.10**c**). In this computer-generated analysis, the higher the number, the better the comparative ranking is to women of her same skin type and age. This "spot" analysis represents a 17% improvement in undesirable brown spots. In addition, due to the hypervascularity in the periorbital region, the light energy delivered to the skin penetrates into the dermis, targeting the deeper vasculature. This creates an inflammatory process, which leads to neocollagenesis and a 17% improvement in fine skin wrinkles[7] (▶ Fig. 8.10**d,e**).

Skin rejuvenation encompasses more than just an improvement of unwanted dyschromia. Although it is not an exact science, the VISIA device provides analytical information that supports patient's statements of an improvement in the quality of one's skin following photorejuvenation therapy. Three months after her fifth photorejuvenation treatment, this woman had an improvement of her spots (69%) (▶ Fig. 8.11**a**), skin pores (84%) (▶ Fig. 8.11**b**), texture (167%) (▶ Fig. 8.11**c**), and skin wrinkles (30%) (▶ Fig. 8.11**d**).

Photorejuvenation is an excellent adjunct to surgical procedures. When performed correctly, it is safe to do such treatments on darker skin types. This Asian woman did not like the appearance of her eyelids, neck, and skin (▶ Fig. 8.12**a,b**). She underwent an endoscopic browlift, lower blepharoplasty, and facelift. During her recovery period, she received a series of five, full-face photorejuvenation treatments. An advantage of performing such skin treatments after surgery is that the facial skin is relatively numb, eliminating the need for topical anesthetics for skin treatments. Three months after her last photorejuvenation treatment, she had a significant improvement in the appearance and condition of her skin. She had a reduction in undesirable hyperpigmentation and hypervascularity without any hypopigmentation complications. Her reduction in unwanted brown spots was confirmed by VISIA analysis, which shows more than a 25% improvement in her unwanted brown spots (the higher the number reflects a better appearance) (▶ Fig. 8.12**c**).

Treating both the face and adjacent neck regions when the patient has significant sun damage in both regions may provide a more complete "rejuvenation." In such clinical settings, only correcting the undesirable dyschromia on the face would leave the patient with a "sun-damaged" neck adjacent to a more rejuvenated face. This woman wanted an improvement in her facial skin laxity as well as the quality of her skin (▶ Fig. 8.13**a**). Six months after receiving an endoscopic brow lift, upper and lower blepharoplasty, lip augmentation, and facelift, she has a more youthful appearance and was started on her photorejuvenation treatments of her face and neck (▶ Fig. 8.13**b**) Three months after her last skin treatment and 1 year after her surgery, her skin color parallels the improvement in her skin laxity, reflecting a more complete, youthful appearance photo (▶ Fig. 8.13**c**).

Improving the appearance of nonfacial skin is important to many patients. In addition to improving the skin on the neck, photorejuvenation can improve areas such as the chest and hands. This woman was concerned about the appearance of her chest skin (▶ Fig. 8.14**a**) Analysis of her skin revealed both vascular and pigment problems. Immediately after treatment, she had redness on her chest that resolved within 6 hours (▶ Fig. 8.14**b**). One week after her first treatment, she has the expected "speckling" of the treated region (▶ Fig. 8.14**c**) This is not a complication but rather part of the treatment recovery process. Six months after her fifth session, she has an improvement of the appearance of her chest skin (▶ Fig. 8.14**d**).

After undergoing facial surgery and skin rejuvenation, the appearance of one's hands may be a concern. The skin wrinkling and hyperpigmentation may not parallel the rejuvenated, facial transformation. After undergoing a facelift, this patient was concerned that her hands looked aged due to the brown spots (▶ Fig. 8.15**a**) Six months after having five photorejuvenation treatments, the appearance of her hand skin is better (▶ Fig. 8.15**b**)

Combining modalities is helpful. Injecting a "filler" to replace volume loss beneath the skin of one's hand and treating the skin discoloration is complementary to the individual's overall rejuvenation process. This patient had previous facial surgery

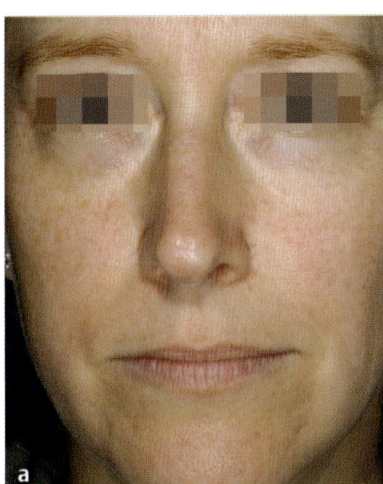
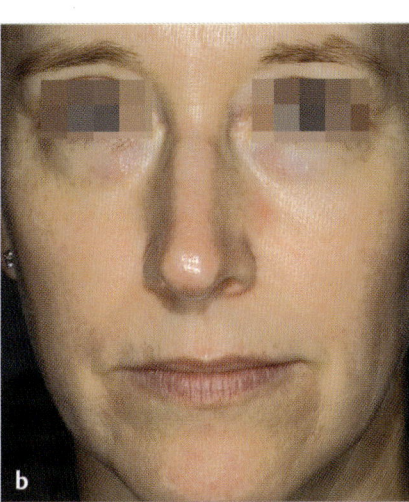

Fig. 8.10 (**a**) Prior to treatment. (**b**) Three months after having five IPL treatments. (*continued*)

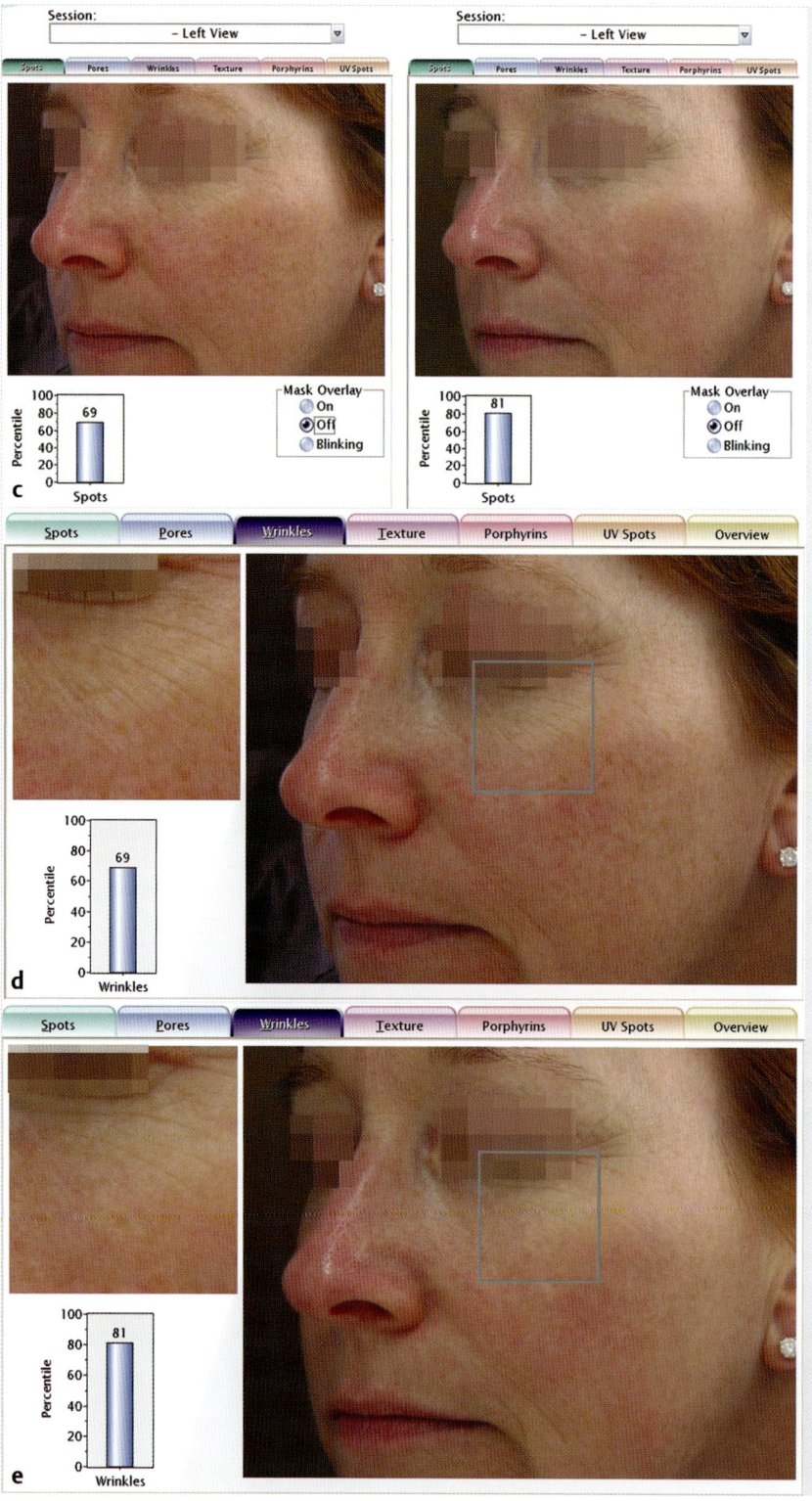

Fig. 8.10 (*continued*) **(c)** Using Canfield's spot analysis method of image capture analysis, the higher percentile number reflects an improvement in skin spots in the posttreatment image on the right. **(d)** Canfield wrinkle analysis. Prior to treatment. The small inset image illustrates the fine wrinkles in the periorbital region prior to treatment. **(e)** Canfield wrinkle analysis. Three months after five IPL treatments without any other intervention including neurotoxins, there is an improvement in periorbital skin wrinkling.

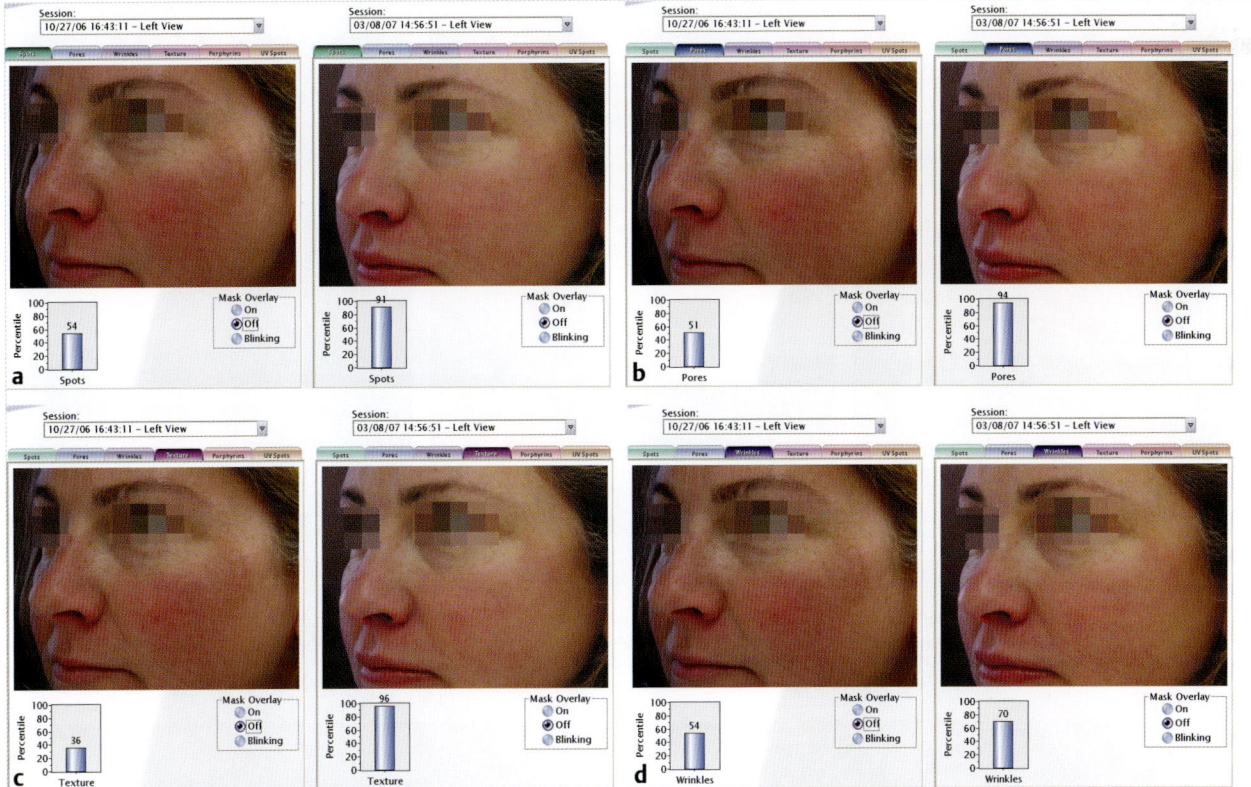

Fig. 8.11 Three months after her fifth photorejuvenation treatment, this woman had an improvement of **(a)** her skin spots, **(b)** her skin pores, **(c)** her skin texture, and **(d)** her skin wrinkles.

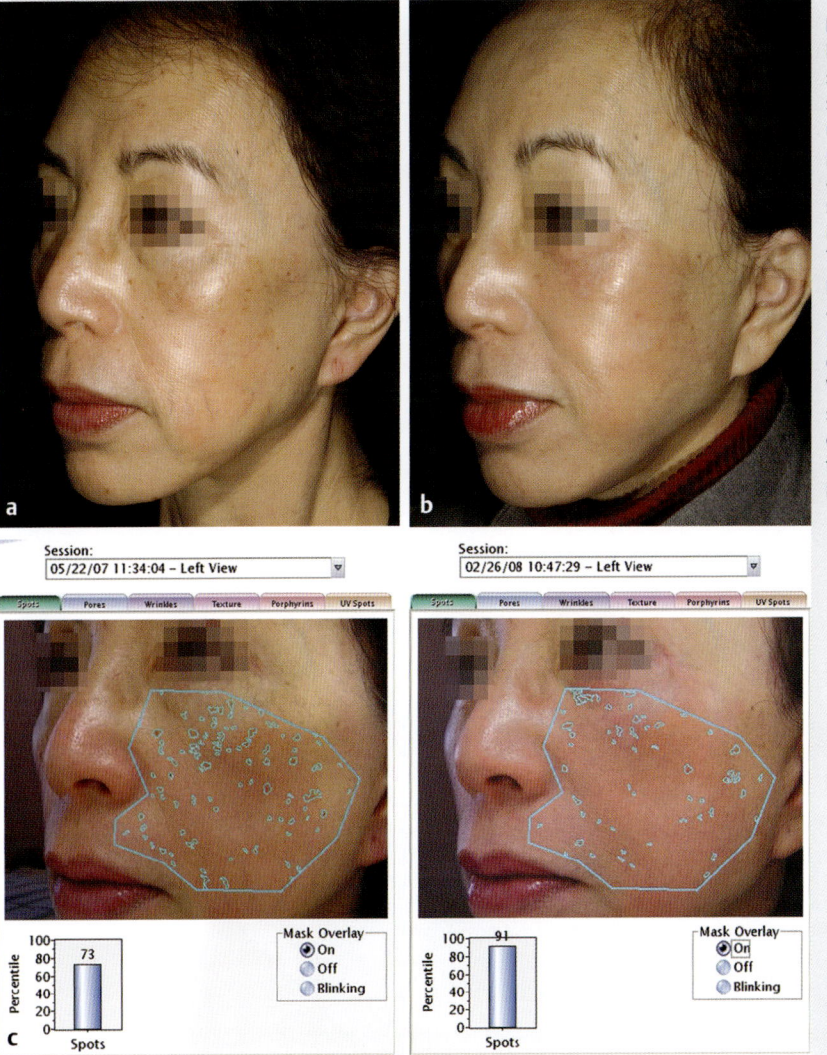

Fig. 8.12 (a) This Asian woman wanted a surgical improvement as well as an improvement in her skin appearance. **(b)** She received her facial surgery and IPL treatments during her surgical recovery. Three months after her last photorejuvenation treatment, she has a better appearance of her skin tone, as taken by a standard digital camera. Her surgical procedure improved the positioning of her facial/eyelid skin. The postoperative treatment of her skin with photorejuvenation treatments improved the appearance of her skin. **(c)** This before-and-after photograph screen shot demonstrates the comparable zone of analysis by the VISIA system. Within the outlined region of analysis, one can see that there are fewer identified "spots" depicted as blue color outlines in the post-IPL treatment zone, reflecting a 25% improvement in brown spots.

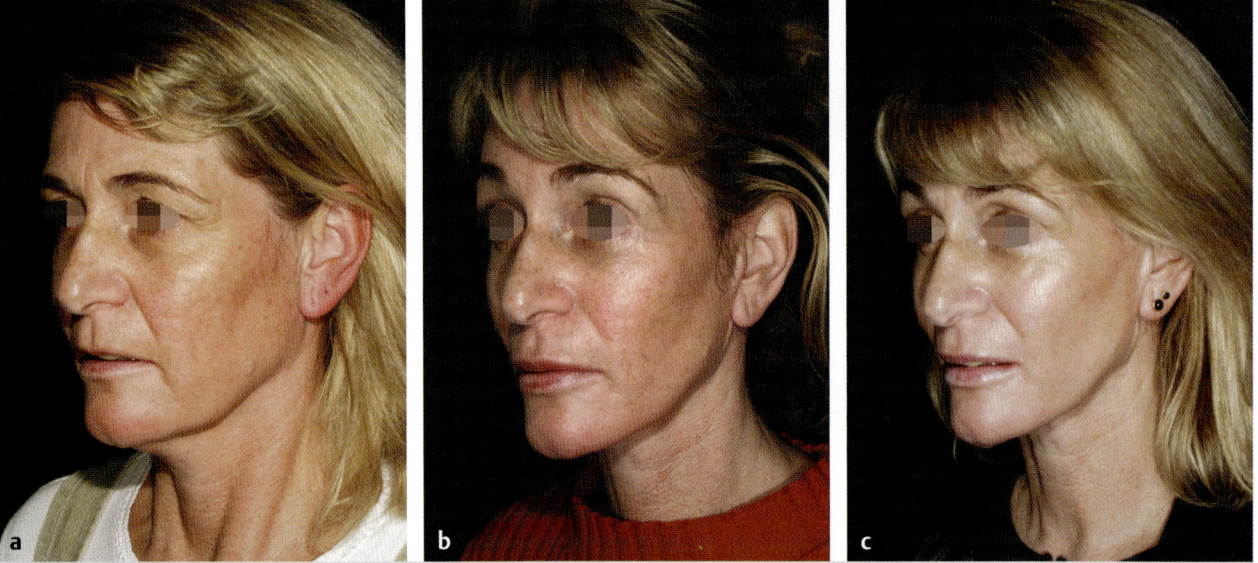

Fig. 8.13 (a) This woman in her forties did not like the appearance of her face. This included the extra skin, fat, and the quality of her skin due to sun damage. (b) Six months after her surgical procedures (an endoscopic brow lift, upper and lower blepharoplasty, lip augmentation, and facelift), she has a more youthful appearance. However, she felt that her sun-damaged skin did not reflect the rejuvenation process she was wanting. (c) Three months after her last photorejuvenation treatment and 1 year after her surgery, she has both an improvement in the skin position and the appearance of the skin in terms of reducing unwanted dyschromia of her face and neck.

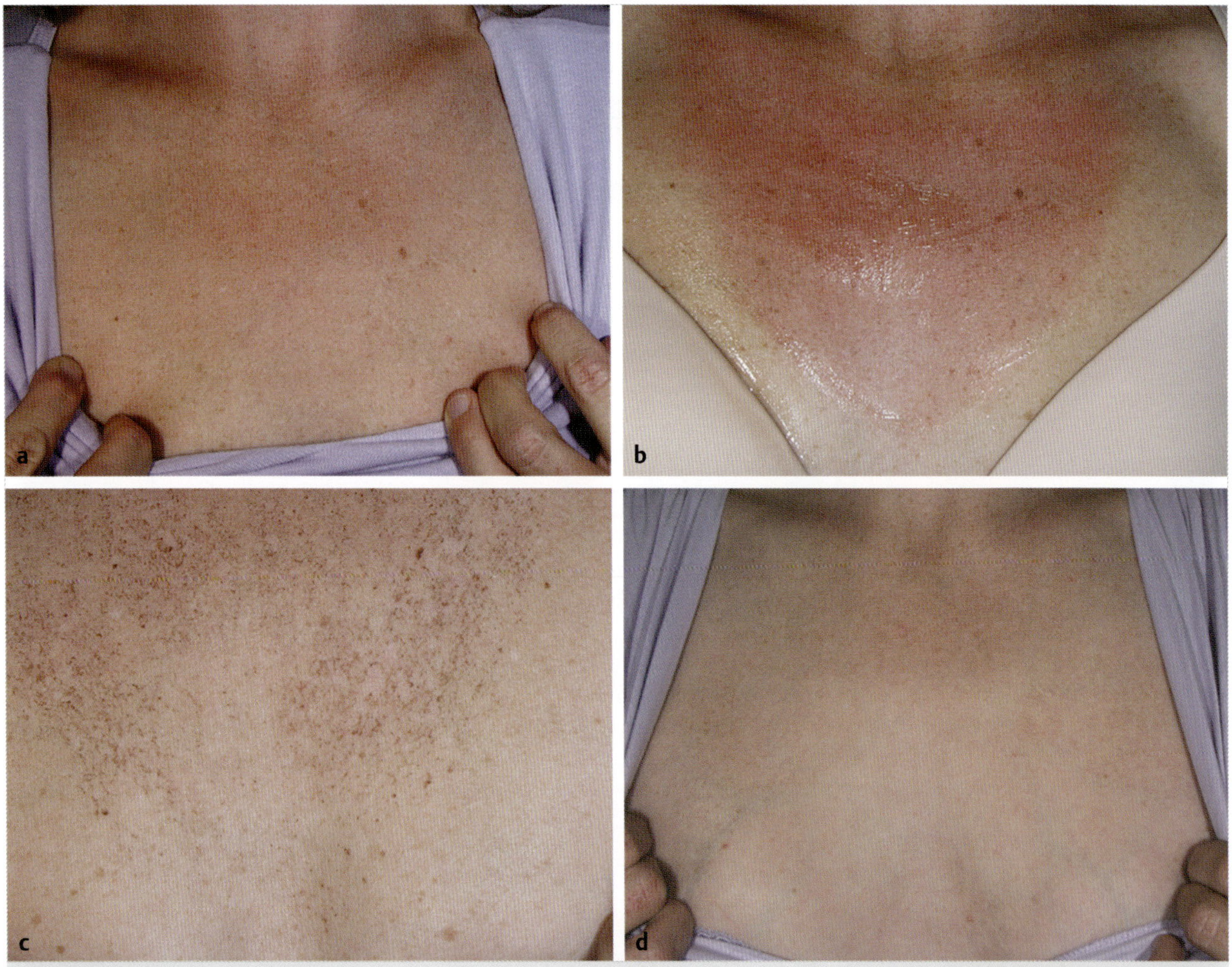

Fig. 8.14 (a) Prior to treatment, this woman had diffuse sun damage. Defining the region of treatment is important in terms of patient expectations. Treating the "decolletage" region requires the treater to have good "blending skills," because the adjacent regions also have sun damage but would not be treated. (b) Immediately after treatment. This is the color of the skin that represents a good therapeutic treatment. Subsequent treatments may reveal less redness even with an increase in energy delivered as the undesirable chromophore is removed. (c) One week after treatment. This type of skin appearance demonstrates a confluent reaction to photorejuvenation in the treatment region. The epidermis appearance is reacting as anticipated. Subsequent treatments should not have such a posttreatment dark specking appearance even as the light energy is increased, because the light energy will be focused on the underlying hypervascularity as the epidermal damage sloughs. The result of "blending" the primary treatment area to the adjacent sun-damaged skin depends on the treater's skill. (d) Six months after the fifth session. She has an improvement in her chest skin appearance without a line of demarcation between the primary treatment region and the adjacent chest skin.

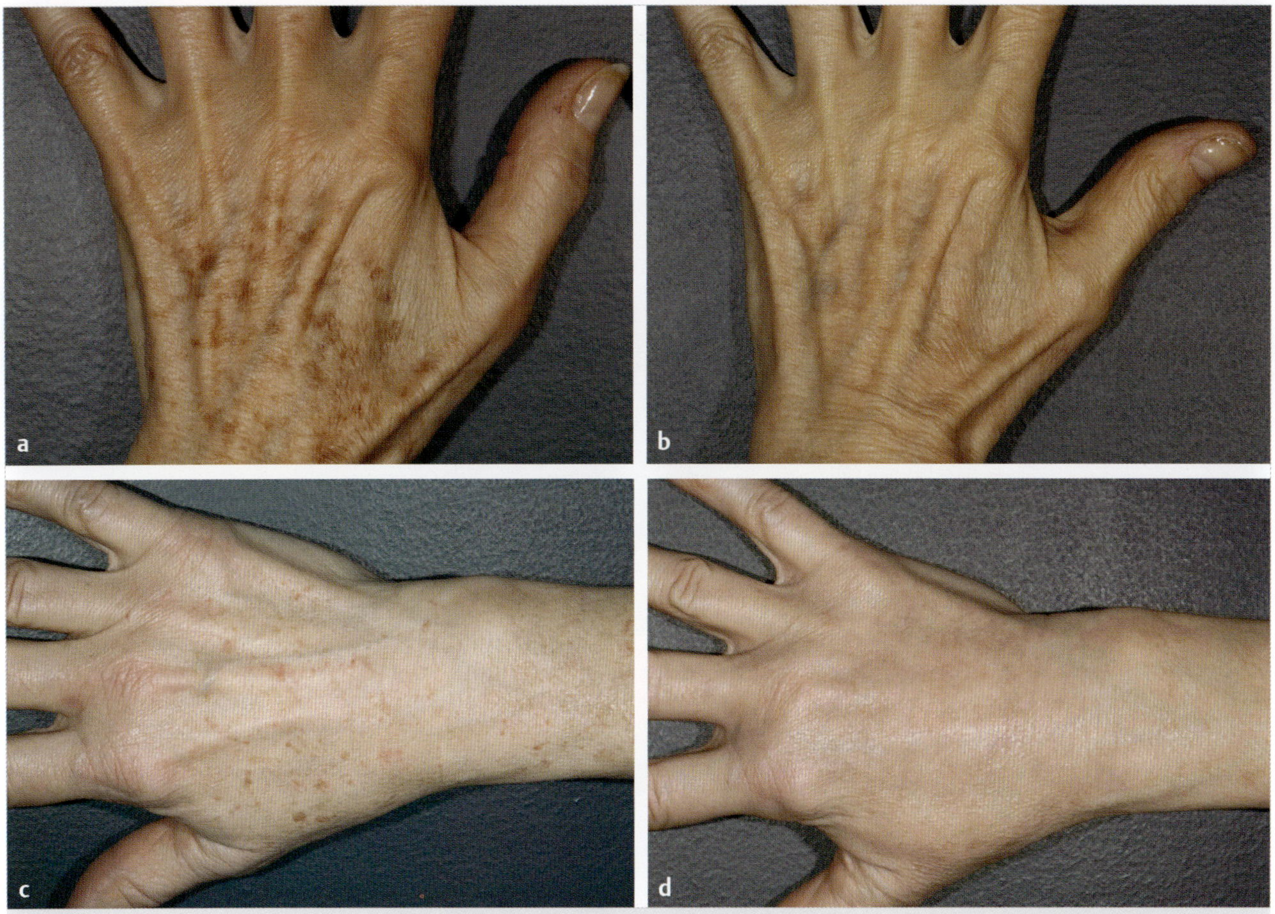

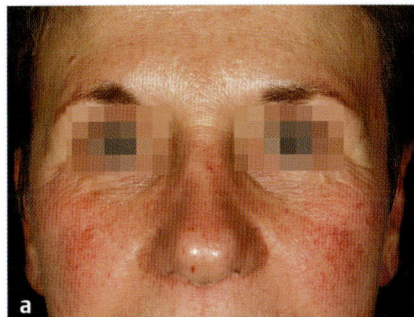
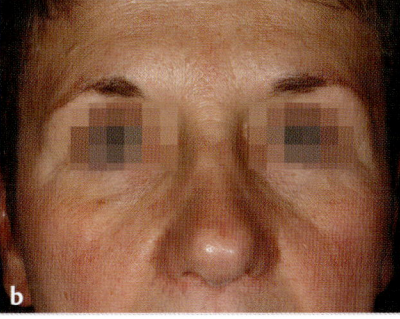

Fig. 8.15 (a) This patient was concerned about the brown spots on her hands. (b) Six months after photorejuvenation. (c) Following facial rejuvenation, she felt that her hands did not parallel her facial presentation. (d) Six months after the last photo rejuvenation session. She underwent fat injections to fill the volume void in her hands. She also underwent IPL skin treatments to improve the skin color.

Fig. 8.16 (a) This patient had severe rosacea across her malar and periorbital region. (b) Six months after five IPL treatments. She has improvement of her rosacea and fine skin wrinkles.

and expressed concerns that her hands did not match her more youthful facial appearance (▶ Fig. 8.15c). She initially received fat injections beneath her hand skin, and during the recovery process of her fat injection, she received five topical photorejuvenation treatments to her hands. Six months after her last photo rejuvenation skin treatment, her hands look more youthful because of an improvement in both contour and skin appearance (▶ Fig. 8.15d).

Photorejuvenation should not be viewed as a primary LAEBT for treating fine skin wrinkling. However, in certain clinical settings, a considerable improvement can be obtained in terms of skin contour where there was a significant amount of hypervascularity within the region of fine wrinkling. The energy provided to reduce the hypervascularity creates an inflammatory process within the dermis that leads to neocollagenesis and skin smoothening. This patient had severe rosacea across her malar and periorbital regions (▶ Fig. 8.16a) Six months after having five IPL treatments without having any neurotoxins injected, she has a smoothening of her skin as well as an improvement of her rosacea and dyschromia (▶ Fig. 8.16b). This gentleman had considerable facial dyschromia and fine skin wrinkling in the periorbital region (▶ Fig. 8.17a-d). The brown/yellow hyperpigmentation masked the underlying hypervascularity. One year after five IPL treatments and no use of neurotoxins, he has improvement of the dyschromia and skin contour.

Use of Light- and Energy-Based Therapies with Cosmetic Surgery

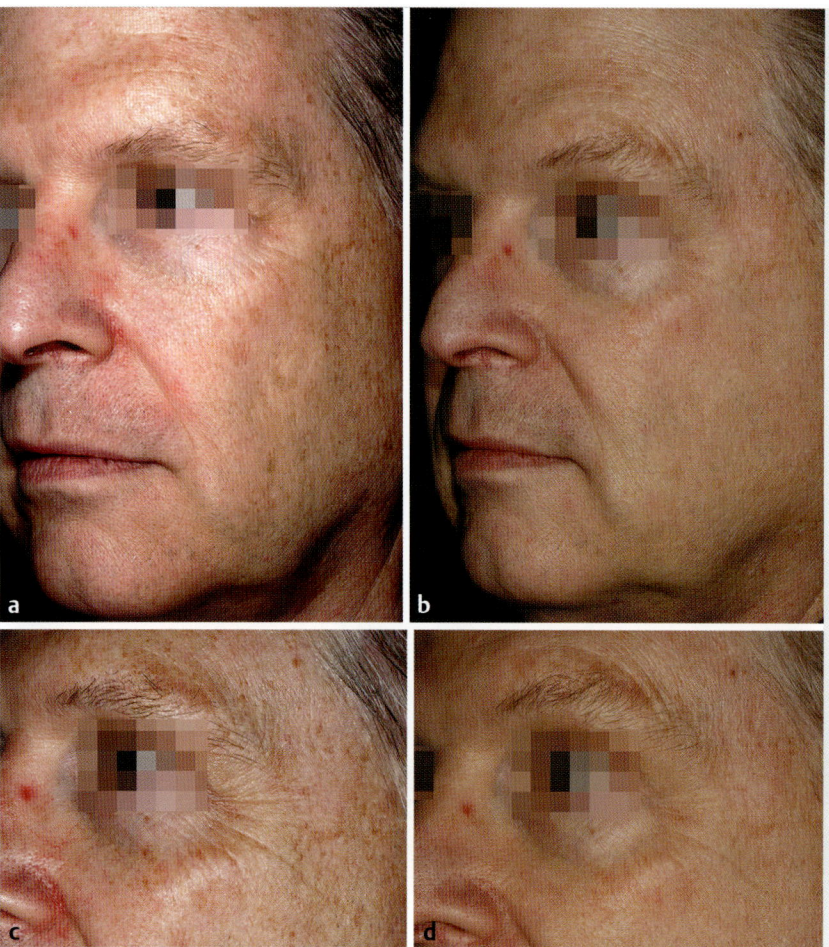

Fig. 8.17 (a) This gentleman had considerable facial dyschromia and fine skin wrinkling in the periorbital region. (b) One year after having five IPL treatments (c) Pretreatment closeup of the periorbital region (d) One year after having five IPL treatments.

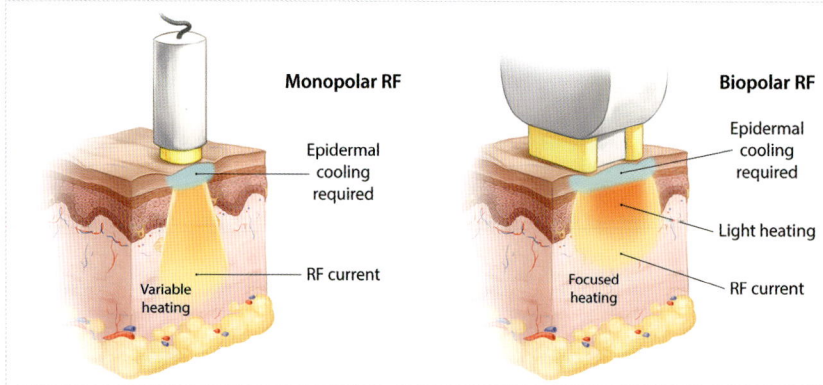

Fig. 8.18 Monopolar and bipolar radiofrequency (RF) devices delivering RF energy to the dermis. Each device needs to have epidermal cooling. The monopolar handpiece needs to have a grounding pad. The bipolar device has light energy that comes from the central crystal, which actually touches the skin, allowing the physician to adjust the depth of the RF current. The heating pattern from the monopolar device is variable in terms of dermal penetration. Monopolar RF energy requires an energy exit portal placed elsewhere on the skin, similar to an electrocautery device. A bipolar device does not require this.

8.4.4 Nonablative Radiofrequency

In the early 2000s, manufacturers responded to patients' desire to receive skin tightening without surgical intervention or ablative treatment. Delivery of transcutaneous, RF energy provided an option that fit these patients' desires. The goal of this technology was to deliver energy beneath the skin surface to create neocollagenesis.[13,14] The RF energy delivered to the skin travels from one electrode to the other, raising the temperature of the dermis beneath the active electrode (▶ Fig. 8.18). The subsequent inflammatory process stimulates new collagen formation within the dermis, which improves skin texture.

Unless RF energy is directed to the epidermis, it is blind to a patient's Fitzpatrick skin color typing and can be used on all skin color types without the need for pretreatment or posttreatment skin bleaching creams. Various delivery systems are available and range from monopolar to bipolar devices. Treatment end points are based on manufacturers' recommendations, which are based partially on posttreatment skin color and the patient's response to each treatment. Typical facial

Use of Light- and Energy-Based Therapies with Cosmetic Surgery

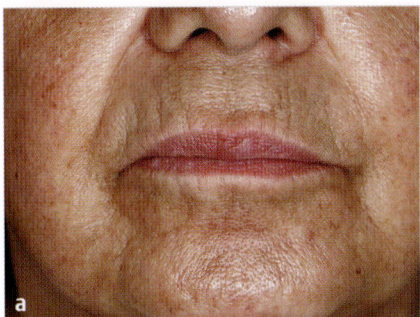
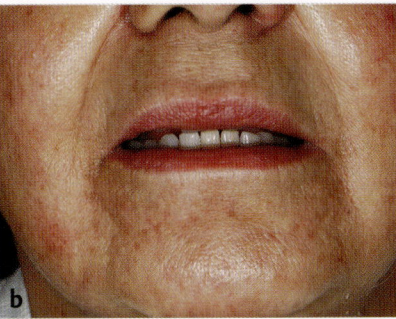

Fig. 8.19 (a) Prior to treatment, this patient was concerned about her perioral wrinkles. (b) After eight perioral bipolar RF treatments.

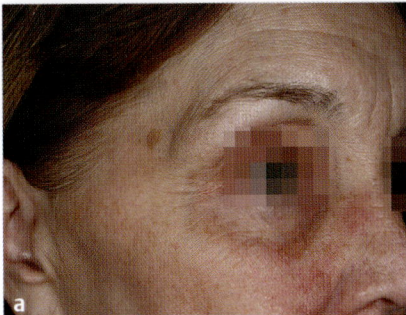
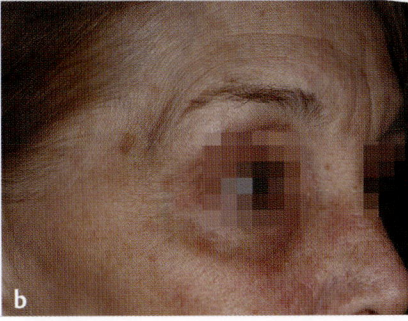

Fig. 8.20 (a) This woman wanted improvement in the wrinkles around her eyes and forehead. (b) Six months after three full-face RF treatments with the Polaris device, she had improvement in the periorbital wrinkles. However, her forehead lines did not show much improvement.

recovery includes mild to moderate swelling for 1 to 3 days and transient skin redness for less than 24 hours, depending on the device settings and energy delivered. In general, such a recovery is needed to provide improvement in skin contour. In my experience, whereas lower energy settings require only topical anesthesia, higher settings often require regional nerve blocks to obtain good clinical results and to provide optimal patient comfort. A series of treatments, often between three and five treatments, are required. Although there is no predictable correlation, the more treatments provided, the better the clinical results. Plastic protective eye goggles must be worn during treatment. Due to the reflection of energy, device settings may need to be reduced over bony regions such as the forehead and malar/zygomatic arch. When treating the perioral region, it is prudent to insert a protective barrier between the mucosa of the lips and the underlying teeth. The ideal patient is younger and is not looking to have this technology parallel the result of a facelift or ablative therapy, so he or she is not expecting this technology to correct unwanted redness or hyperpigmentation.

Clinical Results

The device used to obtain the following results has a bipolar RF delivery handpiece. (Polaris, Syneron). It also provides laser energy, 900 nm, which helps focus the RF energy. With multiple sessions, the laser energy can make slight improvements in hyperpigmentation. This woman received a rhytidectomy. She was still concerned about her perioral wrinkles (▶ Fig. 8.19) Wrinkle improvement could have been obtained using ablative technology or a chemical peel. However, she was concerned about the potential of hypopigmentation and possible lines of demarcation. She received eight perioral, bipolar RF treatments to her perioral region. Six months after her last treatment, she has an improvement in her wrinkles and there is no line of treatment demarcation.

This woman had deep forehead wrinkles and fine lines around her periorbital region (▶ Fig. 8.20a). Six months after three, full-face treatments, she had minimal change in her forehead wrinkles but a good improvement in her periorbital lines (▶ Fig. 8.20b). Six months after eight, full-face RF treatments, this patient had an improvement in skin laxity as demonstrated by VISIA image capture. She also had an improvement in her perioral wrinkles and her cheek skin texture (▶ Fig. 8.21). Although not scientifically corroborated, patients who are relatively younger in age obtain a more consistent skin tightening with the RF treatment technology utilized. This may be related to an improved physiologic response to dermal heating. This VISIA image capture of a woman in her forties shows a significant improvement on the right oblique image, 3 months after having four bipolar RF treatments (▶ Fig. 8.22).

Further improvements in the delivery of RF energy should add to its efficacy in dealing with skin wrinkling. The evolution of RF energy is currently focused on devices that have very small probes/needles that are coated to protect the epidermis. These small needles penetrate the skin, but the coated portion of the probe should protect the epidermis from the energy delivered. Once under the skin, the energy will be distributed in the dermis and hypodermis. This energy will heat the tissue and create neocollagenesis.

8.4.5 Skin Re-pigmentation

Hypopigmentation of the skin can result from many causes (▶ Fig. 8.23) Unsightly scars and hypopigmented spots are undesirable, and many treatments have been used to try to deal with this aesthetic concern. As with many of the LAEBT, the predictability and consistency of results are a concern. No analgesia is needed for this type of therapy. Studies have not yet identified the "ideal" patient for this type of therapy.

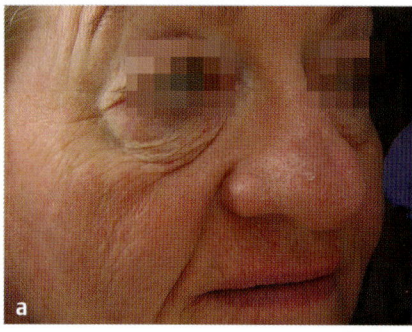 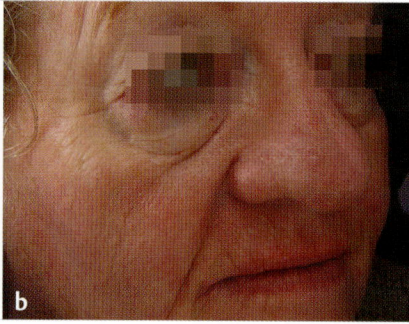

Fig. 8.21 (a) This are side-by-side Canfield VISIA screen shots of a woman in her sixties who did not like the texture of her skin and extra skin. She did not want surgery. (b) Six months after having eight full-face Polaris treatments.

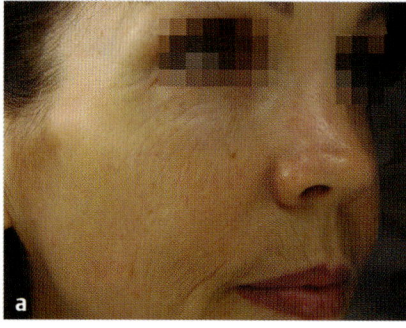 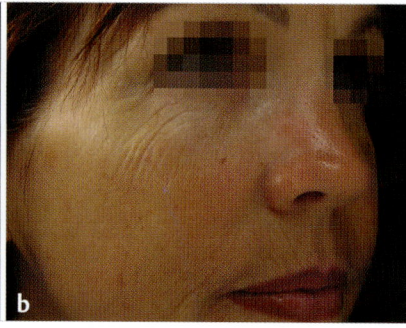

Fig. 8.22 (a) This patient shows improvement in her skin contour at 3 months following four bipolar RF treatments. (b) Pretreatment.

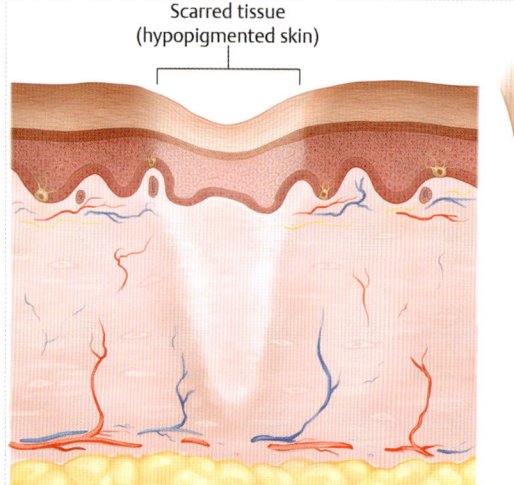 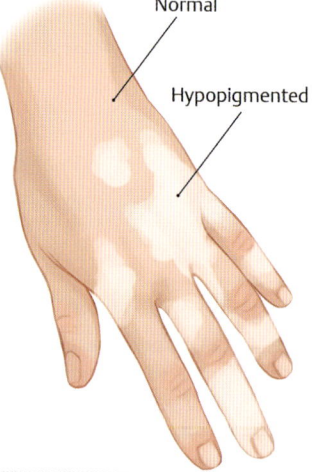 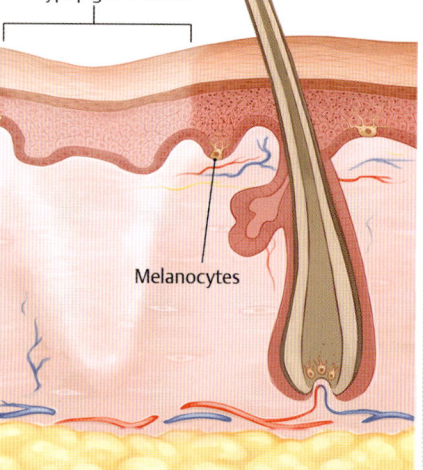

Fig. 8.23 The lack of melanin within the basal layer of the epidermis contributes to hypopigmentation. It can be due to a "scar" or conditions like vitiligo.

I (M.I.K.) have used the ReLume (Lumenis) laser device successfully in treating skin hypopigmentation, and it is FDA approved for such usage. It can be applied to any body location, and treatments with ReLume are not painful. The device produces a narrow-beam, polychromatic, incoherent ultraviolet B (UVB) energy that stimulates melanocytes either in the scar and or the adjacent tissue to produce melanin.

Often the surrounding "normal" skin can become hyperpigmented as a sequel of this therapy, but the hyperpigmentation eventually fades. The initial recovery process is a transient redness (sunburn). Patients need to protect the treated area from sunlight during ongoing therapy. A series of treatments provided one or two times per week, are needed. The length for each treatment depends on the surface area of hypopigmentation. The exact number of treatments to repigment the skin is not predictable due to patient expectations, skin response, and initial color discrepancy. Following the initial series of treatments, improvement in skin color match can be obtained. It is expected that the preliminary skin color improvement will fade and another series of treatments will be required. The longevity of the improvement depends upon the lasting deposition of melanin within the hypopigmented region.

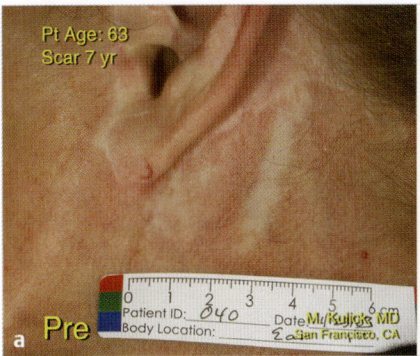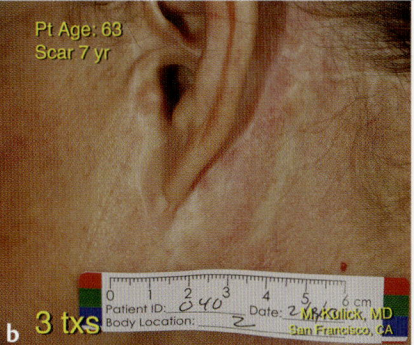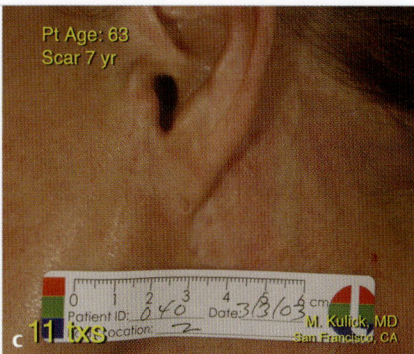

Fig. 8.24 (a) This patient had a previous facelift but did not like her residual hypopigmented scarring. (b) After three ReLume treatments. (c) After 11 treatments.

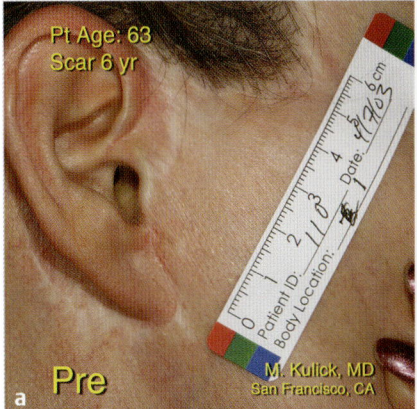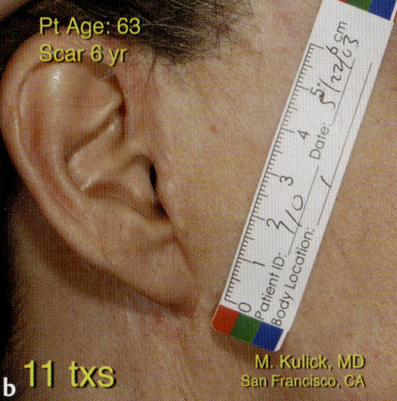

Fig. 8.25 (a) Scarring after facelift 6 years earlier. (b) After 11 ReLume® treatments.

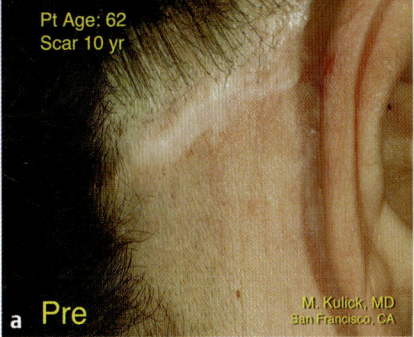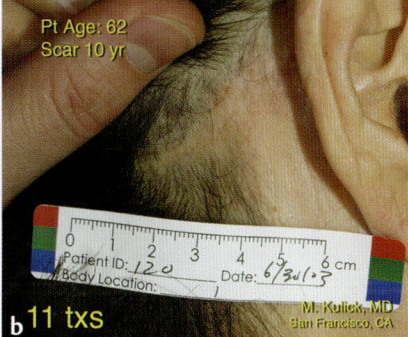

Fig. 8.26 (a) This patient exhibited a wide band of hypopigmentation following a facelift 10 years earlier. (b) After 11 ReLume treatments.

Clinical Results

Seven years prior to ReLume treatment, this woman had a previous facelift by another physician and did not like her residual hypopigmented scarring (▶ Fig. 8.24). After three treatments, she has some improvement in the color of the scars. Her scar color is much better after seven treatments. After 11 treatments, she has a significant improvement in the color of her facial scars.

Another example of an improvement in facial scar color is shown in this patient. The scars were a result from a facelift 6 years prior to her ReLume treatments (▶ Fig. 8.25). Prior to treatment, she had hypopigmented scars. After 11 treatments, it is hard to see where the undesirable scars existed.

Some of the best results are obtained when treating the scars in the retroauricular region. This may be due to the impact of this therapy on the pilosebaceous units within this region. Prior to treatment, this patient had a wide band of hypopigmentation within her hairline following a facelift 10 years prior (▶ Fig. 8.26). After 11 treatments, she had a significant improvement in the color of her scar.

The following examples demonstrate the efficacy of this technology on nonfacial regions. This woman did not like the hypopigmented spots on her chest (▶ Fig. 8.27). After seven treatments, she has improvement in the color of these hypopigmented spots. This patient did not like the "slash marks" on her forearm (▶ Fig. 8.28). After nine treatments, it is hard to see these regions of hypopigmentation.

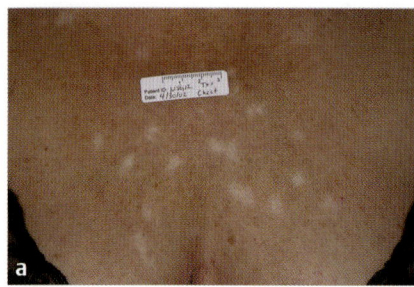 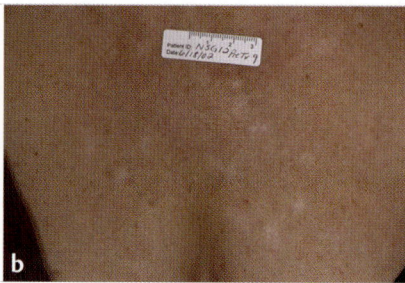

Fig. 8.27 (a) This patient did not like the hypopigmented spots on her chest. (b) After seven ReLume treatments.

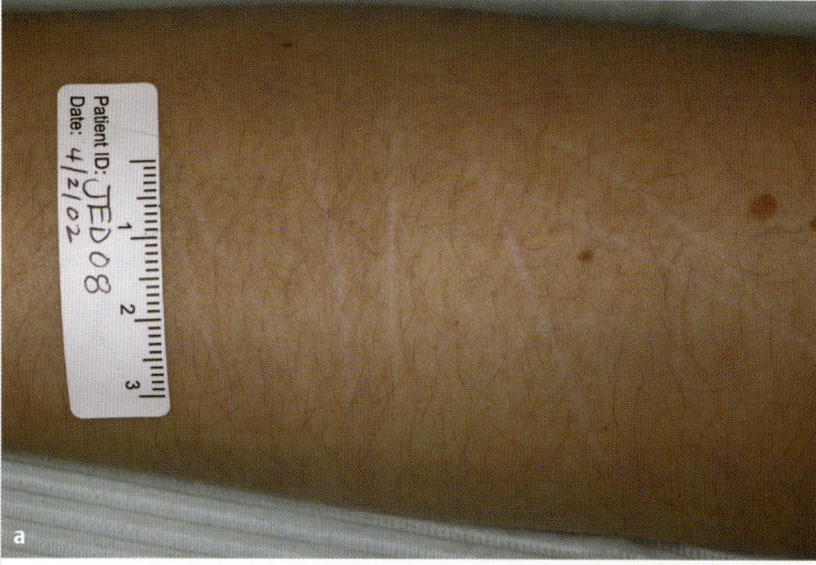
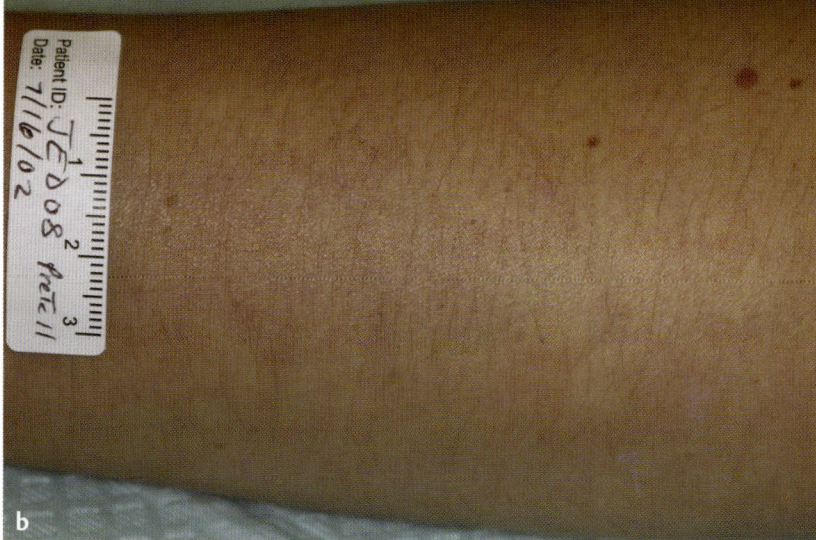

Fig. 8.28 (a) This patient did not like the slashlike marks on her arm. (b) After nine ReLume treatments.

The treatment of hypo-pigmented skin is a significant adjunct to one's practice. Regardless of the cause of the hypopigmentation, making hypopigmented regions less visible contributes to a patient's aesthetic improvement.

8.5 Posttreatment Protocol

Recommendations for aftercare are predicated on the therapeutic impact of the LAEBT on the skin. Therefore, there is no single protocol that is best among the various modalities available. Ablative devices require a greater focus on initial skin healing, because the expected dermal injury requires greater attention to wound healing. The analogy would be the treatment provided to a patient that had a second-degree burn. After the epithelial layer is intact, posttreatment redness can be concealed with topical cosmeceuticals containing a yellow or green base until the recovered redness/pink skin color is no longer a concern. Skin moisturizers are helpful to deal with the expected dryness after treatment. Photorejuvenation devices that impact the epidermis but do not damage the dermis require patient counseling regarding the exfoliation process. This would include a focus on skin care that aids with the removal of the undersirable hyperpigmentation. In contrast, devices that do not injure the epidermis have posttreatment protocols that focus on the initial posttreatment skin redness and edema. Regardless of the modality used, proper skin hygiene, pain management, and the use of topical sunblock and skin-bleaching creams for darker skin types are important factors to incorporate in the posttreatment protocol.

Manufacturers and physician researchers are continually working to improve delivery systems and investigating new energy sources to improve the appearance of the skin. Clinicians and their patients will benefit from this concerted effort.

8.6 Complications and Shortcomings

When treatments are performed correctly, complications are very limited. The informed consent should outline such potential problems that can result from LAEBT treatments. In general, the more ablative the LAEBT device is, the greater the potential for complications. The cause of most of the unwanted outcomes falls into the following categories.

8.6.1 Patient Expectations and Operator Experience

When reviewing patient opinion forums, the most frequent complaint is that patients do not feel that their pretreatment anticipated results were actualized. This can be minimized by not overpromoting the LAEBT therapeutic potential. Currently, photorejuvenation provides the most predictable result of all the modalities described. There is no other peer-reviewed method that can provide a simultaneous reduction in unwanted red, brown color and improve skin contour that lasts for more than 6 months without other therapeutic intervention. Using current RF devices on the forehead and zygomatic arch area often requires a reduction in the energy delivered. An overlap of the second pulse should be avoided, because the skin temperature rise from the initial pulse would make the underlying skin susceptible to a burn. Regardless of the energy source, the potential need for multiple treatments to obtain the patient's desired goal should be confirmed prior to his or her first session. The clinician performing the treatments must understand how to optimize the LAEBT's parameters while maintaining patient safety as the top priority. Attendance at continuing medical education courses provides clinicians with helpful information to optimize patient results.

8.6.2 Device Maintenance

Many devices have handpieces that have a limited lifespan. A new handpiece may provide energy that could have a different impact on the skin surface than the one replaced. Conversely, the energy output from a device may deteriorate with time, resulting in suboptimal energy transfer. Having one's device routinely serviced can mitigate this type of problem.

8.6.3 Creative License

As an operator becomes proficient with a particular device, it provides a comfort zone where the LAEBT may be used beyond the manufacturer's recommendations. Such creativity needs to be balanced with keeping patient safety as the top priority as well as understanding that results obtained on facial skin are based on the blood supply and dermal thickness, which are different when treating nonfacial areas. Simultaneous application of any form of energy to skin that has been surgically treated requires a great deal of experience to avoid complications.

8.6.4 Patient Compliance

All LAEBTs require a pretreatment and posttreatment protocol that the patient should follow, which is customized to the condition at hand and device used. It is important to provide patients with such a template that is reviewed at the pretreatment office visit when the informed consent is signed. Contacting the patient after his or her initial treatment can reinforce these instructions and provide the clinician feedback regarding the patient's recovery. Documentation of this interaction in the patient's medical record is also important.

8.7 Commentary

Julius W. Few Jr.

The authors present a very succinct and effective argument for using multiple forms of light-based energy to address a mixed clinical issue, and this is a first in comprehensive print form. The ability to combine IPL with both ablative and nonablative laser resurfacing is a powerful concept, one that we have also applied to address both superficial and deep dermal–epidermal issues. With such an application, one can apply ablative laser resurfacing to address age-related change while simultaneously address both pre-existing and secondary telangiectasia/redness.

Another major consideration presented is the concept of IPL use in patients of diverse skin pigmentation, which is something that can be fraught with complications if it is not approached carefully and thoughtfully. With the outstanding recommendations presented here, we strongly agree with the authors support of test spot application in skin types and/or presentations that traditionally have higher risk, such as those individuals with darker skin and/or non-Caucasian skin.

The importance of looking at the entire patient history cannot be overstated, and we agree with the warnings presented for treating patients with a history of past connective tissue disorders and related autoimmune conditions that potentially complicate healing after laser and energy treatment.

References

[1] Hernández-Barrera R, Torres-Alvarez B, Castanedo-Cazares JP, Oros-Ovalle C, Moncada B. Solar elastosis and presence of mast cells as key features in the pathogenesis of melasma. Clin Exp Dermatol. 2008; 33(3):305–308

[2] Longo C, Casari A, Beretti F, Cesinaro AM, Pellacani G. Skin aging: in vivo microscopic assessment of epidermal and dermal changes by means of confocal microscopy. J Am Acad Dermatol. 2013; 68(3):e73–e82

[3] Chan NP, Ho SG, Yeung CK, Shek SY, Chan HH. The use of non-ablative fractional resurfacing in Asian acne scar patients. Lasers Surg Med. 2010; 42(10):710–715

[4] Chan NP, Ho SG, Yeung CK, Shek SY, Chan HH. Fractional ablative carbon dioxide laser resurfacing for skin rejuvenation and acne scars in Asians. Lasers Surg Med. 2010; 42(9):615–623

[5] Verdier-Sévrain S, Bonté F, Gilchrest B. Biology of estrogens in skin: implications for skin aging. [Review]. Exp Dermatol. 2006; 15(2):83–94

[6] Fitzpatrick TB. The validity and practicality of sun-reactive skin types I through VI. Arch Dermatol. 1988; 124(6):869–871

[7] Biesman BS. Fractional ablative skin resurfacing: complications. Lasers Surg Med. 2009; 41(3):177–178

[8] Few J. "Facial Aesthetic Surgery in Skin of Color." The Art of Aesthetic Surgery Principles & Techniques. 2nd ed. 2011:88–113

[9] Tierney EP, Hanke CW. Ablative fractionated CO2, laser resurfacing for the neck: prospective study and review of the literature. [Review]. J Drugs Dermatol. 2009; 8(8):723–731

[10] Sadick NS, Malerich SA, Nassar AH, Dorizas AS. Radiofrequency: an update on latest innovations. J Drugs Dermatol. 2014; 13(11):1331–1335

[11] Sadick NS, Nassar AH, Dorizas AS, Alexiades-Armenakas M. Bipolar and multipolar radiofrequency. [Review]. Dermatol Surg. 2014; 40 Suppl 12:S174–S179

[12] Larouche D, Kim DH, Ratté G, Beaumont C, Germain L. Effect of intense pulsed light treatment on human skin in vitro: analysis of immediate effects on dermal papillae and hair follicle stem cells. Br J Dermatol. 2013; 169(4):859–868

[13] Kulick M. Evaluation of a combined laser-radio frequency device (Polaris WR) for the nonablative treatment of facial wrinkles. J Cosmet Laser Ther. 2005; 7(2):87–92

[14] Kulick MI, Gajjar NA. Analysis of histologic and clinical changes associated with Polaris WR treatment of facial wrinkles. Aesthet Surg J. 2007; 27(1):32–46

9 Blending Nonsurgical Treatments with Surgery for Facial Rejuvenation

Lawrence S. Bass, Jason N. Pozner, and Barry E. DiBernardo

Summary

Nonsurgical therapy can be a prelude to cosmetic surgery for patients not yet ready for surgery, either as an adjunct to surgery or after surgery. The goal of using the blending of surgical and nonsurgical treatments is to obtain a more complete correction than what can be achieved through surgery alone.

Keywords: Botox (onabotulinumtoxinA, Allergan, Inc.) injection, chemical peel, hyaluronic acid filler injection, laser hair removal, laser skin resurfacing, microdermabrasion, nonsurgical, facial rejuvenation, nonsurgical skin tightening, photorejuvenation, pulsed light hair removal, surgical

Key Points

- Surgical and nonsurgical approaches are commonly combined in modern-day facial rejuvenation.
- Nonsurgical treatments may precede surgical intervention or be used concomitantly or subsequently for maintenance or additional correction.
- Some nonsurgical techniques address issues that are separate from surgical treatments, such as intense pulsed light (IPL) therapy for age spots and facelifting for laxity.
- Some nonsurgical and surgical techniques represent alternative approaches to treating the same problem, such as microfocused ultrasound and facelifting for laxity, or injectable filler and fat injection for volume loss.
- Nonsurgical techniques and technologies are undergoing rapid development and are taking the lead in the care of the aging face.

9.1 Introduction

Surgical rejuvenation of the face has been the mainstay of therapy for many years, but many nonsurgical options and adjuncts have been introduced recently. Data from the American Society of Plastic Surgeons (ASAPS) collected annually since 1997 have shown the rapid rise of nonsurgical options for facial rejuvenation[1] (▶ Table 9.1). Nonsurgical therapy can be a prelude to cosmetic surgery for patients who are not yet ready for surgery, or it can be an adjunct to surgery or performed after surgery. There are many publications dedicated to nonsurgical therapy. This book is dedicated to the blending of surgical and nonsurgical treatments, so adjuncts to surgery and postsurgical procedures will be discussed in this chapter. The goal of using adjuncts is to obtain a more complete correction than what can be achieved through surgery alone. While surgery performs the bulk of correction in cases of laxity in aging faces, certain areas of the face are notorious for persisting, to the chagrin of surgeons and patients together.

9.2 Adjunctive Treatments During Facial Rejuvenation Surgery

Facial rejuvenation surgery includes brow lifting, eyelidplasty, midface lifting, and facelift. Nonsurgical or minimally invasive procedures may be used alongside these procedures or as a replacement for some of these procedures while in surgery. Postsurgical adjuncts will be discussed in the next section.

9.2.1 Browlifting

In the mid-1990s, the procedures for browlifting underwent a change in many plastic surgeons' practices from coronal or

Table 9.1 ASAPS Top 10 for 2015

Rank	Nonsurgical Procedure	Number of Procedures	Percent Change 2015 vs 2014
1	Botox (onabotulinumtoxinA, Allergan, Inc.) injection	4,267,038	18.9
2	Hyaluronic acid filler injection	2,148,326	26.6
3	Hair removal (laser or pulsed light)	1,136,834	37.2
4	Chemical peel	603,305	24.6
5	Microdermabrasion	557,690	33.7
6	Photorejuvenation (IPL)	483.792	30.3
7	Nonsurgical skin tightening (including Ulthera System [Ulthera, Inc.], Thermage [Solta Medical, Inc.], Pellevé [Cynosure])	471,759	58.2
8	Full-field ablative laser skin resurfacing	326,120	-20.2
9	Sclerotherapy	322,170	2.0
10	Nonsurgical fat reduction (including CoolSculpting [ZELTIQ Aesthetics, Inc.], Vaser Shape [Solta Medical, Inc.], Liposonix [Solta Medical, Inc.])	160,763	18.7

(Data from http://www.surgery.org/sites/default/files/ASAPS-Stats2015.pdf. Accessed February, 2017)

hairline incisions to endoscopic techniques. Recently there has been an aesthetic shift toward a more natural, less elevated brow, and many surgeons have limited their use of browlifts to those patients with very significant brow ptosis. For patients who need just a small amount of brow elevation, the question that now arises is what techniques could be used as an adjunct when other procedures (i.e., facelift) are performed. Several useful options are discussed.

9.2.2 Laser Resurfacing

In addition to creating a fresh epidermal surface and smoothing of the dermal rhytids, laser resurfacing may be used to elicit some brow elevation. This is most likely due to collagen remodeling and new collagen and elastin deposition. Although there has not been a formal study of this phenomenon, the elevation seems to persist and needs further study (▶ Fig. 9.1).

Microfocused Ultrasound

Microfocused ultrasound has had FDA approval for brow elevation since 2010. This procedure is generally used in lieu of surgery for patients who require only a modest improvement in brow elevation or to improve brow symmetry. However, microfocused ultrasound can also be performed in the operating room while the patient is under anesthesia for another surgical procedure for the face, which avoids the discomfort that is often experienced during the treatment as a standalone.

Microfocused ultrasound has the ability to focus on different areas of the brow that may not be successfully elevated by the particular brow procedure being utilized by the surgeon. This provides more complete correction or can amplify the correction applied to brow ptosis or brow asymmetry, which is currently not completely addressed by any procedure.

Fillers and Fat Grafting

Filling of the upper periocular area or brow with fillers or fat may be used to elevate the eyebrow or fill the brow to give the illusion of an elevated brow. This can easily be performed simultaneously with other facial surgery. Such contouring can also correct hollowing of the upper eyelid sulcus resulting from overresection of orbital fat during previous upper eyelid surgery or caused by aging changes.

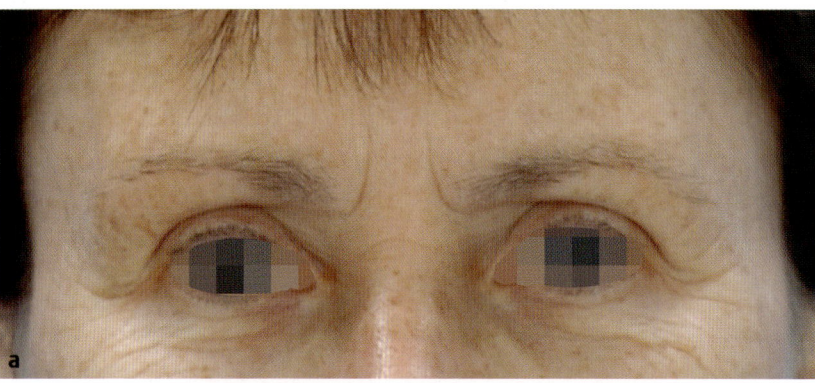

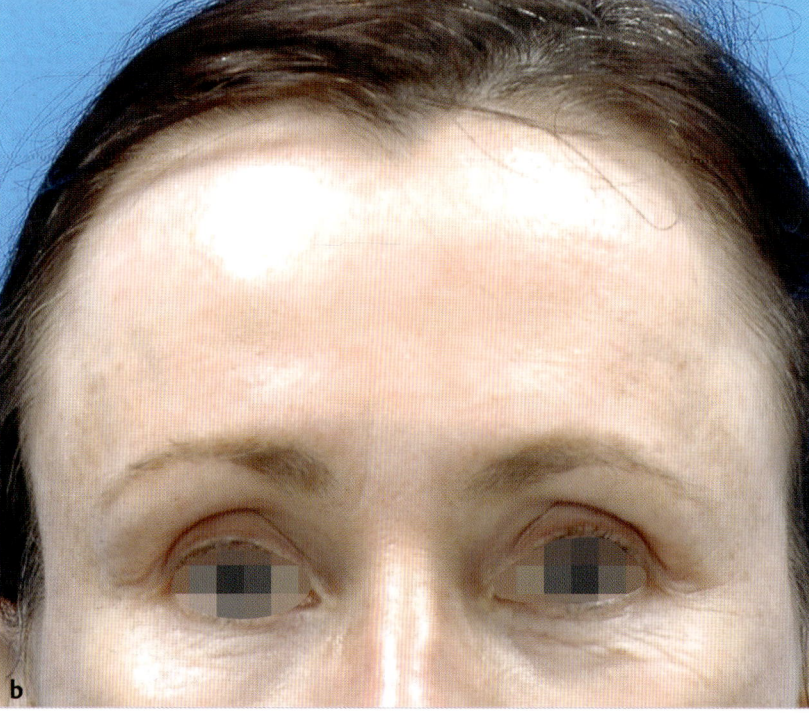

Fig. 9.1 (a) Before and (b) 1 year after full-face laser resurfacing, Note the brow elevation.

Botulinum Toxins

Botulinum toxins can be used to modify the upper face musculature. Conceivably, they may be administered during facial rejuvenation surgery either to provide immediate correction or on the theory that blocking animation during healing improves the "take" of the correction. Although this theory is appealing, there is no meaningful data to support or refute the efficacy of such an approach. We prefer to use botulinum toxins after surgery when the patients can animate, allowing more precise placement and dosing.

Other Tightening or Lifting Devices

Radiofrequency (RF) microneedling has anecdotally proved to be useful for smoothing mild skin laxity (see Chapter 7). Although there is no formal FDA approval at this time, these devices may be used during other facial surgery for brow elevation.

9.2.3 Eyelidplasty

Eyelid surgery is a very common procedure in plastic surgery, with just under 170,000 surgeries being performed by core physicians in the United States in 2015.[1] Trends in eyelid surgery are for a more natural, less operated look. For this reason, current techniques for upper eyelid surgery involve less removal of orbital fat to avoid hollowing. Occasional volume replacement is needed, even in primary cases and especially in older patients.

Lower lid techniques increasingly use the transconjunctival approach, avoiding skin excision or limiting skin excision to a skin-only pinch. This amplifies the need to address skin texture, redundancy, and laxity issues in the lower lid. There are many nonsurgical adjuncts that can be used along with more traditional surgical techniques.[2]

Laser Resurfacing

Laser resurfacing is the mainstay of our nonsurgical facial adjunctive techniques. There are a variety of lasers that may be used for eyelid rejuvenation, but our preference is to use the variable pulse-width erbium laser (Sciton, Inc.) in a nonfractional full-field mode. This laser may be used on the upper and lower eyelids as a replacement for excisional techniques or along with excisional techniques. It is very common in our practices to perform traditional excisional upper lid blepharoplasty with laser resurfacing of the area from the incision line to the inferior portion of the eyebrow. This achieves additional elevation and correction of some skin laxity (▶ Fig. 9.2).

A widespread approach for lower eyelid rejuvenation is laser resurfacing.[3] This is often combined with transconjunctival fat removal and with a skin pinch for those cases with marked skin excess. Skin muscle flaps or subcutaneous lower blepharoplasties should not be resurfaced simultaneously to avoid skin necrosis and an increased risk of lid retraction. Aside from surgical interventions, multiple nonsurgical modalities are available to rejuvenate periocular skin. Microfocused ultrasound has a role in the periocular area, but it cannot be used within the confines of the orbit itself for fear of damaging the globe.[4]

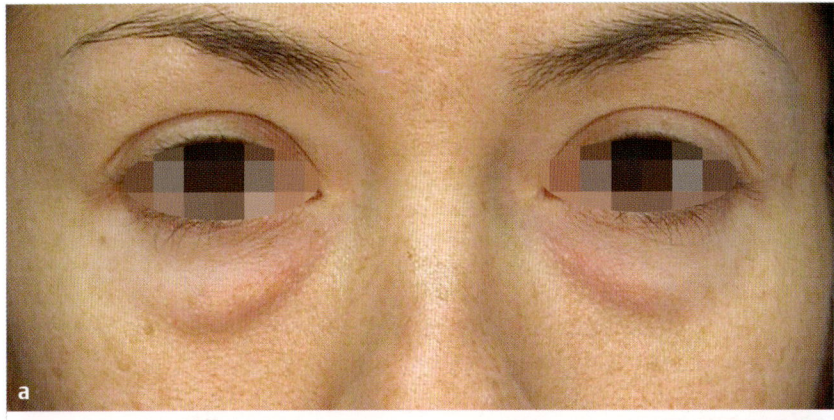

Fig. 9.2 (a) Before and (b) 13 years after tranconjunctival blepharoplasty and laser resurfacing.

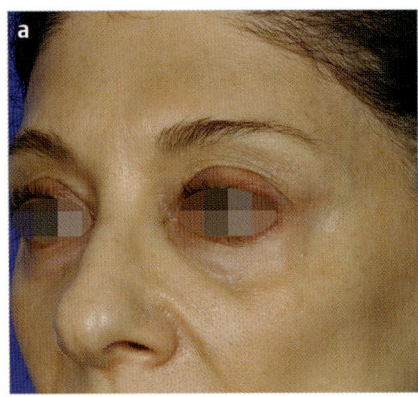 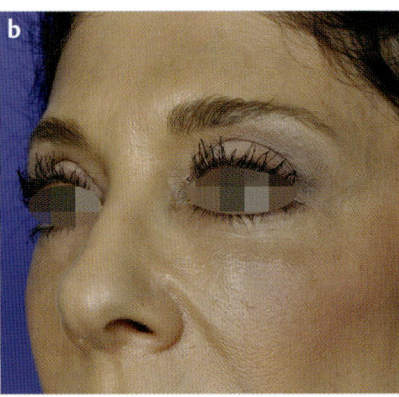

Fig. 9.3 (a) Before and (b) after nanofat injections.

Fat Grafting and Fillers

It is very common to fat graft the periocular area during other facial surgery. Lateral brow filling or tear trough filling with minimal fat aliquots is considered a standard procedure at this time. The use of nonfat fillers, such as hyaluronic acids in the periocular area, is possible but probably better off performed postoperatively for increased accuracy. Controversy exists over the best techniques for fat harvest, processing, and grafting. Micrograft processing or harvesting techniques (sometimes called nanofat grafting), those designed to produce very small graft particles, are more likely to be employed when grafting in the periocular area. Whether this improves the percent of graft take or reduces the risk of visible nodules in this treacherous area is unknown at this time[5](▶ Fig. 9.3).

Botulinum Toxins

Botulinum toxins (Botox, OnabotulinumtoxinA, Allergan; Dysport, abobotulinumtoxinA, Balderma Laboratories LP; Xeomin, incobotulinumtoxinA, Mert North America, Inc.) are routinely used in the periocular area, but most plastic surgeons would perform these injections either as a precursor or after surgery. There is no advantage to using botulinum toxins during a facial surgical procedure. There is a theoretical advantage to having an area resurfaced for rhytides in an adynamic state during healing to provide the best result, although substantiating evidence for this benefit is lacking.

9.2.4 Midface

Surgical options for the midface are lifting or volumizing with the use of implants. Endoscopic or open midface lifting techniques were very common in the past, but they have fallen out of favor with the increased use of fat grafting. This is true for several reasons:

1. Endoscopic and midface techniques were typically used in younger patients with mild laxity or shape change (flattening) in the midface area.
2. For mild laxity, volume addition with fat grafting or fillers can restore shape, and such re-expansion of the soft tissue space greatly reduces or eliminates mild laxity of the skin envelope in this area.
3. The recovery time and risk associated with fat grafting is substantially less than that associated with midface lifting and with endoscopic facelift, both of which were also notorious for undercorrection or incomplete correction deficiencies despite the significant recovery.
4. Patient perceptions of the relative degree of invasiveness of fat grafting compared to mini-facelift variants may also be driving the end results in procedure selection.

Cheek implants have also been supplanted largely in recent times with fat grafting or off-the-shelf filler injections. Cheek implants can create a larger and certainly more-defined shape than fat grafting or lifting procedures. A role for these treatments remains, particularly in the patient who desires a durable result.

Suture Lifts

The use of barbed sutures to lift the cheeks was a common procedure a few years ago as an alternative procedure for facial rejuvenation, but some surgeons used them during facelift as an adjunct to elevate the midface. Now, however, the use of permanent barbed sutures for midface lifting has been pretty much abandoned. Recently, a new absorbable suture with cones was introduced for facial lifting (Silhouette Instalift, Sinclair Pharma plc). This procedure is intended for those patients who are not yet ready for a more extensive facial lifting procedure or for those patients who are not considered to be good candidates for surgery (**see Videos 2.6, 2.7, 2.8 and 2.9**). The absorbable barbed threads last approximately 2 years but also cause some filling of the area due to a stimulation of tissue growth. These sutures could conceivably be used as an adjunct to facelift to achieve more midface elevation or for the SMAS/platysma tissues to more evenly distribute the tension along the suspension.

Fat Grafting and Fillers

Fat grafting is now considered a routine option during surgical facial rejuvenation for many plastic surgeons. The midface is the area most suitable for facial volume restoration, and we routinely perform fat grafting during facelifts in patients who manifest moderate or severe volume depletion. As previously mentioned, many plastic surgeons have abandoned the use of cheek implants or midface lifting techniques in favor of fat grafting.

Specific features that can be modified include projection of the malar eminence, inferomedial cheek curvature, and submalar hollowing. Additional fill in the prejowl sulcus, nasolabial folds, marionette lines, and temples are also commonly employed. The use of nonfat fillers, as with the periocular area, may be used during the facelift but probably is more accurate and easier after healing occurs.

Laser Resurfacing

Laser resurfacing during facelift surgery is routinely employed. This serves as a way to improve the quality of the aging skin that redraping alone is unable to accomplish, bringing the patient to a more complete correction. Skin surface features like rhytides, solar lentigines, and assorted pigmentary and textural issues can be addressed, while initiating a protracted period of increased collagen synthesis in the skin. The resulting skin, which looks and biologically acts more like youthful skin, is an important component of meaningful facial rejuvenation.

When laser resurfacing is undertaken during facelift alone, central areas of the face such as the forehead, glabella, and periorbital and perioral regions may be resurfaced in a fashion similar to that used as standalone procedures. Full-face laser resurfacing during facelifting allows the entire block of facial skin to be addressed in one step. However, significant modifications in technique are required over the undermined flaps to allow full-face laser resurfacing to be performed concomitantly with facelift.[6,7] Full-field resurfacing using a variable pulse Erbium:YAG laser (Sciton, Inc.) with limited fluences over the medial nonundermined cheek and use of the profractional (fractional erbium) component with very superficial settings over the undermined flap, minimizes risks of flap necrosis and healing delay (see Product Index (p. 176)). Resurfacing may be delayed until after the facelift heals to allow a much more aggressive resurfacing to be performed. This approach will be discussed in the Postoperative Care, Complications, and Shortcomings section (p. 102).

9.2.5 Perioral Area

This is an area routinely rejuvenated with complementary techniques during facial surgery. The problems are usually loss of volume with or without skin laxity or wrinkling issues.

Fat Grafting and Fillers

Fat grafting to the perioral area is a routine part of facial rejuvenation surgery. The lips and marionette lines are routinely fat grafted if indicated. A state-of-the-art facelift is capable of creating mild improvement in these features but will never produce complete correction without unwanted facial distortion. An additional technique must be employed to obtain optimum correction. As in the other areas, the use of nonfat fillers to the perioral area is possible but easier if done preoperatively or postoperatively.

Laser Resurfacing and Chemical Peels

The use of laser resurfacing of the periocular area is routine during facelift. As with the other areas, the variable pulse erbium laser (Sciton, Inc.) is used in the periocular area and there are no changes in technique or fluences for laser resurfacing performed prior, during, or after facelift. Certainly, a single recovery period has advantages for the patient if procedures are performed concurrently. Safety precautions must be taken to avoid combustion of supplemental oxygen in this area. If no closed airway is present, oxygen should be discontinued several minutes before laser exposure. For endotracheal tubes or laryngeal mask airways, additional shielding must be employed unless the tube is specifically designated as a laser-safe tube.

Similarly, deep chemical peels (or light) may be used in the perioral area during facelift. The debate over the relative merits of laser resurfacing versus chemical peeling has gone on for the past two decades and is beyond the scope of this chapter. Ideally, surgeons select the technique that works best in their hands based on their training and experience. Compared to laser resurfacing, chemical peeling results are more heavily dependent on the skill and experience of the provider (▶ Fig. 9.4).

9.2.6 Neck

There are a number of aging changes present in the neck that are not well addressed by surgical skin redraping but are increasingly treatable with a variety of nonsurgical, energy-based techniques.

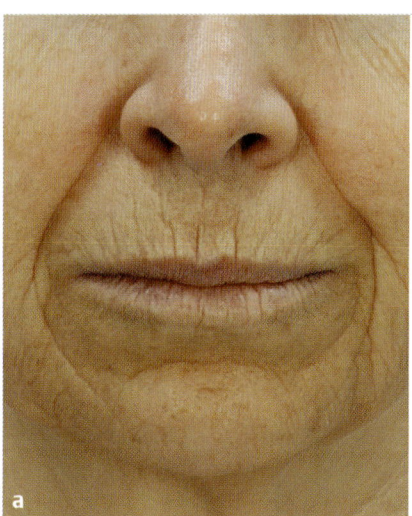
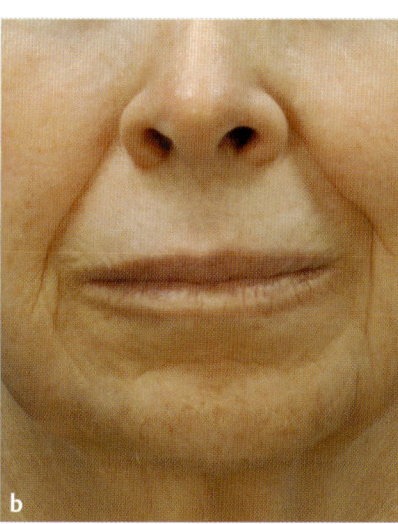

Fig. 9.4 **(a)** Before and **(b)** 6 years after laser resurfacing.

These can be used during surgery in some cases, but neck skin is considerably less forgiving and slower healing than facial skin, having typically 1000-fold fewer adnexal structures, which can act as a reservoir of healing cells for epithelialization.

The risk of scarring with more aggressive energy treatments in the neck requires the surgeon to tread cautiously in undermined areas or defer energy treatments altogether until after the surgery is well healed. Crepiness, and transverse neck rhytids typically seen inferior to the level of the thyroid cartilage, are two features that are being increasingly treated before, during, or after facelift. Patients having facial procedures, such as eyelidplasty, browlift, facial laser resurfacing, or facial fat grafting, may have mild neck skin laxity that is not yet extensive enough to warrant surgical lifting but can be addressed with a nonsurgical lifting device. In facelift patients, mild skin laxity in the lower neck skin that may not be adequately addressed by the surgery, can be treated at the time of facelift or afterward. The common and frustrating recurrence of mild visible laxity at the cervicomental angle in the first year or two after facelift can be treated with a nonsurgical lifting device in lieu of revision surgery in some patients.

Nonsurgical Laxity Reduction and Lifting

What is commonly referred to as skin "tightening" (a term for which the FDA has not found a meaningful definition) really relates to the ability to nonsurgically reduce visible skin laxity or redundancy. As of this writing, microfocused ultrasound (Ulthera System, Ulthera, Inc.) is the only technology that has specific FDA clearance to lift the skin of the neck and under the chin noninvasively (see Product Index (p. 185)). Various other technologies are being used off-label to produce tissue coagulation and collagen deposition during healing to create similar effects. Technologies approach this "outside-in" through transcutaneous energy application or "inside-out" with energy delivered subcutaneously through a fiber, needle, or probe (**see Video 2.11**).

Outside-In

There are many devices that are marketed for transcutaneous neck tightening including RF, lasers (Nd:YAG), and pulsed-light devices that provide full-field exposure through multiple treatments, with little to no discomfort, making them easy to perform before or after facial surgery. Microfocused ultrasound and RF microneedling are the two device classes that could be used while the patient undergoes other facial surgery, both of which create discreet (fractionated) thermal zones in the dermis, making them safe enough to perform on skin adjacent to undermined skin with typical parameters.

Microfocused Ultrasound

As mentioned earlier in this chapter, microfocused ultrasound is first used to map skin thickness and then to place discreet thermal zones in or under the dermis. The significant discomfort of the procedure leads some patients to elect treatment with this device while undergoing other facial surgery. Microfocused ultrasound is safe and efficient to combine with other facial surgery but it must not be performed in the undermined skin flaps. Modest additional skin tightening can be produced in the neck if this is not part of the surgical field, and this can be combined with fractionated resurfacing for more complete rejuvenation of the neck skin.[8,9]

Radiofrequency Microneedling

RF microneedling devices are further classified into insulated needles, which only allow energy to the discreet thermal coagulation zone at the tip, and noninsulated needles, which allow energy throughout the exposed needle. The authors prefer the insulated needles for precision of the depth of thermal zone placement. Most patients receive a series of three RF microneedling treatments, and we see no problem with incorporating one of these into a surgical plan. In fact, it is common to use these devices on the face or other body area when other nonfacial surgical procedures are performed.

Inside-Out

Other technologies apply energy under the skin to create tissue coagulation and collagen deposition/remodeling during healing. Historical approaches applying laser energy to the underside of undermined skin flaps in the face or neck produced an unacceptable risk of complications. Current approaches involve the deposition of energy beneath nonundermined skin, sometimes to be followed by liposuction of the area. Although controversial, there is a growing body of evidence that laser liposuction (e.g. Smartlipo, Cynosure, Inc.) can amplify skin laxity reduction compared with liposuction alone.[10] In patients with early skin laxity who are having midfacial or eyelid procedures performed, the early neck changes can be addressed with laser liposuction.

Separate from any removal of fat, the neck skin can be treated with a subcutaneously delivered exposure to RF energy (Thermi products, ThermiGen, LLC) (see Product Index (p. 195)). An insulated needle is passed back and forth under the skin, with concomitant monitoring of the tissue temperatures produced in proximity to the needle combined with skin-surface-temperature optical monitoring. This feedback monitoring insures that the target temperature believed to be adequate to achieve a result is obtained and maintained for an adequate interval, and it safeguards against overexposure or temperature excess, which could create complications including burns.

Laser Resurfacing

Laser resurfacing should be performed with caution, if at all, on undermined neck tissue. On nonundermined tissue, a very superficial full-field fractional or hybrid fractional laser procedure may be performed to achieve texture and pigment blending but not to aggressively reduce neck rhytides. Overaggressive treatments can lead to tissue necrosis, protracted healing, erythema, or hypertrophic scarring (▶ Fig. 9.5).

Botulinum Toxins

Use for platysmal bands is not recommended in asleep or IV-sedation patients, because contraction of the neck musculature is important for accuracy of placement (**see Video 2.3**).

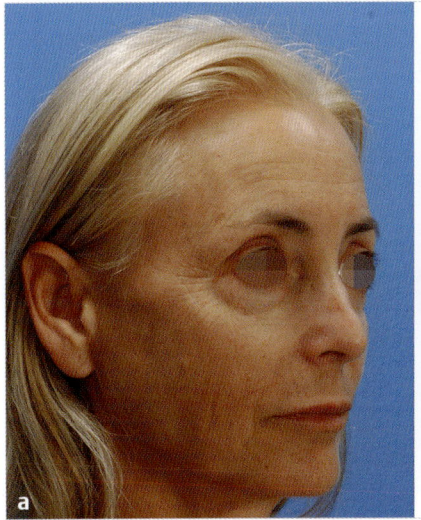 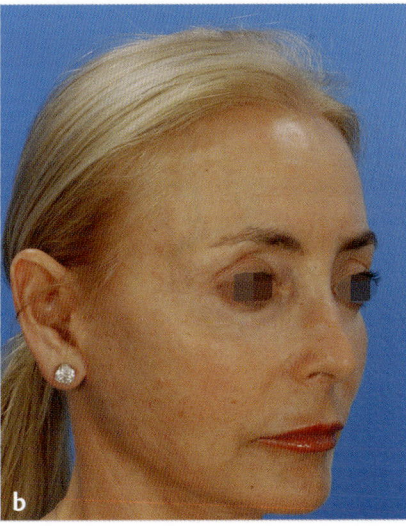

Fig. 9.5 (a) Before and (b) 1 year after facelift, fat grafting, and laser resurfacing.

9.3 Adjuncts After Facial Rejuvenation Surgery

Patients often have difficulty understanding why the facelift does not "fix" everything, eliminating the need for botulinum toxin, filler, and laser treatments. Education regarding the multifactorial nature of facial aging, and the focused specific improvements resulting from each type of treatment, helps patient decision-making, producing a more complete rejuvenation and higher patient satisfaction. These are often essential steps to complete the rejuvenation and to help maintain it.

In this section, we will address the procedures for the full face rather than separating the face by areas, because there is limited to no difference in technique when these procedures are performed after a healed surgical procedure. The strategy, more than the technique, is what is unique to this time point. Our approach to decision-making and treatment program planning in the early and late postoperative periods will be detailed.

9.3.1 Laser Resurfacing and Chemical Peel

Facelift repositions the skin but leaves the same photodamaged, elastotic skin that was present before the procedure. Laser treatments are essential to create the best appearance of the skin and to induce the skin to behave like younger, more metabolically active skin. A significant resurfacing, followed by a series of maintenance treatments in the following years, is reasonably efficient from financial and downtime perspectives. Some patients with limited photodamage may be treated well with fractional or hybrid treatments, but most patients with enough aging changes to require a facelift will be better served by an initial full-field resurfacing. The depth of an initial resurfacing will vary depending on the severity of rhytides and the patient's available downtime.

When resurfacing is going to be performed as a standalone procedure, 6 weeks postfacelift is a safe interval barring any healing difficulties that would delay the secondary laser treatment. Separating the facelift and laser resurfacing into two staged procedures allows a more complete resurfacing of the face with none of the modifications that are required when the two procedures are performed concomitantly. Also, the facelift scars can be resurfaced at the same time to further blend them. Sometimes, practical considerations, such as no availability of a resurfacing laser in the operating room used for the facelift, dictates separation of the two procedures.

Follow-up maintenance treatments starting 1 or more years later will keep the results fresh. These can be as simple as multiple treatments annually with an intense pulsed light (IPL) source, to annual or biennial fractional nonablative resurfacing, to fractional ablative resurfacing or hybrid resurfacing every few years, depending on the rate of development of rhytides, elastosis, and solar lentigines.

9.3.2 Microfocused Ultrasound and Radiofrequency Microneedling

As previously mentioned, microfocused ultrasound or RF microneedling may be used for facial tightening or lifting after facial surgery. These procedures are often useful for the patient who desires more complete correction of laxity than was achieved with surgery. Conversely, many patients who do not achieve desired tightening/lifting with these devices in lieu of surgery will eventually have a facelift to achieve a better result. This is usually not an early treatment postfacelift but rather a maintenance treatment starting 2 or 3 years after facelift or it is a fix for residual laxity after facelift, typically performed at 6 to 12 months after the procedure (see Chapter 7).

9.3.3 Botulinum Toxins

The use of botulinum toxins in the face postsurgery is very common. It provides softening and/or lifting of specific areas, including many areas that are minimally addressed through surgical lifting. There are many publications outlining the use of botulinum toxins in the brow, for which, further discussion is beyond the scope of this chapter.[11]

9.3.4 Filler Injections

Filler injection has become a mainstay for treatment of early aging changes in the face.[12] The shape changes in the lower lid, nasolabial folds and later marionette lines, prejowl sulcus, and malar areas are well corrected without resorting to surgical intervention. As laxity becomes more visible, filler can be used to reduce laxity, but this only works in the early stages. At some point, laxity becomes great enough, separate from age-related volume loss. The amount of filler needed as a sole treatment would create an unnatural, puffy, or bloated look. Surgical lifting is the appropriate choice if more complete correction is desired by the patient. Neck laxity remains an area where filler plays little to no role in correction, even when performed at an early stage.

When one or two small areas require correction, off-the-shelf filler is usually the best option. When multiple areas or panfacial volumization is required, fat grafting is more cost-effective but requires a trip to the operating room and at least some recovery time. When a trip to the operating room is planned for facelift or any other surgical intervention, fat grafting is the obvious choice if adequate fat stores are available.

Fat is very good at providing large volumes for shape and volume restoration, and it has been speculated to stimulate biological responses in the host tissues that are rejuvenative in other ways that filler is not. However, fat has its limitations. Fat provides a foundation for shape restoration by adding bulk volume, but fine shape is not well provided by fat and the physical properties of the material (softness) and unpredictable percentage of graft survival are further limitations. Volumizing fillers are much better suited to refining shape and fine-tuning the results to a much more perfect and symmetric endpoint. This makes volumizing fillers ideal after facelift or facial fat grafting to complete the correction, refine the shape, and maintain the result. Periodic retreatment over time as the patient continues to age can compensate for changes in fat, ongoing volume loss, and mild recurrent skin laxity. Superficial fillers can address issues for which fat is wholly unsuited, such as any dermal features or surface refinement that may be needed or that remains uncorrected by energy-based surface treatments.

9.4 Postoperative Care, Complications, and Shortcomings

In general, postoperative care is dictated by the surgical procedure and is not modified in a significant way by the addition of nonsurgical treatments. Occasionally, the addition of nonsurgical options may require specific treatment, such as maintenance with ointment or other topical products. However, this may alter the nature of the surgical dressing that can be used. Treatment of the skin surface with lasers may need to be modified to reduce the risk of healing difficulties in undermined or surgically manipulated skin. Protocols for the application of resurfacing lasers at the time of facialplasty mandate the reduction of surface coverage and depth for undermined skin.[6] Increasingly, nonsurgical treatments alone have little or no postoperative care requirements, making them easy to mate with a surgical procedure without modification of typical postoperative care requirements.

Complications associated with combined treatments have not been extensively studied, making it impossible to state with certainty whether there is a significant change in the risk of any specific complication. In general, multitreatment therapy is a daily event in aesthetic practice with customary outcomes and no noticeable increase in complications. There is a general feeling that having more procedures on the face increases the amount of bruising, swelling, and recovery time somewhat, although this has not been quantified in a formal study.

Overall, treatment with multiple concomitant modalities should be considered routine and necessary to obtain the more complete correction that has become the current standard of care. Patients should be counseled realistically about the potential impact of multiple concomitant modalities on recovery time. Performing multiple concomitant procedures generally makes it difficult for the surgeon to focus on the most aggressive treatment with any one modality, perhaps making results slightly more limited than what can be achieved through stand-alone procedures. This needs to be balanced in clinical decision-making against the savings in time, money, recovery, and efficiency gained by completing multiple steps of a rejuvenation plan in one sitting.

9.5 Conclusion

Single-modality approaches provide focused correction to facial aging changes. Because aging occurs in a multifactorial way with myriad manifestations, a combination approach is standard as of this writing to achieve the most complete rejuvenation. The best blend of treatments, which treatments, and when to perform them is an increasingly complex but essential skill for the surgeon, combining an understanding of the capabilities of the various options, and a detailed analysis of the patient's condition and the patient's aesthetic priorities.

9.6 Commentary

Julius W. Few Jr.

We live in a world that has limitless connectivity. With social media outlets like RealSelf and other media outlets, we have seen a relative revolution to the way patients voice their thoughts and desires, even immediately after a given cosmetic procedure. It is more important than ever to have adjuncts to facilitate recovery and address undesirable outcomes. The authors of this chapter have created a dynamic and effective way to address the surgical patient both before and after cosmetic surgery. Many of these applications and strategies have been employed in our clinical setting, and the power is almost limitless.

The versatility of microfocused ultrasound in the operating room setting in nicely illustrated in this chapter, and we have seen its usefulness in the patient who is undergoing periorbital surgery but does not want to have a surgical facelift. We have employed blepharoplasty rejuvenation with microfocused ultrasonic lifting to achieve true synergy. We have also incorporated Ulthera with corset platysmaplasty to achieve a dynamic, robust lift with defined neck tightening, without formal facelifting in the operating room, lending this approach to a treatment algorithm of less than 90 minutes and a 2-day recovery (see Product Index (p. 185)).

Neuromodulators allow the surgeon the opportunity to address early postsurgical asymmetry throughout the face but especially for the brows, as the authors point out. They provide a dynamic approach that can be used both early and late in the postsurgical setting (**see Video 1.1**).

The expansion of fillers, especially hyaluronic acid-based fillers, have allowed for significant enhancement during the intermediate and long-term postoperative visit, making a good result great. This approach can be bundled into the surgical package easily and effectively, with a hyaluronic acid midface volumizer such as Juvéderm Voluma or Restylane Lyft (see Product Index (p. 167) and **Videos 2.1, 2.2 and 2.3**).

I personally credit Dr. Pozner for applying ablative laser resurfacing to the upper eyelid skin at the time of or after upper blepharoplasty, to achieve optimal periorbital rejuvenation without the natural risk of skin overresection in an attempt to smooth the skin.

The ability to incorporate energy-based, tissue-heating options, such as laser lipolysis to unwanted neck fat while performing a facelift, allows for augmented tissue tightening. The authors have also nicely illustrated the power of micro-invasive RF in limiting the extent of a traditional facelift dissection while achieving excellent results.

References

[1] http://www.surgery.org/sites/default/files/ASAPS-Stats2015.pdf
[2] Langelier N, Beleznay K, Woodward J. Rejuvenation of the upper face and periocular region: Combining neuromodulator, facial filler, laser, light and energy-based therapies for optimal results. Dermatol Surg. 2016; 42 Suppl 2:S77–S82
[3] Pozner JN, DiBernardo BE. Laser resurfacing: full field and fractional. Clin Plast Surg. 2016; 43(3):515–525
[4] Pak CS, Lee YK, Jeong JH, Kim JH, Seo JD, Heo CY. Safety and efficacy of ulthera in the rejuvenation of aging lower eyelids: a pivotal clinical trial. Aesthetic Plast Surg. 2014; 38(5):861–868
[5] Buckingham ED. Fat transfer techniques: general concepts. Facial Plast Surg. 2015; 31(1):22–28
[6] Scheuer JF, III, Costa CR, Dauwe PB, Ramanadham SR, Rohrich RJ. Laser resurfacing at the time of rhytidectomy. Plast Reconstr Surg. 2015; 136(1):27–38
[7] Bass LS, Pozner JN. Discussion–Laser Facial Resurfacing. In: Cohen M, Thaller S, eds. The Unfavorable Result in Plastic Surgery. 4th ed. St. Louis, MO: CRC Press; in press
[8] Oni G, Hoxworth R, Teotia S, Brown S, Kenkel JM. Evaluation of a microfocused ultrasound system for improving skin laxity and tightening in the lower face. Aesthet Surg J. 2014; 34(7):1099–1110
[9] Woodward JA, Fabi SG, Alster T, Colón-Acevedo B. Safety and efficacy of combining microfocused ultrasound with fractional CO2 laser resurfacing for lifting and tightening the face and neck. Dermatol Surg. 2014; 40 Suppl 12: S190–S193
[10] DiBernardo BE. Randomized, blinded split abdomen study evaluating skin shrinkage and skin tightening in laser-assisted liposuction versus liposuction control. Aesthet Surg J. 2010; 30(4):593–602
[11] Monheit G. Neurotoxins: current concepts in cosmetic use on the face and neck –upper face (glabella, forehead and crow's feet). Plast Reconstr Surg. 2015; 136(5) Suppl:72S–75S
[12] Bass LS. Injectable filler techniques for facial rejuvenation, volumization and augmentation. Facial Plast Surg Clin North Am. 2015; 23(4):479–488

10 Blending Nonsurgical Treatments with Surgery for Skin Lifting on the Body

Lawrence S. Bass, Barry E. DiBernardo, and Jason N. Pozner

Summary

The aesthetic treatment of body areas poses unique challenges. Surgical lifting procedures such as thigh lifts, buttock lifts, abdominoplasty, brachioplasty, and body contouring after massive weight loss continue to be popular treatments. However, significant downtimes and incidences of complications and unfavorable results make nonsurgical options and minimally invasive options the wave of the future, and nonsurgical corrective options must be blended with surgical corrective options.

Keywords: broadband light (BBL), cellulite, cryolipolysis, intense pulsed light (IPL), microfocused ultrasound, nonablative fractional resurfacing, radiofrequency-assisted liposuction (RFAL), skin excision procedures, skin laxity, striae

> **Key Points**
> - Nonsurgical skin lifting and smoothing has unique biological and commercial challenges compared to comparable facial treatments.
> - Currently, nonsurgical treatments principally address skin surface smoothness, whereas surgical approaches address major skin laxity along with cellulite.
> - Nonsurgical approaches are useful to reduce small amounts of fat or to make small revisions in surgical results.
> - Skin smoothing requires multiple treatments, creating small incremental changes.
> - Pharmacologic and biological approaches hold promise for the future either alone or in combination with energy-based treatments.

10.1 Introduction

Aesthetic treatment of body areas poses unique challenges to the surgeon. After addressing body shape and size with surgical and nonsurgical options for contouring, the skin itself must be addressed. Skin laxity and a variety of issues of skin smoothness need to be treated. Surgical lifting procedures have historically been the only useful options. Thigh lift, buttock lift, abdominoplasty, and brachioplasty have been able to tailor out skin redundancy to a productive degree. While this continues in growing numbers, particularly in body contouring after massive weight loss, the significant downtime associated with the procedures, the significant incidence of complications, and the occasional unsatisfactory aesthetic tradeoffs such as widened scars, put momentum behind the search for alternative approaches. Separate from laxity per se are various issues of skin smoothness such as cellulite, striae, and skin crepiness. They represent specific changes resulting from aging, skin injury, and photodamage, respectively, that represent unique morphologic/anatomic manifestations and pathophysiology.

These differences color the specific treatment approaches needed for each of them. Skin tailoring surgery has not addressed these issues well, nor has classical liposuction. Nonsurgical options and minimally invasive options are the mainstay of treatment currently and for the foreseeable future and must be blended with surgical corrective options.

Significant progress has been made in the past few years developing treatment modalities that consistently and durably create improvement in these unwanted features. Nonetheless, at this writing, the ability to create the degree or completeness of improvement that most patients desire has remained an elusive challenge. The active modern lifestyle places patients in more revealing clothing more often than ever before. This shift has made body skin smoothing much more central to the modern scope of aesthetic medicine.

10.2 Why Is Body Smoothing a Hard and Unsolved Biological Issue?

There are many issues relating to the development of "loose skin" in body areas. The skin itself is undergoing all of the aging changes that have been described for facial areas. The amount, density, integrity, and organization of structural proteins has degraded along with the amount of glycosaminoglycans in the skin. This is due, in part, to the slowing of metabolism and the reduction in vascularity associated with a more aged appearance to the skin, which is more pronounced in body areas than in the face due to the lower baseline turnover/metabolic rate and vascularization. Such changes are exacerbated by controllable factors such as ultraviolet light exposure and smoking.

Skin in the body is exposed to gravitational forces across much larger areas than the face. A complex network of connective tissue fibers supports the skin in place so that it does not sag to the bottom of the trunk or appendage in the direction of the current gravitational pull. Such support undergoes changes in the organizational pattern of the fiber direction, and in vascularity, and it is distorted by the weight- and surface-distorting effects of fat from weight gain and/or loss. The amount of weight in the skin flap and the amount of laxity that can develop is much greater in magnitude than that associated with most aging faces.

Medical treatments that produce modest improvements in skin density or support, which can be clinically useful in the face when cumulated over the area of the face and neck, can be less productive when attempting to treat the body because of the larger magnitude of the changes present and the greater degree of correction needed to achieve desirable aesthetic outcomes. Adding more energy to most treatments simply does not further amplify the biological response obtained, but it does increase the risk and recovery time.

The ability to create fractional wounding over large areas with safety and a reasonable time course of healing has also been challenging. This represents the principal challenge in taking treatments that were developed for the face and adapting them for use on body sites.

10.2.1 Economic Issues

Whereas the treatment for skin smoothing was originally designed for the face and requires the use of a disposable with an additional cost for the provider, there has been an additional economic challenge. The cost of treatment is adapted for coverage of the face and neck areas. Treating larger body areas with the same technology becomes cost prohibitive. Some manufacturers have overcome this by creating a handpiece or disposable that is adapted for body use, but it must be configured in a way that prevents use on the face to avoid cannibalizing the more lucrative facial revenue stream. These kinds of economic challenges have limited the use of some technologies on the body. Other technologies are equally suited to use in a wide variety of anatomic sites or are developed specifically for body site treatment. The size of the applicators used in facial rejuvenation are often so small that treatment times on body sites are lengthy, further adding to the cost and tedium of cross-purposing the device for body treatments (**see Video 2.11**).

10.2.2 Basic Approach of Energy

Energy-based treatments take several approaches, from heating to create a biological expression of various cytokines or some other mechanism of upregulating synthetic or metabolic activity in cells, to cell shock yielding apoptosis, to frank coagulation at one or more defined depths in the skin or subcutaneous tissues.[1] During the healing response that ensues with the latter approach, new collagen is deposited that may change the thickness, biomechanical properties, or relationship of the skin relative to its associated tissues, thereby improving its appearance. This sort of tissue remodeling has some inherent limitations. Most treatments deliver an empirically determined set of energy parameters in the hope of producing a desired tissue temperature/time/spatial distribution profile. To the extent that any individual patient differs from the average in the study group used to validate the technology, the endpoint achieved in practice may vary significantly. This may be further exacerbated by technique differences from provider to provider, and further modulated by patient discomfort tolerance issues.

Some of the more advanced options currently available offer feedback to help ensure that the proper endpoint is attained. Even ensuring that the target tissue effect is perfectly achieved does not guarantee a particular outcome. These techniques, unlike invasive surgery, do not make a major anatomical or mechanical change in patient tissue, but they push the tissue by creating a controlled injury and then rely on the healing response to provide the clinical improvement. The problem is that the tissue response varies widely from individual to individual even among patients who appear to be ideal candidates for treatment. There will always be a proportion of patients that will generate a subclinical response (nonresponders). Efforts to accurately predict which patients will behave in this fashion have so far been unsuccessful, necessitating careful patient counseling and a realistic perspective on the part of providers about the current state of the art and its associated limitations.

Treatments whose endpoint stops short of coagulation seem to produce somewhat less of a response than the more aggressive treatments. However, the mean result and range of results of these two approaches have not been studied in a comparative manner. The degree of improvement may be only modestly different in most patients. A baseline level of energy exposure is necessary to reach the onset of a clinical response. Increasing the exposure beyond this seems to provide only modest improvements in results. Bulk heating or any treatment that produces bulk tissue necrosis is clearly associated with significant recovery time and adverse events, including tissue tethering, distortion of contour, nodules, and induration, which can take months to resolve or leave permanent sequelae. There is a certain sweet spot where improvement is optimized with few if any adverse events. "Dialing up the energy" adds little clinical improvement but greatly increases the incidence of adverse events.

10.2.3 Basic Approach of Pharmacology

A variety of medications have been used topically to stimulate skin synthetic activity. Due to the difficulty of getting biologically active molecules into the skin topically, changes to deep skin and subcutaneous structures have not been well addressed in this fashion. Office-based treatments have been attempted to drive medications or serums into the skin using ultrasound, microdermabrasion, fractional resurfacing, and iontophoresis, among others.

The observation that fillers stimulate collagen replacement has prompted some investigators to attempt broad-based placement of small amounts of diluted filler under the affected skin. Using active dermal matrix fillers, which stimulate a controlled inflammatory response, this may result in enough collagen deposition to restore some of the support and texture of youthful skin.[2] This is analogous to the energy-based devices that produce tissue coagulation and an inflammatory healing response to produce new collagen and aesthetic improvement. Other investigators have attempted to control the direction of skin smoothing or redraping with linear injection of filler oriented along the intended vector(s) of redraping.[3] Massive-weight-loss patients have a greater diversity and severity of aesthetic issues that need correction and are beyond the scope of this chapter.

10.3 Selecting Surgical and Nonsurgical Options Based on Patient Findings

During surgical planning, an analysis must be performed of the effect of each procedure on the various anatomic layers of the surgical site, such as skin, fat, muscle, and fascia.[4] Surgery may not address a layer at all, or surgery may improve one aspect of the aesthetic problems in a tissue layer but not others. For example, skin laxity may be reduced but the surface texture and biological functioning of the skin and its intrinsic elasticity remain unchanged. If skin is pulled tighter, there is no change

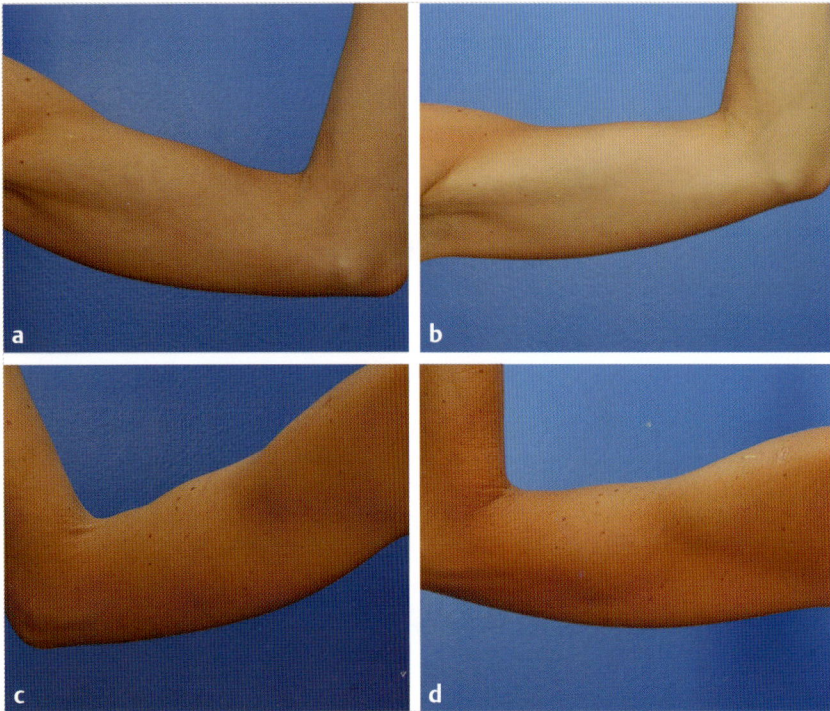

Fig. 10.1 (a,b) A 74-year-old patient with skin laxity. **(c,d)** Six months after one liposuction with needle-based RF (ThermiRF, ThermiGen, LLC) to arms.

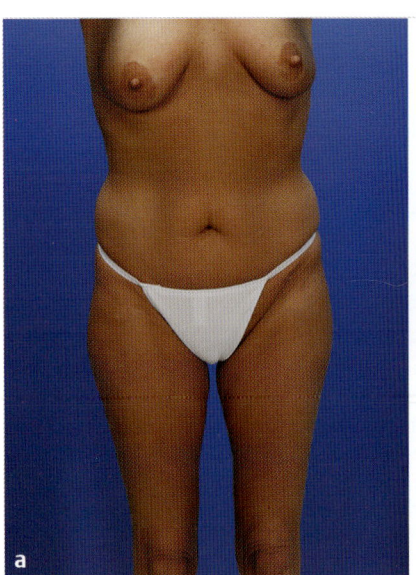
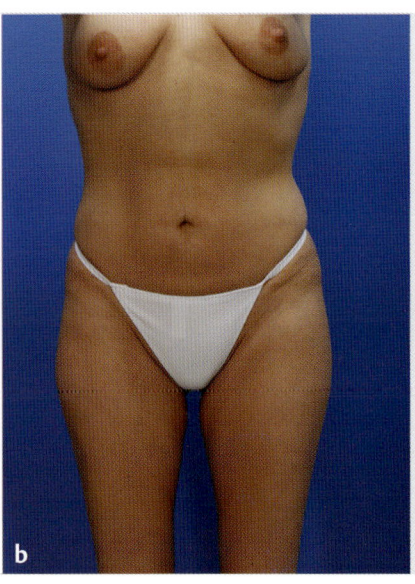

Fig. 10.2 (a) A 64-year-old with skin laxity. **(b)** 1 year after radiofrequency-assisted liposuction (RFAL).

in the aging composition of the skin itself. Energy-based devices stimulate the production of collagen and elastin, resulting in skin that more closely resembles youthful skin in histology, composition, and metabolism. In the adipose layer, minor postsurgical irregularities are common. A "touch-up" can be performed using liposuction, but noninvasive body-contouring devices produce just as good an improvement in a more efficient fashion. Surgical body-contouring procedures make shape and size changes but have little or no impact on the overall appearance of the skin surface. Liposuction alone can reduce fat with little or no change in skin laxity and a frequent loss of smoothness. Energy-based devices can achieve a more meaningful combination of reduced fat and tightened skin. These devices may be used at the time of surgery in conjunction with liposuction (▶ Fig. 10.1 and ▶ Fig. 10.2). Alternatively, there are energy-based modalities that can be used after a surgical or nonsurgical contouring procedure (▶ Fig. 10.3). These principles form the basis for planning combinations of surgical and nonsurgical approaches to achieve more complete aesthetic improvement.

Blending Nonsurgical Treatments with Surgery for Skin Lifting on the Body

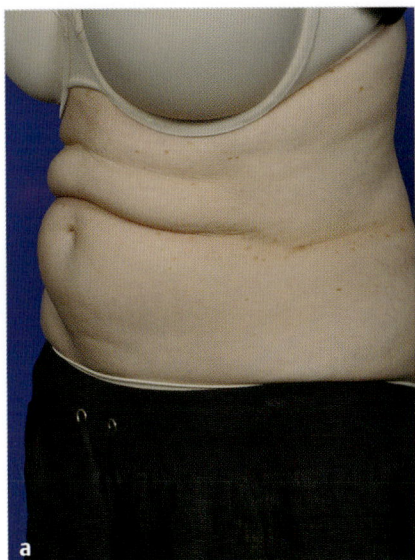
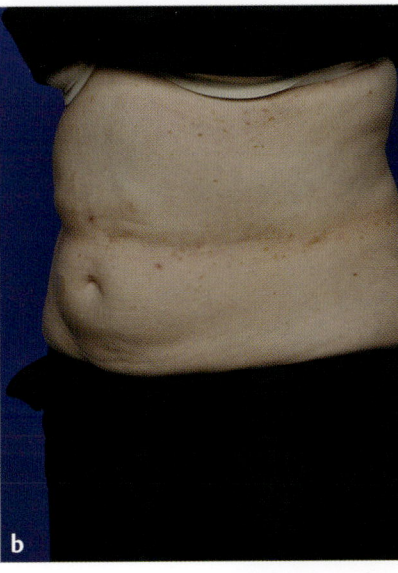

Fig. 10.3 (a,b) A 74-year-old woman who had cryolipolysis to abdomen. (b) Three months posttreatment.

10.3.1 Laxity

The next set of considerations in treating body skin is an assessment of the combination and magnitude of changes present. Laxity in minor form may be addressable with nonsurgical lifting devices. Whereas these devices have not currently been expressly created or optimized for body skin, minor improvement can be effected with a variety of the "outside-in" techniques that directly expose the skin surface to energy using laser light, multiwavelength light, radiofrequency (RF) energy delivered in a variety of fashions, and microfocused ultrasound.[5,6,7,8,9] More significant laxity more likely to be adequately addressed with "inside-out" techniques dumps large amounts of energy under the skin, exposing the skin and fibrous septae between the skin and fascia to energy, often with some form of feedback to limit overexposure or to ensure that adequate tissue temperatures are achieved. These techniques use laser light or RF delivered transcutaneously either as a standalone procedure or in conjunction with a surgical procedure such as liposuction.[10,11,12,13,14] As a standalone, laxity alone is addressed. In conjunction with liposuction or another surgical procedure, these techniques can enhance the contour reduction, address the skin smoothing or laxity reduction needs that were pre-existing patient problems, or minimize the production of these issues simply because of the surgical treatment (e.g., liposuction producing increased skin laxity due to large amounts of fat removal).

RF energy in particular has found significant use for skin laxity in the body and breast using a RF needle delivered through a 1-mm skin puncture (Thermigen, LLC) (▶ Fig. 10.4). Major degrees of skin laxity will require surgical-lifting (skin excision) procedures such as abdominoplasty, thigh or buttock lift, brachioplasty, mastopexy, and others.

The role of injectable therapies alone or in conjunction with energy-based therapies to reduce skin laxity is tantalizing but remains largely unexplored. Creating studies that combine commercial products from different companies are not sponsored and are fraught with the complexities of sorting out the contribution of each treatment to the clinical results (**see Video 1.1**).

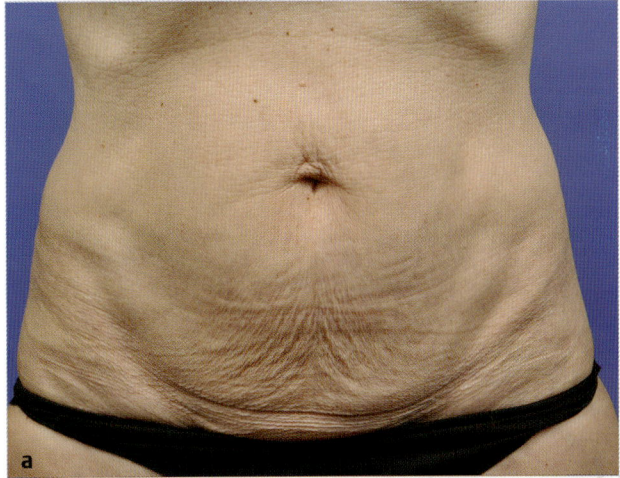
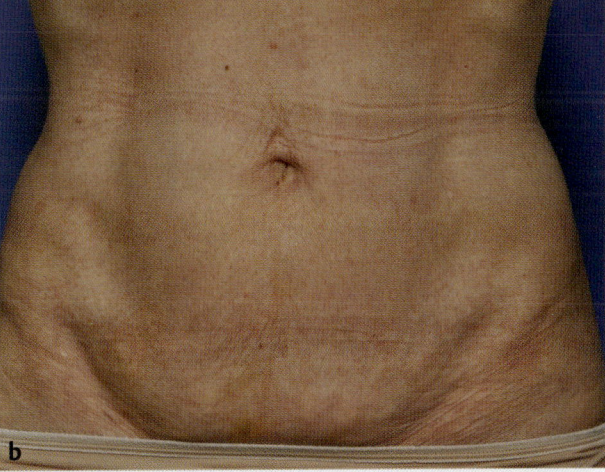

Fig. 10.4 (a) This patient underwent liposuction several years prior to a single treatment with needle-based feedback-controlled RF (ThermiTight, ThermiGen, LLC) to lax abdominal skin. (b) Three months after treatment.

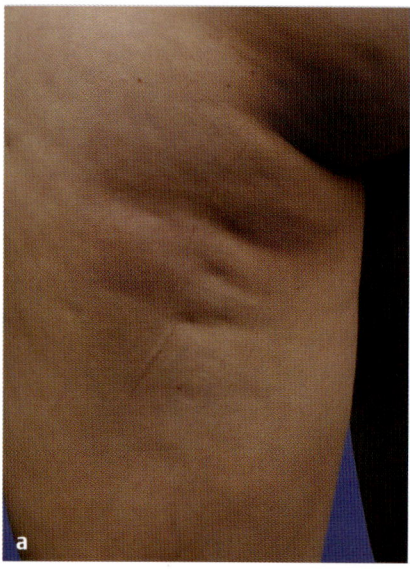
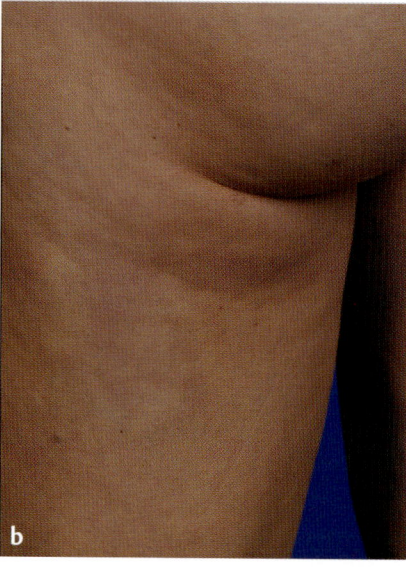

Fig. 10.5 (a) Patient treated with Cellulaze (Cynosure, Inc., 1440 nm side firing fiber subcision) treatment for skin smoothing/cellulite reduction, and then (b) 6 months later underwent Sculpsure (Cynosure, Inc., 1060 nm diode laser hyperthermia) treatment for contour reduction.

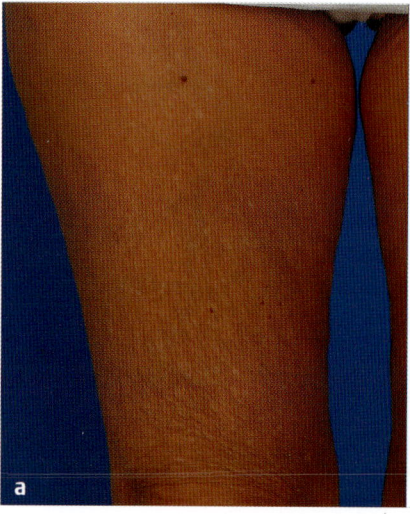
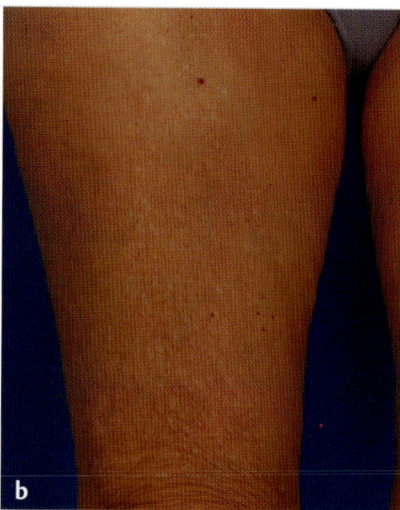

Fig. 10.6 (a) Before and (b) 3 months after two microneedle RF treatments to leg skin for the smoothing of crepiness.

10.3.2 Skin Surface Contour Irregularities

Surface-texture attributes on the skin include crepiness, rhytides, striae, and cellulite. Because full-field ablative resurfacing is usually not possible on body sites, fractional energy delivery strategies must be employed, often in a series of treatments to produce the desired improvement. Combination treatments are common (▶ Fig. 10.5). Superficial chemical peels, microdermabrasion, or similar techniques may also play a role but are less commonly employed. Mild changes often respond to outside-in techniques using the same modalities that apply to facial features but with reduced parameters, more treatments, and less complete clearance. Nonablative fractional resurfacing, microfocused ultrasound using superficial transducers, and RF are most often used. RF energy can be delivered using large electrodes or in a fractionated fashion noninvasively or using insulated or noninsulated needles that are introduced intradermally (▶ Fig. 10.6). These outside-in approaches are more common for surface features than inside-out approaches.

Pharmacologic treatments have been used for skin smoothing and fat reduction for decades in Europe.[15] Such mesotherapy treatments often involve a cocktail of a dozen or more ingredients. Recent studies have identified two predominantly active ingredients in many formulations—the bile salts deoxycholic acid and phosphatidyl choline—both of which can produce adipocytolysis, or the breakdown of the membrane of the adipocyte with cell death. An intense inflammatory reaction ensues, producing thickening of the dermis and fibrosis in connective tissue septae, all of which contributes to a smoother and less lax skin contour.[16,17] Additional agents such as salmeterol, a beta agonist, are also in testing for fat reduction.[15]

Combinations of pharmacologic and energy-based treatments are finding increasing use to produce a process of skin maintenance and smoothing, although there is no data to support a particular sequence or selection of technologies.[1] Similarly, outcomes data on efficacy, particularly with any quantitative component, are lacking for many therapies as standalone treatments and even more so for combination approaches, even though these combination approaches are widely employed in clinical medicine today.

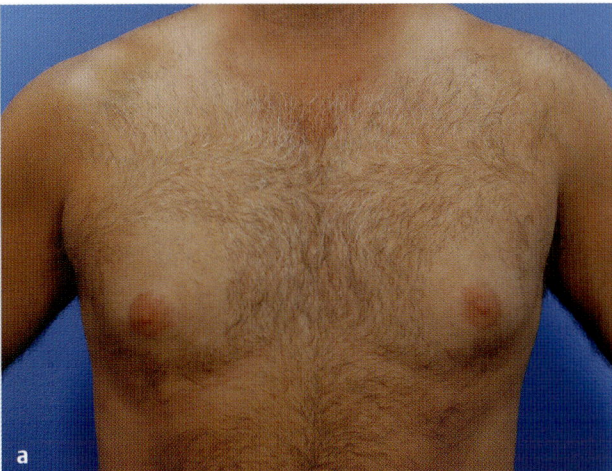

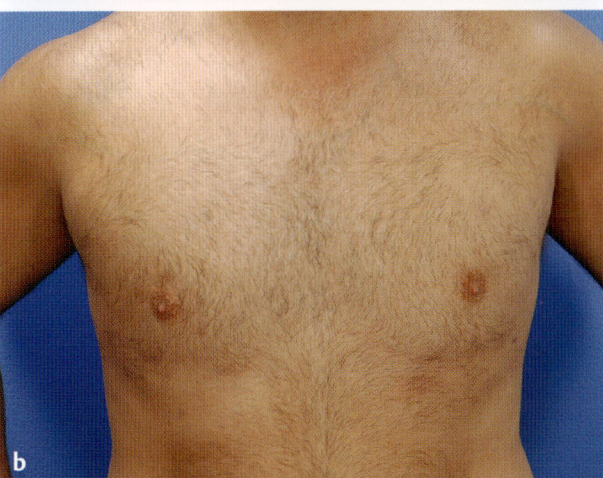

Fig. 10.7 (a) Before and (b) 1 month after three BBL treatments to the chest for pigment clearance.

10.3.3 Dyspigmentation

Pigment change in the skin as a result of ultraviolet damage or inflammatory processes can be blended or cleared. Vascular changes in the form of telangiectasias, angiomas, and more general plethoric changes in the skin can all be addressed. Laser light (typically 532- and 1064-nm wavelengths) and high-intensity multiwavelength light (intense pulsed light [IPL]) (e.g., BBL, Sciton, Inc.) are most commonly employed (see Product Index (p.176)) (▶ Fig. 10.7).

10.4 Summary

Aging changes in the skin are multifactorial and typically large in magnitude. Treatment is made more difficult by the large surface area, the magnitude of the changes, and the diminished healing capacity of the skin compared to comparable facial areas. Combination or multimodality treatment is almost always needed to obtain the most complete correction. Many modalities are available and continue to evolve to create incremental improvements in the ability to address body skin laxity, aging and photodamage issues.

10.5 Commentary

Julius W. Few Jr.

I have respected and followed the work of the authors of this chapter for more than a decade. They are to be congratulated for producing thought-provoking considerations with significant, reproducible results. The authors show high-level consideration for one of the most difficult components of body contour, skin management. The technology that ultimately address, in an absolute fashion, loss of skin tone with aging has affectively captured one of the number-one complaints I hear in practice. Currently, due to the extreme complexity of treating atrophic skin and the scar challenges of traditional surgical options, combination strategies are critically important to achieve results that compete with surgery in a meaningful way. Surgery remains the gold standard, but combination therapies can be very effective in well-selected patients.

This chapter brings up the important issue of practicality and financial consideration. Several facial-based solutions work extremely well but have a high utilization cost, because of disposables and the relative amount of supply needed to render a treatment. To this end, we have also utilized approaches that address the external and internal components of the skin, often using laser, focused ultrasound, and RF to achieve predictable skin tightening and improved external tone and clarity. We have utilized hyper-dilute fillers, hyaluronic acid-based, with an admixture of 10 to 20:1 with preservative containing saline and lidocaine plain. The intradermal tumescence of the skin does seem to create a lasting effect, in terms of collagen stimulation and enhancing the effect of energy-based technology. In particular, the filler is placed just before laser resurfacing to create a local effect, making the treatment painless while enhancing the laser effect. It is critical to not use epinephrine in this combined simultaneous approach to allow for monitoring of the desired end points.

Finally, as has been shown by other authors in this book, the ability to offer an effective nonsurgical salvage liposuction induced skin laxity and/or other iatrogenic side effects of plastic surgery, which dramatically expands the treatment capability of the plastic surgery.

References

[1] Jerdan K, Fabi S. A noninvasive approach to off-face skin laxity and tightening: a review of the literature. Semin Cutan Med Surg. 2015; 34(3): 118–128

[2] Yutskovskaya Y, Kogan E, Leshunov E. A randomized, split-face, histomorphologic study comparing a volumetric calcium hydroxylapatite and a hyaluronic acid-based dermal filler. J Drugs Dermatol. 2014; 13(9):1047–1052

[3] Cogorno Wasylkowski V. Body vectoring technique with Radiesse(®) for tightening of the abdomen, thighs, and brachial zone. Clin Cosmet Investig Dermatol. 2015; 8:267–273

[4] Kreuger N, Sadick N. Three-dimensional rejuvenation of the photoaged body. Cosmet Dermatol. 2011; 24(8):381–387

[5] Weiss RA. Noninvasive radio frequency for skin tightening and body contouring. Semin Cutan Med Surg. 2013; 32(1):9–17

[6] Elman M, Vider I, Harth Y, Gottfried V, Shemer A. Non-invasive therapy of wrinkles and lax skin using a novel multisource phase-controlled radio frequency system. J Cosmet Laser Ther. 2010; 12(2):81–86

[7] Alster TS, Tanzi EL. Noninvasive lifting of arm, thigh, and knee skin with transcutaneous intense focused ultrasound. Dermatol Surg. 2012; 38(5):754–759

[8] Gold MH, Sensing W, Biron J. Use of micro-focused ultrasound with visualization to lift and tighten lax knee skin (1.). J Cosmet Laser Ther. 2014; 16(5):225–229

[9] Rokhsar C, Schnebelen W, West A, Hornfeldt C. Safety and efficacy of microfocused ultrasound in tightening of lax elbow skin. Dermatol Surg. 2015; 41(7):821–826

[10] DiBernardo BE. Randomized, blinded split abdomen study evaluating skin shrinkage and skin tightening in laser-assisted liposuction versus liposuction control. Aesthet Surg J. 2010; 30(4):593–602

[11] Sasaki GH. Quantification of human abdominal tissue tightening and contraction after components treatments with 1064-nm/1320-nm laser-assisted lipolysis: clinical implications. Aesthetic Surg. 2010 Mar

[12] Dudelzak J, Hussain M, Goldberg DJ. Laser lipolysis of the arm, with and without suction aspiration: clinical and histologic changes. J Cosmet Laser Ther. 2009; 11(2):70–73

[13] Theodorou S, Chia C. Radiofrequency-assisted liposuction for arm contouring: technique under local anesthesia. Plast Reconstr Surg Glob Open. 2013; 1(5):e37

[14] Duncan I. Nonexcisional tissue tightening: creating skin surface area reduction during abdominal liposuction by adding radiofrequency heating. Aesthet Surg J. 2013 Nov

[15] Chen DL, Cohen JL, Green JB. Injectable agents affecting subcutaneous fats. Semin Cutan Med Surg. 2015; 34(3):134–137

[16] Duncan D, Rotunda AM. Injectable therapies for localized fat loss: state of the art. Clin Plast Surg. 2011; 38(3):489–501, vii

[17] Park EJ, Kim HS, Kim M, Oh HJ. Histological changes after treatment for localized fat deposits with phosphatidylcholine and sodium deoxycholate. J Cosmet Dermatol. 2013; 12(3):240–243

11 Nonsurgical Salvage and Enhancement of a Surgical Result

David A. Sieber, John E. Hoopman, and Jeffrey M. Kenkel

Summary

The principle of thermal disruption of collagen fibers is the basis for many nonsurgical aesthetic treatments, such as intense pulsed light (IPL), radiofrequency (RF), high-intensity focused ultrasound (HIFU), and skin care with peeling agents. All of these treatments cause skin tightening. Understanding wavelength, power, spot size, pulse width, and cooling help optimize outcomes and reduce unfavorable results.

Keywords: ablative, downtime, CO_2 laser, Er:YAG laser, facial rejuvenation high-intensity focused ultrasound (HIFU), intense pulsed light (IPL), microthermal zones (MTZs), nonablative, radiofrequency (RF), skin laxity, soft tissue deflation

> **Key Points**
> - Proper patient selection and realistic expectations are key for optimal nonsurgical results.
> - Thermal energy is responsible for skin tightening.
> - Patients should be treated at the lowest energy able to produce a response.
> - All nonsurgical devices carry risk for significant complications.

11.1 Introduction

Nonsurgical aesthetic medicine continues to be a growing field, with an increase of 22% in the number of nonsurgical procedures performed in 2015.[1] Demand for minimally invasive options is increasing due to the increase in the popularity of nonsurgical procedures and the industry's focus on direct-to-consumer marketing. The nature of these types of procedures allows for patients to continue to cycle through a practice and may ultimately lead to surgical conversion for some patients in the future. Techniques such as nonablative and ablative lasers, intense pulsed light (IPL), radiofrequency (RF), high-intensity focused ultrasound (HIFU), and skin care with peeling agents may also be used in conjunction with surgery to optimize the patient's overall aesthetic results.

Each of these technologies relies on a similar principle of thermal disruption of collagen fibers. Collagen is a polymer held together by hydrogen bonds, and it is these cross-links that attribute to the collagen strength. Thermal energy causes a denaturing of the collagen while the heat-stable intramolecular cross-links are preserved.[2] Skin tightening occurs due to a physical shortening of the collagen fibers with preservation of the intramolecular hydrogen bonds, possibly increasing the elastic properties of the skin.[3,4] With increased delivery of thermal energy (i.e., increased tissue temperature), there is a greater degree of collagen denaturation and thus resultant tissue tightening. Thermal injury also induces local fibroblasts to produce new collagen as a part of the wound-healing response. Balancing appropriate thermal injury without causing tissue necrosis remains the greatest challenge as the demand for improved efficacy and reproducible treatments rise.

Changes within the collagen occur in a time- and temperature-dependent manner, meaning that both short exposures to high temperatures or prolonged exposure to lower temperatures will both create a degree of collagen shortening. Bozec and Odlyha[5] demonstrated that denaturing of collagen fibrils occurs at approximately 65 °C, with initial collagen injury occurring around 58 °C. Additional studies agree that disruption and denaturing of collagen occurs in the 60 to 65 °C range, with a greater degree of denaturation occurring at higher temperatures.[2,3,6,7] It is this initial collagen insult along with the resulting neocollagenesis that triggers the healing response responsible for the observed thermal tightening. However, the burn literature suggests that extensive cell membrane breakdown begins to occur at temperatures above 45 °C.[8]

As with any device, the user must understand the parameters of the device not only to optimize outcomes, but also to reduce possible treatment-related complications. Understanding and manipulation of five key parameters allow the user to master the laser device at hand instead of being at the mercy of preset manufacturer protocols.[9]

> **Five Parameters for Operating a Laser Device**
> 1. Wavelength: determined by the target chromophore and its location within the tissue
> 2. Power: the amount of energy delivered to the tissue target
> 3. Spot size: used in correlation with the power to determine the power density
> 4. Pulse width: the delivery or exposure time of selected energy delivered to the tissue target
> 5. Cooling: allows for maximal depth of injury without harming more superficial tissue

Only through a complete understanding of the interplay of these five parameters is the user able to adequately treat the target tissue with lasers without unnecessarily damaging the collateral tissue in the process[10] (▶ Table 11.1). With each

Table 11.1 Ideal Pulse Width versus Vessel Diameter

Size	200 um	300 um	400 um	500 um	600 um	700 um	800 um	900 um	1.0 mm
P/W	15 ms	20 ms	25 ms	30 ms	35 ms	40 ms	45 ms	50 ms	55 ms
(< 100um = 10 ms)									

Nonsurgical Salvage and Enhancement of a Surgical Result

subsequent treatment, the patient's tissue is uniquely changed and will thus present differently for each subsequent treatment. This leads to a need for slight modifications to the treatment parameters with each procedure.

11.2 Laser and Intense Pulsed Light Therapies

Nonsurgical laser devices may be divided into two categories, nonablative and ablative, which share a similar goal of making skin-surface changes. When evaluating patients for laser or light therapy, the correct device needs to be chosen to address the specific skin disorder being treated, the target chromophore, and it must have acceptable downtime (▶ Table 11.2) The most commonly used nonablative, ablative, and light-based devices in our practice are the

- Fractionated 10,600 nm CO_2.
- 2940 nm erbium:yttrium-aluminum-garnet (Er:YAG) laser.
- Full-field Er:YAG.
- 1064 nm neodymium-doped:yttrium-aluminum-garnet (Nd:YAG) laser.
- 532 nm potassium titanyl phosphate (KTP) laser.
- IPL device.

When using laser and light therapy, there are three main target chromophores within tissue: hemoglobin, melanin, and water.

Table 11.2 Choice of Devices Based on Treatment Issue and Associated Downtime

	Downtime	
	Hours	Weeks
Pigment	IPL, KTP (532)	Erbium
Redness	IPL, YAG (1064), KTP (532)	
Wrinkles	Botox, Fillers	TCA, Erbium, FCO_2
Acne	Fillers	Excision, Erbium, FCO_2
Laxity	Ultrasound, RF	Surgery

Hemoglobin has three peaks at 400 nm, 532 nm, and 577 to 600 nm, with 577 nm being the most selective for this chromophore. Melanin is found in a wider spectrum—between 400 to 1100 nm of light—with the ranges of 400 to 475 nm and 630 to 810 nm being the most selective. Ablative lasers rely on water molecules stored within the tissue target (▶ Fig. 11.1).

In our hands for skin resurfacing, the full ablative 2940 nm Er:YAG laser has the most dramatic effect on skin resurfacing at the cost of increased downtime. The Er:YAG laser has largely replaced the previous generation of CO_2 lasers because of the Er:YAG's precise depth of ablation without the undesirable collateral tissue heating commonly seen with traditional CO_2 devices. Total ablative Er:YAG resurfacing has a much more significant recovery than any of the nonablative lasers. However, the Er:YAG is able to provide very predictable results with

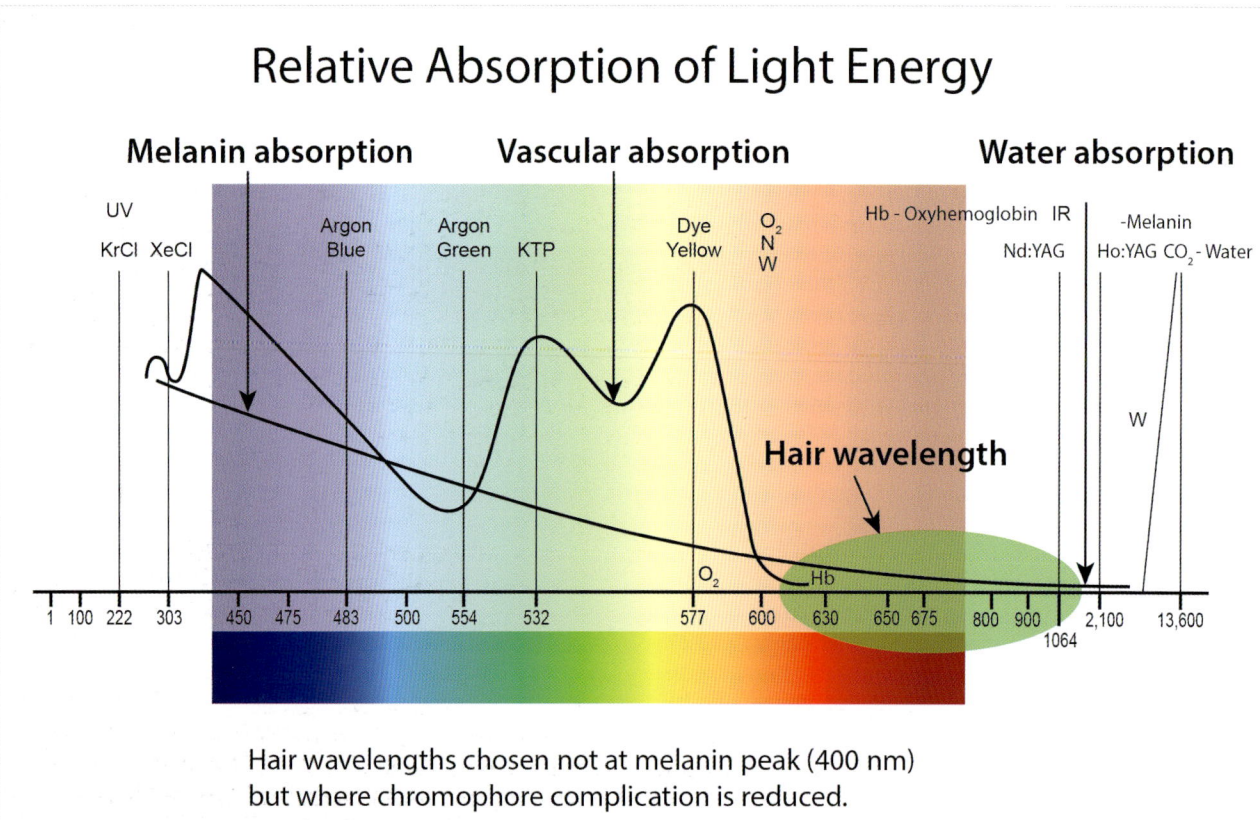

Fig. 11.1 The wavelengths chosen for hair reduction are not at the melanin absorption peak (400 nm) but at longer wavelengths to minimize complications.

visible end points. This is in part due to the Er:YAG's high absorption by water, which is 13 times greater than that of the CO_2 laser. Heating of this water with suprathreshold fluences leads to immediate cellular heating, resulting in instant tissue vaporization. A high absorption by water allows for a more precise suprathreshold ablation, with less subthreshold collateral damage to the surrounding tissue. The main downside to the Er:YAG is the prolonged recovery, usually requiring 7 to 10 days for complete re-epithelialization as compared to nonablative modalities. Patients typically have prolonged redness for at least 2 to 3 months posttreatment, and it may persist for up to 6 months. This may be shortened by use of IPL vascular treatments to reduce redness after a few weeks postresurfacing.

Fractionated lasers were developed with the hope of achieving an end result similar to that of the fully ablative CO_2 and Er:YAG lasers while allowing the patient a quicker recovery with less downtime. Fractionated devices use extremely high fluences to deliver focused columns of energy into the tissue, resulting in microthermal zones (MTZs) of injury. Areas surrounding these MTZs only reach sublative temperatures, yet they still undergo significant protein denaturation, tissue coagulation, and apoptosis.[11] The thermal injury sustained generally extends 200–300 μm, although it can go deeper, into the dermis, leading to the previously mentioned cascade of heat-induced collagen shortening and neocollagenesis. By delivering a discontinuous, segmental injury to the tissue, reservoirs of healthy tissue remain to speed healing and to act as a source of keratinocyte migration.[12] Theoretically, these MTZs should produce sufficient injury to create a tissue response similar to that of the fully ablative CO_2 and Er:YAG lasers, yet this has not been the results experienced in our clinic.[13,14]

Doubling the frequency of a 1064 nm laser by way of a KTP crystal is what makes the higher-energy 532 nm KTP laser possible. One specific advantage of 532 nm over 1064 nm are that treatment energies for 532 nm are one order of magnitude less for the same chromophore (arteries or oxygenated hemoglobin), meaning that when treating superficial telangiectasias located in the superficial dermis, less energy is needed to see a response. Whenever treating patients, the goal is to use the minimum effective dose of energy at which a desired clinical end point is still evident, which prevents the delivery of excess energy into target tissue and lessens the risk of subsequent adverse events.[14,15,16] A downside of the 532 nm laser is that it only has a very superficial absorption length and is typically much less effective for vessels larger than 500 μm.[17] Additionally, the use of the 532 nm laser in darker skin types must be approached very cautiously, because melanin competes with hemoglobin at this wavelength.

The 1064 nm, on the other hand, is able to adequately treat deeper tissue and larger vessels, to a depth of 5 to 6 mm and a diameter up to 2 to 3 mm. However, this comes at the cost of increased fluences caused by a decrease in the absorption coefficient, resulting in more discomfort for the patient.

Although surgery remains the gold standard for facial rejuvenation, surgery alone is only able to address skin laxity and soft tissue deflation. Global facial rejuvenation must address the skin surface as well. Years of sun exposure may result in static and dynamic rhytides, poor skin texture, and multiple dyschromias. Although initially there was some hesitancy to perform laser skin resurfacing at the same time as or as an adjunct to surgery, it has since been shown to be safe in select patients using moderate settings.[18,19,20] Despite its safety, many practitioners still prefer to wait 3 to 6 months after surgery before performing full-face laser skin resurfacing.

11.2.1 Intense Pulsed Light

IPL is our most commonly performed office procedure and has high patient satisfaction. Although commonly referred to as a laser, IPL is a flash lamp device, not a laser. This technology works by generating a polychromatic light and most commonly has an output spectrum between 400 nm to 1400 nm within the electromagnetic spectrum. What differentiates IPL from a laser is that a laser most often emits a single wavelength, whereas IPL delivers an entire spectrum of light at the same time. IPL works by passing light through specific filters to block unwanted wavelengths, thus tailoring the emitted wavelengths for a desired chromophore. Although the perception remains that because this is not a laser it is inherently a safer device, the opposite is true, because it emits up to 1,000 different wavelengths and the precise treatment of every chromophore is sometimes difficult to control. Simply put, this is a device that scans for every chromophore due to the spectrum of light emitted, and wavelength-limiting filters are used in an effort to regain some control. These filters are commonly high-pass filters that block wavelengths below the number indicated on the filter while allowing longer wavelengths to pass through to tissue. Shorter wavelengths are absorbed in the more superficial targets, and this allows targeting the deeper dermis without damaging upper skin structures. IPL therapy may be used for the correction of photoaging and the treatment of pigment of vascular lesions, erythema, or acne.

11.3 Patient Selection for Laser And Light-Based Devices

532 nm KTP lasers are best suited for the treatment of small veins, pigment, tattoos, port-wine stains, and for nonablative dermal remodeling.[21] Similar to the KTP laser, the 1064 nm Nd:YAG is commonly used for nonablative facial resurfacing, hair removal, treatment of acne, leg veins, pigmented lesions, and vascular anomalies.[22,23,24,25,26,27,28,29,30] Patients needing aggressive skin resurfacing for select pigments, skin texture, or rhytides are best treated with Er:YAG.[31,32,33,34,35] IPL is the most versatile of the devices due to the broad range of wavelengths it produces. It may be used for the treatment of telangiectasias, dyschromias, and hair reduction[24,36,37,38,39] (▶ Table 11.3).

An excellent way to enhance facial rejuvenation is through the placement of adipose or hyaluronic acid fillers with the addition of concomitant facial resurfacing (**see Video 1.1**).[40] Facial fat grafting can restore lost facial volume, whereas laser resurfacing addresses superficial and deep rhytides, improving facial contours and skin texture. We have performed upper lid surgery, facial fat grafting, and simultaneous laser resurfacing with excellent results. Laser resurfacing has also been shown to be safe and effective when performed at the same time as lower lid blepharoplasties.[41]

Table 11.3 Lasers and Light-based Devices with Associated Treatment Wavelengths, Target Chromophores, and Common Uses

Laser	Wavelength (nm)	Chromophore	Common Uses
KTP	532	Melanin, Hemoglobin	Benign pigmented lesions, telangiectasias
Nd:YAG	1064	Melanin	Benign pigmented lesions, hair, spider veins, leg veins
Er:YAG	2940	Water	Rhytides, atrophic scars, dermal and epidermal lesions
CO_2	10600	Water	Rhytides, atrophic scars, dermal and epidermal lesions
IPL Device	400–1400	Melanin, Hemoglobin, Water	Pigmented lesions, spider veins, leg veins, body hair

11.4 Technical Steps and Treatment Plan

Many patients undergoing more aggressive in-office procedures may require pretreatment with an anxiolytic agent in addition to an oral narcotic. We commonly use 0.25 to 0.50 mg alprazolam (Xanax, Pfizer Inc.) and oral hydrocodone containing medications such as Norco (Allergan, Inc.) or Lortab (Akorn, Inc.; UCB, Inc.). Pretreatment continues with the application of a topical compound containing benzocaine, lidocaine, and tetracaine (BLT) to all treatment areas. Although topical anesthesia is seemingly innocuous, care must be taken when treating large areas due to the potential risk for lidocaine toxicity.[42,43] Regional nerve blocks are sometimes required depending on the pain associated with the procedure and the pain threshold of the patient. Nerve blocks are typically placed using 0.25 to 1% Xylocaine (lidocaine HCl) plain mixed with bicarbonate. Intraocular shields are often placed for corneal protection when the periorbita is being treated. Procedures such as aggressive fractionated CO_2 and erbium are challenging to manage in the office, so these patients are most comfortable under heavy sedation/anesthesia in a monitored setting.

11.4.1 1064 nm (Nd:YAG) Laser for Vascular Lesions

1. ▶ Table 11.1 Use the least amount of energy to effectively close vascular targets.
2. Use contact dynamic (PPP) cooling at 10 to 20 °C for safety.
3. Start at 80 J/cm^2 and titrate energies in increments of 10 J/cm^2 until a desired response is achieved (stasis).
4. Using a 6-mm spot, regardless of vessel diameter, will ensure that the vessel falls within the effective treatment zone. For 200 um and less and when treating over bone or competing targets such as beard hair in the area, use a 3-mm spot and double-treatment energy range starting at 160 J/cm^2.
5. Keep handpiece 90° to tissue plane.
6. Position patient in supine position to equalize pressures.
7. Use sapphire cooling in light contact. The use of optical coupling gel helps step index the light into the skin and draws heat out postdelivery.
8. You should find that a range of 80 to 120 J/cm^2 for 6 mm spot and 160 to 240 J/cm^2 for 3 mm spot will be sufficient to effectively close most vessels regardless of color and or location.
9. Change only one parameter at a time.
10. Once the fluence (J/cm^2) has been established, pulse width is your key parameter on remaining vessels.
11. Goal:
    - Raise blood above 70 °C.
    - Damage intima.
    - Contract Type I & Type III collagen surrounding vessel.
    - Achieve vessel stasis (no purge and refill).

*Treatment range for 6 mm spot: 80 to 120 J/cm^2
*Treatment range for 3 mm spot: 160 to 240 J/cm^2

11.4.2 Fractionated CO_2

Most fractionated devices have several variables one can control including spot size, density, and fluence. Unfortunately, there are no visible endpoints to determine adequacy of treatment. It should be noted that higher-density treatments should be used with caution in darker skin types.

1. Apply a topical anesthetic of choice.
2. Consider regional and local blocks with lidocaine as desired.
3. If a stamp pattern is used, one should plan for a minimum of two passes to eliminate any gaps or overlap in treatment. For example, if a 20% density is desired, two passes at 10% are recommended.
4. A rolling pattern accounts for density and the number of passes are dictated by the software.
5. A crosshatch pattern should be applied for multiple passes to avoid gaps and stacking of treatments (▶ Fig. 11.2)
6. Following treatment, a light moisturizer is applied and used two to three times a day until peeling is complete.

11.4.3 Er:YAG Technical Steps (Micropeel)

1. Apply topical anesthetic 1 hour before procedure. Additional topical may be reapplied but there is a risk for lidocaine toxicity with additional applications.
2. Using wet 4X4's, thoroughly remove topical and pat dry.
3. Set ablation to desired depth, typically 15 to 50 um (no coagulation).
4. 15 um initial peel accomplishes several goals:
    - Allows assessment of individual erythema response. If patient has strong response, the treatment can be adjusted to match the promised recovery time.
    - Removal of stratum corneum decreases topical uptake time while increasing the depth of topical penetration.
    - A second application of topical helps eliminate the need for oral medication in ablations < 100 um.
    - Doing two to three passes will give a more even coverage and ablation.

Nonsurgical Salvage and Enhancement of a Surgical Result

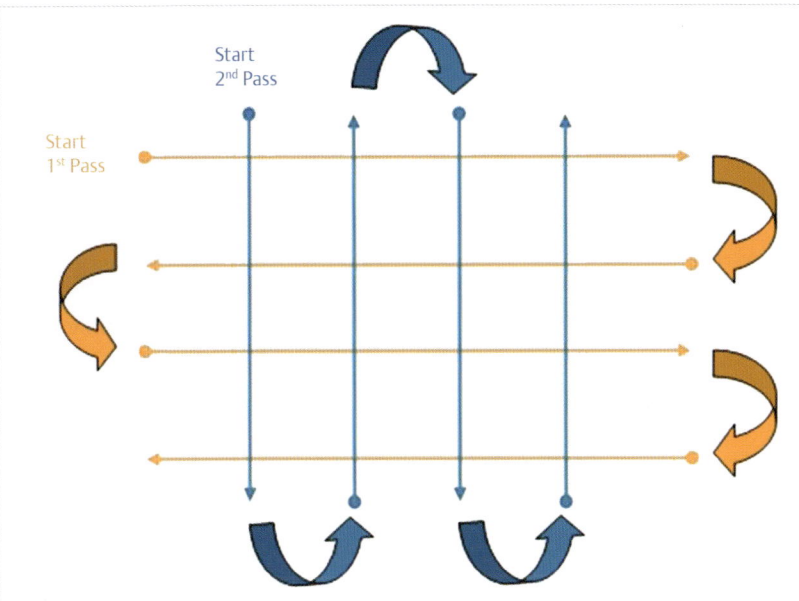

Fig. 11.2 Typical treatment pattern for microlaser peel. (Courtesy John E. Hoopman, Fundamentals of Light presentation.)

5. Set overlap at 50% for first pass.
6. Following first pass, re-apply topical for 10 to 15 minutes to achieve the full effect.
7. Using wet 4X4's, thoroughly remove topical and pat dry.
8. Rotate scanner 90 degrees to form a crosshatch pattern (▶ Fig. 11.2).
9. Set overlap at 50% for the second pass.
10. Select the desired ablation depth not to exceed end points past early reticular bleeding.
11. Wipe off residue and apply topical dressing.
12. Send patient home with postoperative care instructions.

Estimated Recovery Times

As a simple rule, the ratio of epidermal ablation over the original thickness multiplied by 28 days will determine approximate healing time. (Example: 20 microns/110 microns x 28 days = 5 days) Redness is commonly one-third to one-half of that calculated time. Makeup can often be applied in one-quarter to one-third the calculated time (▶ Table 11.4).

11.4.4 IPL For Acne

1. Treatment Basics
   - Apply a 2 to 3 mm layer of colorless gel.
   - Select appropriate settings.
   - Match the trailing edge of one pulse to the leading edge of the next. There should be no overlap between pulses.
   - Pulses should "line up" right next to each other.
2. Parameters (▶ Table 11.5)
3. End Points – There are no definitive end points. The treatment goal is to pack the skin with light. Patients may feel a slight tingling sensation. If the area treated begins to get warm, pause treatment until the area cools down.
4. Posttreatment Care
   - Observation – Possible slight erythema for several hours after treatment.
   - Intervention – Cool compresses or ice packs, though rarely needed, can provide some comfort after treatment.
   - If blistering occurs, aggressive wound-healing measures should be implemented.
   - Intervals – Treatments are performed 1 to 2 times per week. A minimum of 6 treatments are recommended.
   - The destruction of acne continues for a few weeks following the last broad band light (BBL) treatment, and the effects of the treatment will be maintained until bacterial populations rebuild to their initial concentration. Some patients may require a maintenance treatment within 3 to 6 months of the initial series of treatments.

Table 11.4 Estimated Recovery Times

Epidermal Ablation/ Original Thickness	Healing Time	Redness	Makeup Allowed
10 um / 110 um X 28	2.5 Days	1 day	1 day
20 um / 110 um X 28	5 Days	2.5 days	1 day
30 um / 110 um X 28	7.5 Days	3.5 days	2 days
40 um / 110 um X 28	10 Days	5 days	2 days
50 um / 110 um X 28	12.5 Days	6 Days	3 days
60 um / 110 um X 28	15 Days	7 days	4 days

Table 11.5 Broad Band Light Acne Treatment Starting Parameters

Skin Type	Fluence (J/cm^2)	Pulse Width (ms)	Filter (nm)	Cooling (°C)	Passes
I-IV	5	150	420 Blue light	15	2
I-V	15	200	560 Yellow light	15	3*
I-V	15	200	590 Red light	15	6*

Note: Apply 420 nm filter with 2 passes first and then the 560-nm filter with 3 passes and/or the 590-nm filter with 6 passes, except on Skin Type V. Only the 590-nm filter with 6 passes should be used on Skin Type V. On sensitive patients and patients with more severe acne, the use of a small snap-on adapter focused on the individual's acne lesions may help to minimize discomfort and allow for all passes to be completed. This is not recommended for Skin Type VI.

- If performing an acne treatment in conjunction with other procedures such as fractionated treatments, perform the acne treatment first.
- Check with the manufacturer for guidelines on using injectables in conjunction with acne treatments.
- Next pulse application.

Results

Case Example 1

The patient is a 54-year-old woman who presented to the clinic desiring improvement of her acne scars, correction of excess upper eyelid skin, and overall improvement in the texture of skin. The risks and benefits of the various procedures were explained to her, and she elected to undergo in-office management of the previously mentioned issues. She subsequently underwent bilateral upper eyelid blepharoplasty, placement of microionized fat to acne scars, and full-face fractionated erbium laser (Profractional, Sciton) (▶ Fig. 11.3).

Case Example 2

This 56-year-old woman presented to the clinic complaining of a poorly defined jawline, excess skin on her upper eyelids, and poor facial skin texture with fine rhytides. There was a discussion about her surgical versus nonsurgical options. She was not a good candidate for nonsurgical options because of the large amount of skin excess and lipodystrophy in her neck. The patient agreed to pursue upper lid blepharoplasty, neck lift, and full-face erbium resurfacing. Postoperatively, she was treated with serial treatments of IPL. Six months after the initial procedure, she had a treatment with erbium to her lower lids for increased skin tightening. Postoperatively, she still thought there was persistent fullness in her right neck, so this was subsequently treatment with two Ultherapy treatments (Ulthera) to even the lipodystrophy of the neck (see Product Index (p.185)). She underwent upper blepharoplasty, neck lift, and full-face erbium followed by IPL and Ultherapy (▶ Fig. 11.4).

Case Example 3

This 43-year-old man presented to the clinic complaining of unsatisfactory scarring from adolescent acne. He was counseled regarding his treatment options. He ultimately underwent micronized fat injections to the acne scars and 100-micron erbium laser peel in the same setting. He is seen 4 months after treatment in ▶ Fig. 11.5.

11.4.5 Postoperative Care

Light-based and Nonablative Therapy

Recovery is straightforward for these procedures. Patients may display redness for a few hours after the treatment. In patients with pigmentation, there may be accentuation of the pigmentation and ultimately a fine peel in some cases. Moisturizers and sunblock should be used when appropriate. Multiple treatments are usually performed at 3- to 6-week intervals.

Fractionated CO_2 Resurfacing

Patients experience pain and discomfort for 12 to 24 hours until re-epithelialization occurs. A light moisturizer is used 3 times a day to prevent excessive dryness of the skin. Once peeling occurs, patients may experience redness for 4 to 8 weeks posttreatment depending on how aggressive the treatment was. The patient is then transitioned back onto their skin care regimen.

Full-Ablative Erbium:YAG Resurfacing

These patients experience considerable pain until epithelialization occurs somewhere between 2 and 4 days after treatment. Occlusive dressings significantly improve the patient experience and diminish the pain experienced. Dressings are changed at 48 hours so the skin can be assessed. Occlusion is associated with an increased risk for infection, so close monitoring is essential. Once the dressing is removed, then a light moisturizer is used and continued through the peeling process, which lasts approximately 7 to 10 days. The patient is then transitioned back onto their skin care routine.

11.4.6 Complications and Shortcomings

Complications for the 532 nm and 1064 nm devices include hypopigmentation, hyperpigmentation, and/or blistering, which all occur at or near the dermal-epidermal junction. Although seen infrequently, scarring is the most serious complication, occurring when a full-thickness wound is produced with any device. Postinflammatory hyperpigmentation (PIH) is the most commonly see complication across all devices. PIH can sometimes be managed with a skin care regimen of tretinoin or retinol containing products along with hydroquinone. Multiple treatments with a light TCA peel or IPL may also help improve the appearance of PIH. PIH often takes many months to resolve but usually does get better (▶ Fig. 11.6). The main complication from CO_2 or Er:YAG is hypopigmentation due to the permanent destruction of melanocytes at the dermal/epidermal junction (▶ Fig. 11.7). Another short-term issue, which may arise with the use of ablative lasers, is prolonged erythema, which may persist for as long as 6 months posttreatment.

Although seemingly benign, IPL may create serious complications that are usually pigment-related and occur more commonly in patients with Fitzpatrick IV-VI skin. The most common adverse events include hyperpigmentation, hypopigmentation, and blistering, which can be a manifestation of skin type, target density, and device settings. When treating men, some may experience hair loss in their beard distribution from damage sustained by the hair follicle. Treatment of men later in the day creates more chromophores at the surface and may result in complications, so caution should be used.

11.5 Radiofrequency

RF devices utilize alternating electrical currents to polarize tissue within the electrical path using negatively and positively charged electrodes from which the electrical energy conducts. This alternating current causes oscillations in the target tissue ultimately generating heat. As previously discussed, it is this heat that causes collagen breakdown and ultimately neocolla-

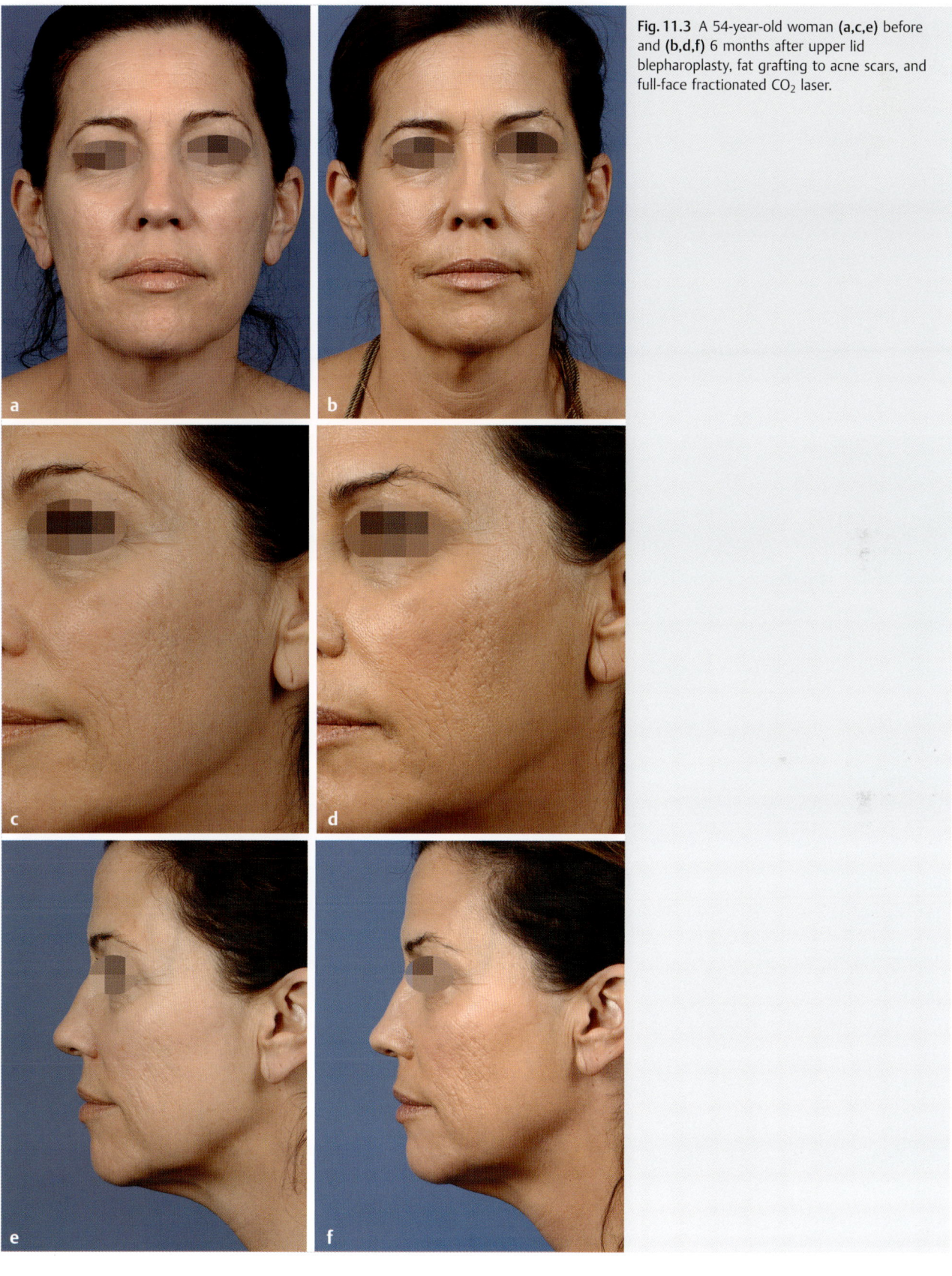

Fig. 11.3 A 54-year-old woman **(a,c,e)** before and **(b,d,f)** 6 months after upper lid blepharoplasty, fat grafting to acne scars, and full-face fractionated CO_2 laser.

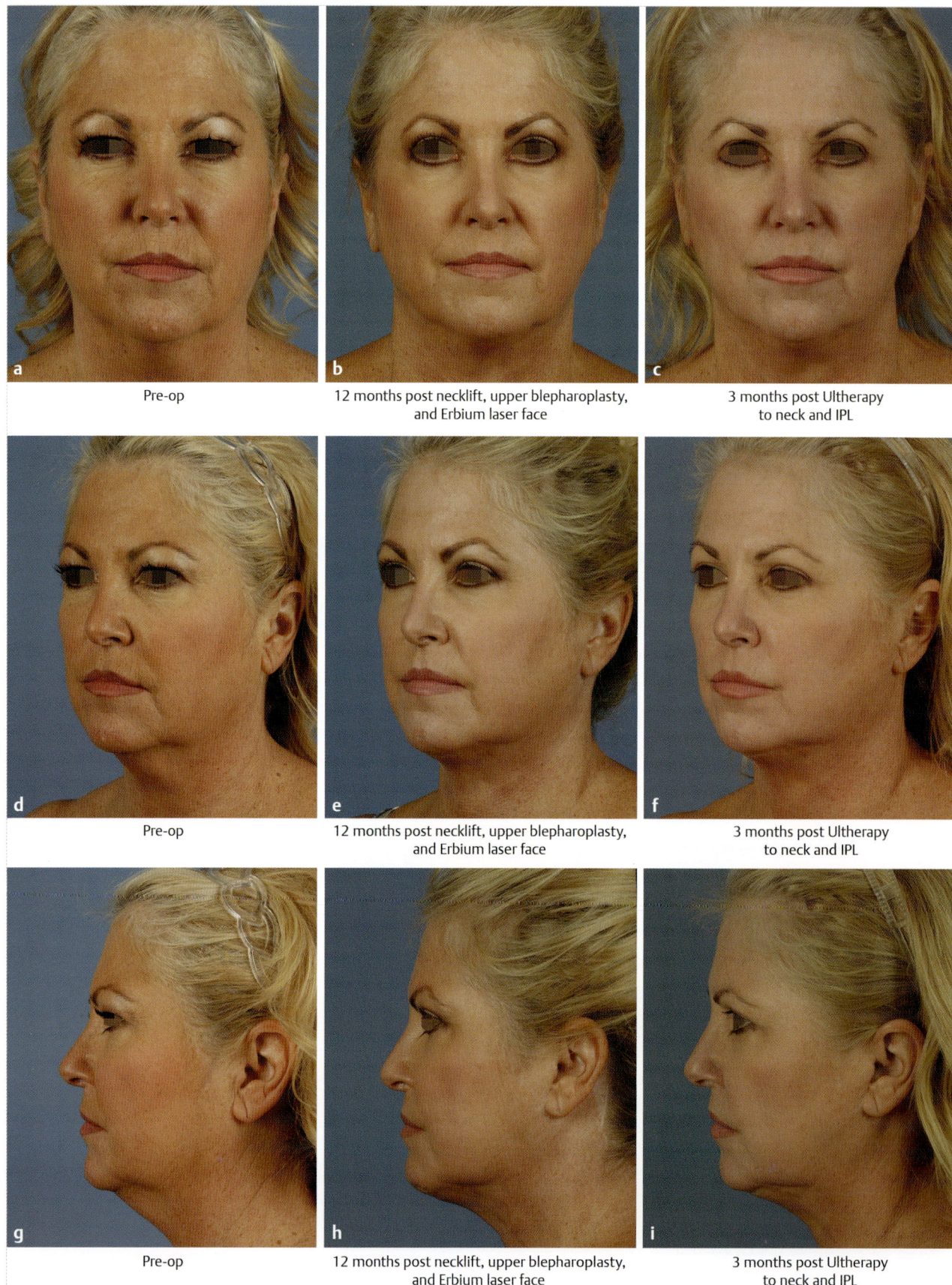

Fig. 11.4 A 56-year-old woman **(a,d,g)** before, **(b,e,h)** 12 months after necklift, upper blepharoplasty, and Erbium laser face, and **(c,f,i)** 3 months after Ultherapy to the neck and IPL.

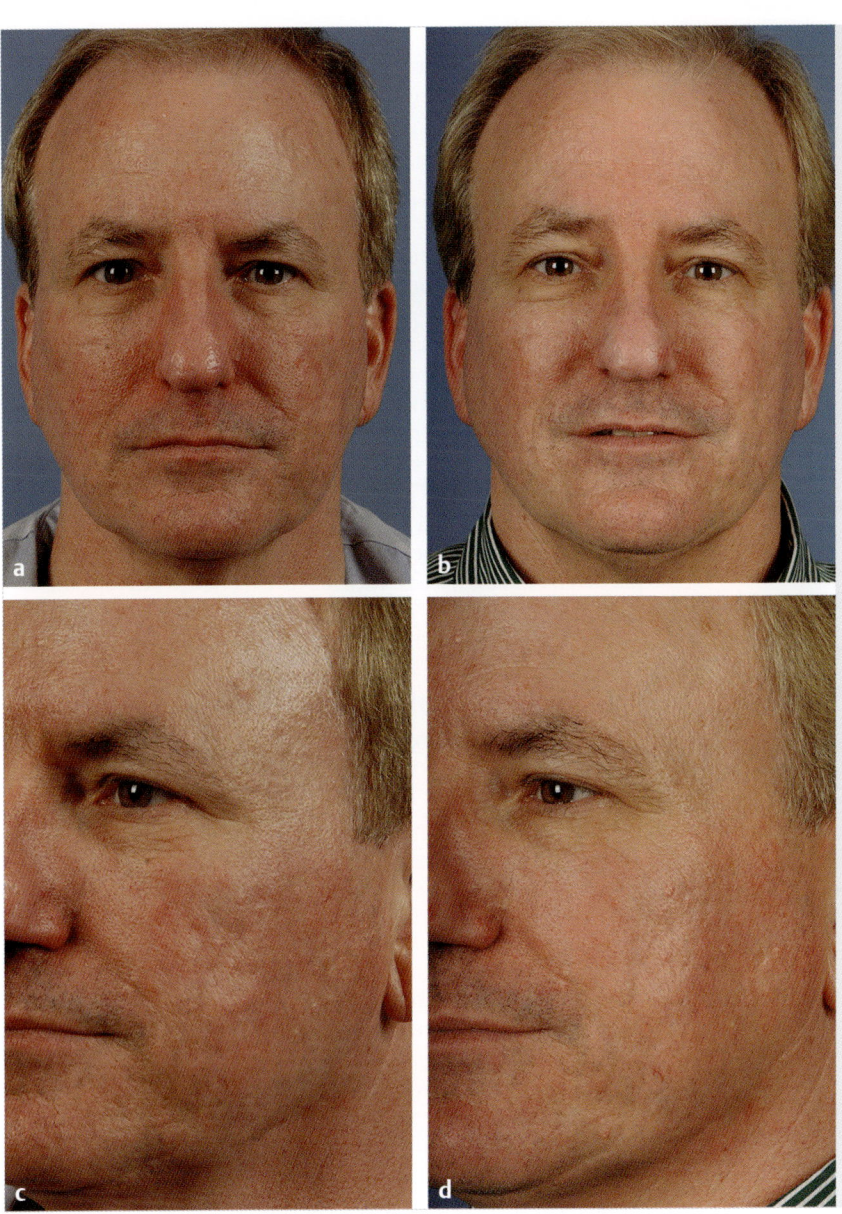

Fig. 11.5 (a,c) A 43-year-old man complained of unsatisfactory scarring from adolescent acne. **(b,d)** Four months after micronized fat injections at the acne scars and 100-micron erbium laser peel.

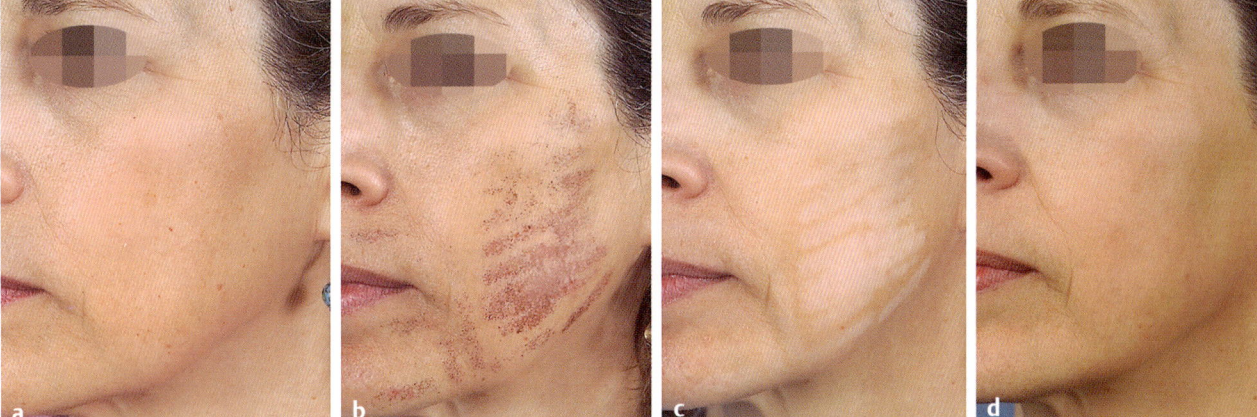

Fig. 11.6 (a) A 48-year-old woman with Fitzgerald type IV skin underwent her third IPL treatment. At the time of treatment, a suntan was not recognized, and **(b)** she subsequently developed localized PIH. The PIH **(c)** was treated and then **(d)** resolved after 6 months with aggressive skin treatment.

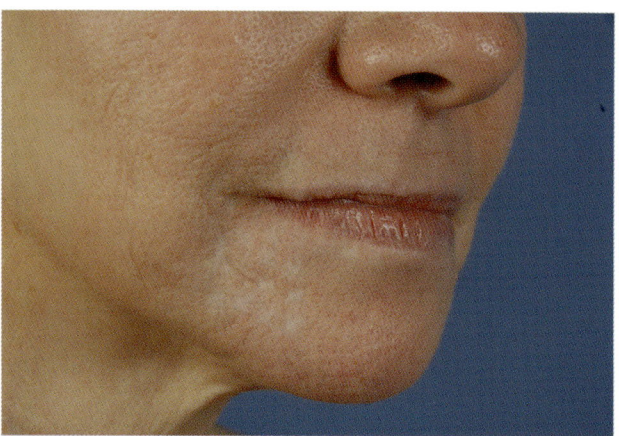

Fig. 11.7 This 54-year-old woman underwent fractionated CO_2 laser resurfacing 9 months previously. She presented with focal areas of hypopigmentation.

genesis with subsequent collagen contraction. Because the RF current is not scattered in the tissue or absorbed by melanin, it is safe to use in patients of all Fitzpatrick skin types.[44]

Four types of RF devices area available: monopolar, bipolar, multipolar, and fractional. Each device requires a specific electrode configuration and generates a different pulse duration and frequency.[45] The nonablative RF devices used in medicine typically have an alternating current between 0.3 and 10MHz.[46] Varying the oscillations of energy delivered changes the target tissue depth, with lower frequencies having longer wavelengths and thus greater depth of penetration.

11.5.1 Patient Selection

RF devices are best used in patients with minimal to moderate skin laxity and lipodystrophy. As with any nonsurgical modality, the patients need to understand that improvement in skin laxity and lipodystrophy, especially in the neck, may lead to other cosmetic deformities such as the exposure of platysmal bands or the uneven correction of adiposity, which may require additional treatments for correction. Patients with severe skin laxity and lipodystrophy are best treated with surgical options.

Contraindications for the use of RF include[47]
- Pregnancy.
- Any implanted electronic device.
- Hip replacement.
- Hip or femur surgery.
- Any implanted metallic device that could be disrupted by RF energy.
- Any active dermatologic or collagen vascular disorder.
- Any active or recent malignancy.
- Any history of disease that may by exacerbated by heat.
- Current use of isotretinoin.
- History of blood coagulation disorders.

11.5.2 Technical Steps and Treatment Plan

As a general rule, we tend to perform simple and less painful procedures first, finishing with the more uncomfortable procedures. If consideration is given to multimodality treatments in a particular area, staging is often performed in the setting of deeper energy-based therapy, because their effect on injectables and fat are unknown.

ThermiTight (ThermiGen, LLC)

1. ½% to 1% xylocaine with epinephrine is warmed and utilized. We place 10-cc syringes in a warmed water bath 15 minutes prior to injection. A room-temperature anesthetic cools the subcutaneous tissues, making treatment longer and more difficult (see Product Index (p. 195)).
2. After waiting 15 minutes, a 16 G needle is used for the access sites. The treatment area is broken down into segments and approached from two sites. The area is homogeneously treated to an internal temperature of 55 to 60 °C and to a temperature of 45 to 47 °C at the surface.
3. Posttreatment, the patients are supported with an elastic chinstrap for a week. Patients do experience swelling for 7 days.

11.5.3 Complications and Shortcomings

Possible complications related to RF therapy include
- Erythema.
- Persistent pain.
- Edema.
- Ecchymosis.
- Burns.

As with all other nonsurgical devices used, approximately one-third of patients have a noticeable positive response, another one-third with minimal change, and a final one-third who do not respond to therapy. Localized fat necrosis may occur in some patients; these typically are self-limiting and get better on their own. Temporary neuropraxia of the marginal mandibular nerve can be seen and is most commonly transient. There are a few shortcomings of current RF and U.S. devices. Oftentimes these devices decrease soft tissue excess to a greater extent than overlying skin laxity. This discrepancy can lead to unwanted contour deformities or exposure of underlying platysmal bands along with persistent skin excess.

11.6 Ultrasound

Ultrasound (US) technology is an acoustic energy-producing modality that can penetrate through tissues to a specific depth while leaving the neighboring tissue relatively unaffected.[48] As the ultrasound travels through the tissue, it is coalesced into distinct areas called *thermal coagulation points* (TCPs). These TCPs form due to a buildup of heat from friction between rapid vibrations of molecules caused by the ultrasonic waves.[49,50] This thermal insult leads down a similar path of collagen damage, collagen shrinkage, and finally neocollagenesis as part of the healing response. Studies have demonstrated clinical tightening and lifting of facial and neck skin.[51,52,53]

11.6.1 Patient Selection

Microfocused ultrasound therapy has FDA approval for lifting of the eyebrows, neck, and submental region. It is also beneficial in the treatment of lines and wrinkles of the décolletage. Two-thirds of patients were satisfied with their treatments, as were 60% of blinded reviewers. One shortcoming of this modality is that it has been found to be less efficacious in patients with BMIs ≥ 30 kg/m2.[54]

A common difficulty with neck rejuvenation is the disappointing longevity of the postoperative neck contours. Even though anterior plastysmaplasty often lasts for many years, the inherent characteristics of skin and soft tissue are not as durable, leading to recurrent skin laxity. Microfocused ultrasound may be able to further tighten recurrent neck skin laxity without requiring additional operative procedures. For those patients unhappy with persistent or recurrent skin laxity, this modality provides a noninvasive alternative that is well tolerated by many patients.

11.6.2 Technical Steps and Treatment Plan

Microfocused Ultrasound

We choose to inject patients with a local anesthetic as our method of analgesia. Our experience with oral narcotics and anxiolytics was not favorable. We feel that a few minutes of "injectable" discomfort is easier for our patients to tolerate than an hour of "procedural" discomfort. It is important to not use epinephrine in your anesthetic, because it tends to eliminate perfusion to the skin and may result in focal heat and skin injury.

Once anesthesia is achieved, we use the scanning ultrasound to interpret the thickness of the skin being treated. We commonly perform two passes, one with the 3.0 mm transducer and the second with the 1.5 mm transducer. We only treat the anterior neck below the hyoid with the 1.5 mm transducer.

Following treatment, some patients may experience dermal swelling that may last for a day or two. We restrict their activities to 4 hours only.

11.6.3 Results

Case Example 4

This 49-year-old woman with a history of chin augmentation presented to the senior author's (Dr. Kenkel's) clinic complaining of excess upper eyelid skin and a prominent tear trough deformity, and she was unhappy with the excess skin and soft tissue along her jawline and neck. After explaining to the patient the various approaches to address her concerns, she ultimately decided to pursue a treatment plan that could be performed locally in the office and with minimal downtime. She subsequently underwent bilateral upper lid blepharoplasty, hyaluronic acid to her tear troughs, and microfocused ultrasound with Ultherapy (Ulthera, Inc.) for treatment of her neck skin laxity and lipodystrophy. Her results are shown in ▶ Fig. 11.8.

Case Example 5

This 55-year-old woman who presented to the clinic was unhappy with the appearance of her excess neck skin and lipodystrophy. She also felt that her tear trough deformities had worsened as she had aged. The patient had heard about Ultherapy for the improvement of neck contours, and she came into the clinic wanting to pursue this treatment option. She was a good candidate for Ultherapy and underwent treatment to her neck while also having hyaluronic acid placed to improve her tear trough deformities. Her results are seen in ▶ Fig. 11.9. She was ultimately not happy with the subtle improvement in her neck contours and went on to have a neck lift performed by Dr. Kenkel.

11.6.4 Postoperative Care

Patients resume their normal skin regimen immediately after treatment.

11.6.5 Complications and Shortcomings

Complications related to ultrasound therapy include
- Procedural and postprocedural pain.
- Ecchymosis.
- Edema.
- Dysesthesia.
- Blisters.
- Erythema at treatment sites.

11.6.6 Skin Care

A well-balanced skin care regimen is crucial for optimizing both surgical and nonsurgical results. All skin care regimens should include sunblock, cleanser, tretinoin/exfoliant, antioxidant, and depigmenting agent when necessary. Much of the superficial skin resurfacing within the epidermis can oftentimes be completed with a good skin care regimen and some patience.

11.7 Combining Surgical and Nonsurgical Modalities

Although surgery is still considered the "gold standard" for the treatment of facial aging, there is a multitude of reasons patients seek out other nonsurgical options, usually related to cost, downtime, or some aversion to surgery. Surgery alone has its own limitations for what is achievable, and this is especially true for central facial rejuvenation and the treatment of sun-damaged skin. Although surgical and nonsurgical modalities are both effective alone for the treatment of many conditions, their combined synergy offers patients a more complete treatment plan to address their concerns.

First and foremost, providers must have a detailed understanding of all nonsurgical devices available. They need to understand the strengths and limitations of these devices, because careless use may lead to irreversible damage to the patient. A safe approach with any new device is to start using it conservatively until a greater knowledge of the device is achieved.

Nonsurgical Salvage and Enhancement of a Surgical Result

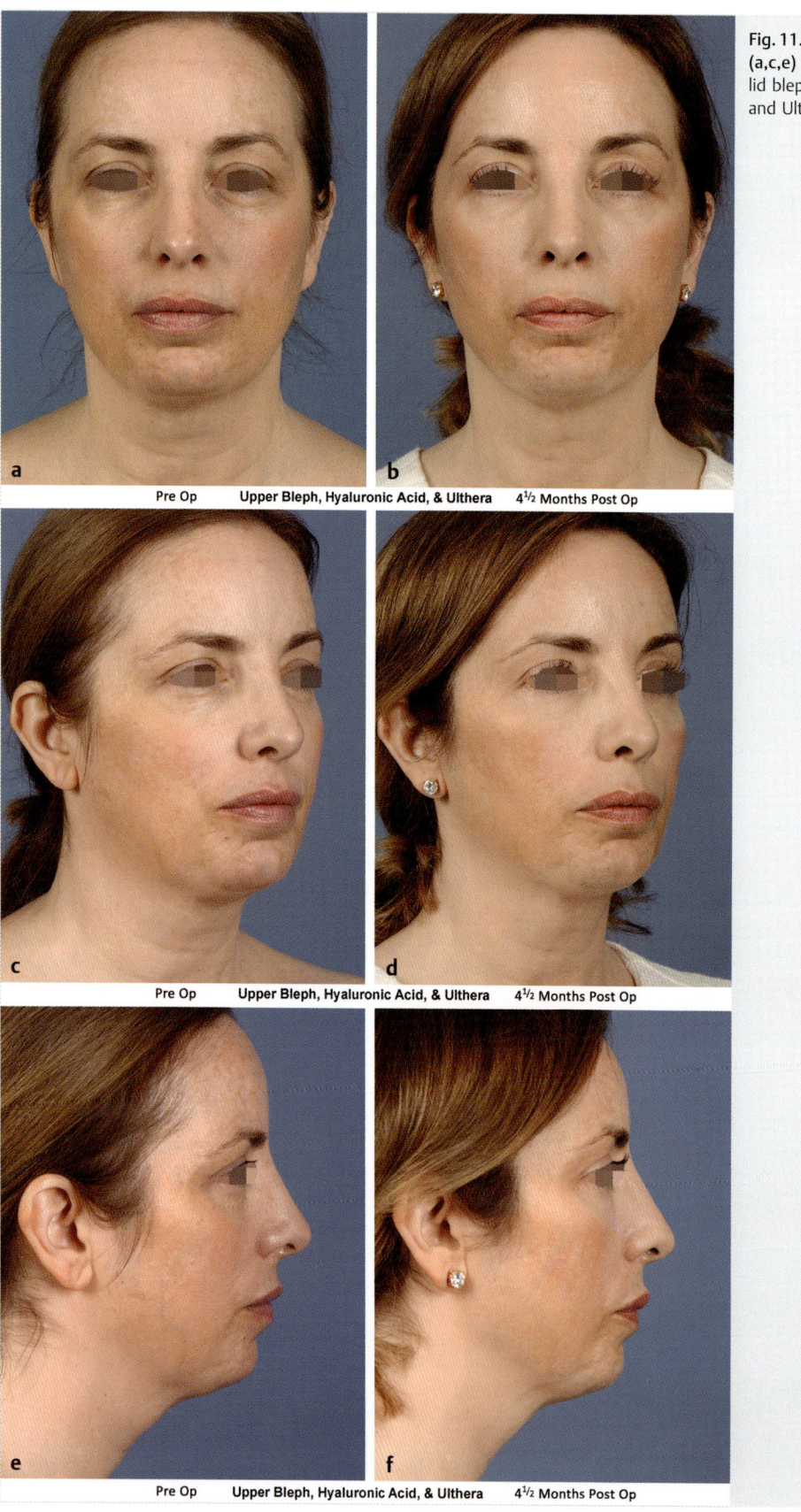

Fig. 11.8 This 49-year-old woman is shown (a,c,e) before and (b,d,f) 4.5 months after upper lid blepharoplasty, HA filler to the malar region, and Ulthera to the neck.

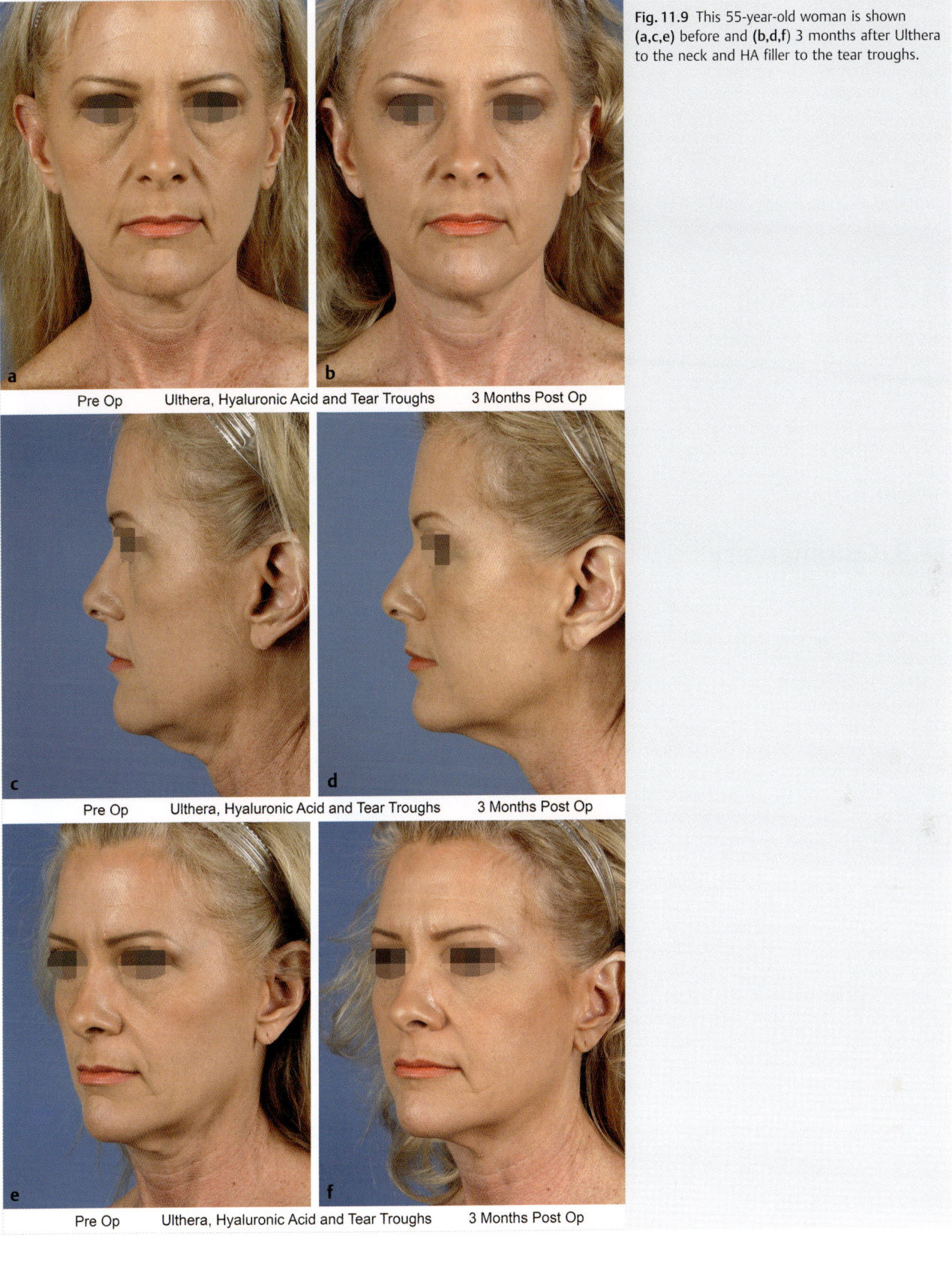

Fig. 11.9 This 55-year-old woman is shown (a,c,e) before and (b,d,f) 3 months after Ulthera to the neck and HA filler to the tear troughs.

Many patients who desire only a subtle change in appearance with minimal to no downtime are ideal candidates for combined therapy. As with any therapy, it is necessary to have a detailed discussion encompassing the patient's desires as well as the limitations of the treatments. Those patients desiring a drastic improvement in skin laxity or lipodystrophy are still better served primarily with surgical options. However, these surgical results may still be optimized through use of the previously mentioned modalities. There are multiple examples in the literature of combining rhytidectomy with laser or chemical facial resurfacing for complete facial rejuvenation.[18,19,20]

11.8 Conclusion

Combining surgical and nonsurgical therapy allows the practitioner to optimize patient results (**Video 11.1**). To maximize the benefits of each device, the provider must have a detailed understanding of the science behind the device. Combined therapy is safe and is well tolerated by many patients in an office-based setting. Although surgery still remains the gold standard, nonsurgical therapy should still comprise a portion of each surgeon's practice.

11.9 Commentary

Julius W. Few Jr.

The authors of this chapter are to be applauded for producing one of the most comprehensive yet practical and concise reviews in publication. This chapter emphasizes controlled damage and inflammation to achieve new collagen formation, based on sound science and principles.

We agree with a preference for the 2940 spectrum for diverse color-friendly applications. With increasing numbers of passes over the skin of the face, more than traditional CO_2, one can achieve more aggressive treatments even when used in a fractional mode of delivery, allowing for great titration ability.

The cases presented are very dynamic and effectively illustrate how, for the plastic surgery patient we all encounter, we want far more but are wanting to avoid surgical intervention due to perceived risk and recovery. The results are excellent, and unneeded surgery was successfully avoided in all patients. The transition is clear, and the treatment strategy is analogous to approaches we have used in our clinic.

The guide in this chapter is not only useful for treatment but also a useful guide for estimated downtimes and management.

Case 1 highlights one of my preferred combinations of micronized fat injection with laser resurfacing while doing periorbital rejuvenation surgery, which can easily be done under local anesthesia with a mild oral sedative.[55]

References

[1] Statistics-American Society of Aesthetic Plastic Surgery. Available at: http://www.surgery.org/media/statistics2016
[2] Arnoczky SP, Aksan A. Thermal modification of connective tissues: basic science considerations and clinical implications. J Am Acad Orthop Surg. 2000; 8(5):305–313
[3] Ross EV, Yashar SS, Naseef GS, et al. A pilot study of in vivo immediate tissue contraction with CO2 skin laser resurfacing in a live farm pig. Dermatol Surg. 1999; 25(11):851–856
[4] le Lous M, Flandin F, Herbage D, Allain JC. Influence of collagen denaturation on the chemorheological properties of skin, assessed by differential scanning calorimetry and hydrothermal isometric tension measurement. Biochim Biophys Acta. 1982; 717(2):295–300
[5] Bozec L, Odlyha M. Thermal denaturation studies of collagen by microthermal analysis and atomic force microscopy. Biophys J. 2011; 101(1):228–236
[6] Lin SJ, Hsiao CY, Sun Y, et al. Monitoring the thermally induced structural transitions of collagen by use of second-harmonic generation microscopy. Opt Lett. 2005; 30(6):622–624
[7] Hsu TS, Kaminer MS. The use of nonablative radiofrequency technology to tighten the lower face and neck. Semin Cutan Med Surg. 2003; 22(2):115–123
[8] Despa F, Orgill DP, Neuwalder J, Lee RC. The relative thermal stability of tissue macromolecules and cellular structure in burn injury. Burns. 2005; 31(5):568–577
[9] Farkas JP, Hoopman JE, Kenkel JM. Five parameters you must understand to master control of your laser/light-based devices. Aesthet Surg J. 2013; 33(7):1059–1064
[10] Ozturk S, Hoopman J, Brown SA, et al. A useful algorithm for determining fluence and pulse width for vascular targets using 1,064 nm Nd:YAG laser in an animal model. Lasers Surg Med. 2004; 34(5):420–425
[11] Geronemus RG. Fractional photothermolysis: current and future applications. Lasers Surg Med. 2006; 38(3):169–176
[12] Manstein D, Herron GS, Sink RK, Tanner H, Anderson RR. Fractional photothermolysis: a new concept for cutaneous remodeling using microscopic patterns of thermal injury. Lasers Surg Med. 2004; 34(5):426–438
[13] Farkas JP, Richardson JA, Burrus CF, Hoopman JE, Brown SA, Kenkel JM. In vivo histopathologic comparison of the acute injury following treatment with five fractional ablative laser devices. Aesthet Surg J. 2010; 30(3):457–464
[14] Oni G, Robbins D, Bailey S, Brown SA, Kenkel JM. An in vivo histopathological comparison of single and double pulsed modes of a fractionated CO(2) laser. Lasers Surg Med. 2012; 44(1):4–10
[15] Major A, Brazzini B, Campolmi P, et al. Nd:YAG 1064 nm laser in the treatment of facial and leg telangiectasias. J Eur Acad Dermatol Venereol. 2001; 15(6):559–565
[16] Clark C, Cameron H, Moseley H, Ferguson J, Ibbotson SH. Treatment of superficial cutaneous vascular lesions: experience with the KTP 532 nm laser. Lasers Med Sci. 2004; 19(1):1–5
[17] Dudelzak J, Hussain M, Goldberg DJ. Vascular-specific laser wavelength for the treatment of facial telangiectasias. J Drugs Dermatol. 2009; 8(3):227–229
[18] Scheuer JF, III, Costa CR, Dauwe PB, Ramanadham SR, Rohrich RJ. Laser resurfacing at the time of rhytidectomy. Plast Reconstr Surg. 2015; 136(1):27–38
[19] Weinstein C, Pozner J, Scheflan M, Achauer BM. Combined erbium:YAG resurfacing and face lifting. Plast Reconstr Surg. 2001; 107(2):593–594
[20] Hollmig ST, Struck SK, Hantash BM. Establishing the safety and efficacy of simultaneous face lift and intraoperative full face and neck fractional carbon dioxide resurfacing. Plast Reconstr Surg. 2012; 129(4):737e–739e
[21] Ha RY, Byrd HS. Septal extension grafts revisited: 6-year experience in controlling nasal tip projection and shape. Plast Reconstr Surg. 2003; 112(7):1929–1935
[22] Cisneros JL, Río R, Palou J. The Q-switched neodymium (Nd):YAG laser with quadruple frequency. Clinical histological evaluation of facial resurfacing using different wavelengths. Dermatol Surg. 1998; 24(3):345–350
[23] Bencini PL, Luci A, Galimberti M, Ferranti G. Long-term epilation with long-pulsed neodimium:YAG laser. Dermatol Surg. 1999; 25(3):175–178
[24] Goldberg DJ. Laser- and light-based hair removal: an update. Expert Rev Med Devices. 2007; 4(2):253–260
[25] Tanzi EL, Alster TS. Long-pulsed 1064-nm Nd:YAG laser-assisted hair removal in all skin types. Dermatol Surg. 2004; 30(1):13–17
[26] Alster TS, Bryan H, Williams CM. Long-pulsed Nd:YAG laser-assisted hair removal in pigmented skin: a clinical and histological evaluation. Arch Dermatol. 2001; 137(7):885–889
[27] Bernstein EF, Kornbluth S, Brown DB, Black J. Treatment of spider veins using a 10 millisecond pulse-duration frequency-doubled neodymium YAG laser. Dermatol Surg. 1999; 25(4):316–320
[28] Sadick NS. Laser treatment of leg veins. Skin Therapy Lett. 2004; 9(9):6–9

[29] Rogachefsky AS, Silapunt S, Goldberg DJ. Nd:YAG laser (1064 nm) irradiation for lower extremity telangiectases and small reticular veins: efficacy as measured by vessel color and size. Dermatol Surg. 2002; 28(3):220–223

[30] Eremia S, Li CY. Treatment of leg and face veins with a cryogen spray variable pulse width 1064-nm Nd:YAG laser–a prospective study of 47 patients. J Cosmet Laser Ther. 2001; 3(3):147–153

[31] Holcomb JD. Versatility of erbium YAG laser: from fractional skin rejuvenation to full-field skin resurfacing. Facial Plast Surg Clin North Am. 2011; 19(2):261–273

[32] Alster TS, Lupton JR. Erbium:YAG cutaneous laser resurfacing. Dermatol Clin. 2001; 19(3):453–466

[33] Sapijaszko MJ, Zachary CB. Er:YAG laser skin resurfacing. Dermatol Clin. 2002; 20(1):87–96

[34] Jimenez G, Spencer JM. Erbium:YAG laser resurfacing of the hands, arms, and neck. Dermatol Surg. 1999; 25(11):831–834, discussion 834–835

[35] Hughes PS. Skin contraction following erbium:YAG laser resurfacing. Dermatol Surg. 1998; 24(1):109–111

[36] Angermeier MC. Treatment of facial vascular lesions with intense pulsed light. J Cutan Laser Ther. 1999; 1(2):95–100

[37] Goldman MP, Weiss RA, Weiss MA. Intense pulsed light as a nonablative approach to photoaging. Dermatol Surg. 2005; 31(9 Pt 2):1179–1187, discussion 1187

[38] Bitter PH. Noninvasive rejuvenation of photodamaged skin using serial, full-face intense pulsed light treatments. Dermatol Surg. 2000; 26(9):835–842, discussion 843

[39] Johnson F, Dovale M. Intense pulsed light treatment of hirsutism: case reports of skin phototypes V and VI. J Cutan Laser Ther. 1999; 1(4):233–237

[40] Ransom ER, Antunes MB, Bloom JD, Greco T. Concurrent structural fat grafting and carbon dioxide laser resurfacing for perioral and lower face rejuvenation. J Cosmet Laser Ther. 2011; 13(1):6–12

[41] Kim EM, Bucky LP. Power of the pinch: pinch lower lid blepharoplasty. Ann Plast Surg. 2008; 60(5):532–537

[42] Oni G, Brown S, Kenkel J. Comparison of five commonly-available, lidocaine-containing topical anesthetics and their effect on serum levels of lidocaine and its metabolite monoethylglycinexylidide (MEGX). Aesthet Surg J. 2012; 32(4):495–503

[43] Oni G, Brown S, Burrus C, et al. Effect of 4% topical lidocaine applied to the face on the serum levels of lidocaine and its metabolite, monoethylglycinexylidide. Aesthet Surg J. 2010; 30(6):853–858

[44] Sadick N. Tissue tightening technologies: fact or fiction. Aesthet Surg J. 2008; 28(2):180–188

[45] Weinkle AP, Sofen B, Emer J. Synergistic approaches to neck rejuvenation and lifting. J Drugs Dermatol. 2015; 14(11):1215–1228

[46] Sadick NS, Makino Y. Selective electro-thermolysis in aesthetic medicine: a review. Lasers Surg Med. 2004; 34(2):91–97

[47] Belenky I, Margulis A, Elman M, Bar-Yosef U, Paun SD. Exploring channeling optimized radiofrequency energy: a review of radiofrequency history and applications in esthetic fields. Adv Ther. 2012; 29(3):249–266

[48] Kennedy JE, Ter Haar GR, Cranston D. High intensity focused ultrasound: surgery of the future? Br J Radiol. 2003; 76(909):590–599

[49] White WM, Makin IR, Barthe PG, Slayton MH, Gliklich RE. Selective creation of thermal injury zones in the superficial musculoaponeurotic system using intense ultrasound therapy: a new target for noninvasive facial rejuvenation. Arch Facial Plast Surg. 2007; 9(1):22–29

[50] Gliklich RE, White WM, Slayton MH, Barthe PG, Makin IR. Clinical pilot study of intense ultrasound therapy to deep dermal facial skin and subcutaneous tissues. Arch Facial Plast Surg. 2007; 9(2):88–95

[51] Fabi SG, Goldman MP. Retrospective evaluation of micro-focused ultrasound for lifting and tightening the face and neck. Dermatol Surg. 2014; 40(5):569–575

[52] Alam M, White LE, Martin N, Witherspoon J, Yoo S, West DP. Ultrasound tightening of facial and neck skin: a rater-blinded prospective cohort study. J Am Acad Dermatol. 2010; 62(2):262–269

[53] Kenkel J. Evaluation of the Ulthera System for achieving lift and tightening cheek tissue, improving jawline definition and submental skin laxity. Paper presented at: American Society for Laser Medicine and Surgery, 2013; Boston, MA

[54] Oni G, Hoxworth R, Teotia S, Brown S, Kenkel JM. Evaluation of a microfocused ultrasound system for improving skin laxity and tightening in the lower face. Aesthet Surg J. 2014; 34(7):1099–1110

[55] Butz DR, Gill KK, Randle J, Kampf N, Few JW, . Facial aesthetic surgery: the safe use of oral sedation in an office-based facility. Aesthetics Society Journal. 2016; 36(2):127–131

12 Integrating Technology in Facial Plastic Surgery

Jonathan M. Sykes and Amir Allak

Summary
This chapter discusses the role of technology in facial plastic surgery. We will analyze the methods and influences that affect physician and patient choices and discuss the role of industry and the Internet in educating and biasing patients. We will also consider the many factors that influence every practitioner, such as economics, ego, industry advertising, and skill level.

Keywords: adipocytolysis, advertising, biases, cryolipolysis, decision-making, deoxycholic acid, direct-to-consumer advertising (DTCA), facial analysis, hair restoration, laser technology, lipolysis, liposuction, online marketing, patient expectations, push marketing, social media, technology, ultrasonic energy therapy

> **Key Points**
> - An essential element of a facial plastic surgery practice is the ability to critically evaluate newer and emerging technology and the resulting investment.
> - An effective marketing strategy is critical to support the success of a facial plastic surgeon.
> - Direct-to-consumer advertising and social media can influence patients and have changed the means of exposure to new companies and devices.

12.1 Introduction

Each time that a facial plastic surgery patient requests alteration in facial appearance and/or function, the practitioner faces a decision-making process that includes several factors: the wants and desires of the patient, the facial analysis, the psychological composition of the patient, and the inherent biases and skills of the surgeon.

Of course, the specific requests of an individual patient are of paramount importance in shaping the discussion regarding procedure choice. The change(s) that the patient is seeking should always be the most important factor in deciding which recommendations to make. After considering the patient's goals, the surgeon should then discuss the therapeutic treatment options. This dialogue is important in educating and empowering each patient. The communication that occurs during the initial consultation plays a significant role in determining whether the patient's expectations can be met and if the procedures suggested will accomplish the patient's desires. This process is as important a factor in determining patient satisfaction as is the performance of the procedure itself.

The best therapeutic option for any patient may be a single procedure or a combination of procedures and technologies. The practitioner's individual skill, comfort level, and personal bias influence what procedure(s) is recommended. It is the duty of each practitioner to use the best evidence regarding any procedure or technology before suggesting this to any patient. It is only after being presented this evidence that the patient can make an informed choice on any given procedure.

This chapter will discuss the role of technology in facial plastic surgery. Specifically, the methods and influences that affect physician and patient choices will be analyzed. The role of industry and the Internet in educating and biasing patients will also be discussed. Finally, the factors that influence every practitioner—economics, ego, industry advertising, and skill level—will be considered.

12.2 Patient Desires

The Internet has been a vehicle to globalize facial plastic surgery. It has contributed to the increase in the frequency of procedures, has improved access to patient education, and has allowed plastic surgeons to advertise their skills and market their practices. Physicians realize that patients relish the ability to research their doctor and his or her practice. Patients often cannot discriminate between fact and fiction, and the information provided on the Internet is not monitored for reliability or accuracy.

Patients commonly request new procedures, products, or technologies. They often feel that what is new is desirable. To many patients, recently adopted procedures with marketed names afford an advantage over more established procedures and technologies. It is common for a plastic surgery patient to ask their practitioner, "Do you have anything new?" or "Are there any new techniques that you are using?" Patients are frequently persuaded by physicians who market their new or "special" technique, or by the industry that markets their product as "the best." The combination of the patient wanting the "latest and greatest" and the physician wanting to sell their product and/or services often makes the patient prey to misleading predictions of outcomes.

12.3 Physician Advertising

Advertising and marketing is an important component of practice in plastic surgery. Individuals who practice any aspect of cosmetic medicine realize that success in their practice is related to their ability to advertise their products and to market their skills. Aesthetic surgery and related aesthetic services are "created wants," not needs. Advertising makes patients aware of the services offered and is an avenue for physicians to educate the public about the credentials and experience of the physician. The Internet is also a tremendous vehicle to disseminate information and to describe new technologies and services.

Two main strategies exist in advertising aesthetic products and services: push and pull marketing campaigns. Each of these strategies is well suited for certain types of offerings provided by facial plastic surgeons and can also be inefficient and unproductive uses of valuable resources when applied in the wrong setting.

Push marketing is defined as the advertising of products or services to potential customers without having considered the good/service before being exposed to the campaign. Examples of push marketing include television or print advertisements, mailing flyers, billboards, and certain types of social media and online marketing. This is what most would consider to be traditional advertising. Push marketing has a high exposure level to a broad population; however, the yield of actual purchases is often proportionally low. The ideal service/product to market with the push design would be targeted toward a patient population that would not normally frequent an aesthetic practice or not be aware of the offering and/or its advantages. An example would be for robotic or micrograft hair transplant. Male patients do not often visit facial plastic surgeons for other purposes and therefore would not necessarily have exposure to hair transplant options without some external promotion.

In pull marketing strategies, consumers who are already engaged in a relationship with the seller are given information about products during ongoing consultation. This is a more familiar archetype for facial plastic surgeons, because the discussion of options for facial rejuvenation often lends itself well to an introduction of new products or procedures. Examples include introducing a patient to a new facial filler or skin resurfacing device while weighing rejuvenative options. Because patients will often see not only the surgeon but also the aesthetician and clinic staff, it is imperative that all staff are aware of the new offerings and can introduce them when relevant. The penetrative exposure of pull marketing is low, but the yield is higher than with push marketing and it has the additive ability to foster trust and build the surgeon–patient relationship.

Both pull and push marketing are useful to inform patients of the goods and services provided in facial plastic surgery. The ideal blend varies based on the spectrum of offerings, the degree of establishment of a practice, and the age and demographics of the clientele, and it can even vary geographically. This is also based on the practice blend of each individual office. Offices that provide cash-based facial aesthetic services in addition to functional insurance-based services will likely find that a different strategy is beneficial to that of a full-time cosmetic practice. Hybrid practices may use more push marketing, because the patients there may not be aware of these services, and sometimes this can be as simple as displaying flyers or providing educational materials in the clinic waiting room. Full-time aesthetic practices will likely have relatively more pull marketing, because patients are already presenting for rejuvenation, but these practices should also employ push marketing to a certain degree to attract new clientele to the office. Regardless of the approach, it is imperative to continually re-evaluate the efficacy of a practice's marketing strategy to ensure that resources are not being wasted and that the return on investment of advertising is acceptable. See ▶ Table 12.1 for a summary and comparison.

12.4 The Role of Industry

Medical device companies play an important role in plastic surgery practices. They fund technology that creates new devices, which expand the services provided to patients. Increasing technology positively impacts physicians' practices, and can improve the overall aesthetic results for patients. Creating these new technologies requires funding that would not be possible without companies willing to raise capital in an effort to capitalize on these technologies.

Of course, the main goal of medical device companies is profit. The process for companies to create profit is to stimulate a new idea, to create and fund the technology, and then to market and sell it. Selling the technology involves marketing the device to the physician and direct-to-consumer advertising (DTCA).

In some ways, DTCA by industry can benefit the aesthetic surgery market and individual physician practices. However, it is common for drug and device companies to inflate the efficacy and downplay the safety issues related to their drug or device. Industry in medicine often gets a product FDA-approved and then markets the product without an adequate scientific basis. The model—the product, followed by marketing, then followed possibly by science—can be deceptive to the public. Physicians cannot rely on the statements of manufacturers to ensure the validity of claims often made by companies to sell products. It is the responsibility of the physician to not just repeat the manufacturer's party line, but also to confirm the accuracy of their claims. This is done by carefully analyzing aesthetic outcomes and monitoring patient satisfaction from new devices and procedures.

12.5 Skin Tightening and Fat Reduction

For many years, the only means to reduce fat volume was with a surgical procedure. In the body, this required liposuction (with or without abdominoplasty or other body lift). In the neck, submental liposuction with or without neck lifting or facelifting was the only treatment. More recently, devices and injectable drugs that create lipolysis and tighten the soft tissues have been designed, giving the patient and practitioner alternatives to surgery (**see Video 2.11**).

Table 12.1 A Summary and Comparison of Marketing Strategies

	Push Marketing	Pull Marketing
Visibility/exposure	High	Low
Yield (patients who pursue product/service based on marketing)	Low	High
Target audience	Those who have not considered/are unaware of procedure/product	Patients already seeking aesthetic improvement
Ideal practice	Both hybrid practices and pure aesthetic	Pure aesthetic

12.5.1 Deoxycholic Acid

An injectable form of deoxycholic acid, Kybella (keoxycholic acid, Allergan, Inc.) has been FDA approved for infiltration into the preplatysmal fat for the reduction of submental fat (see Product Index (p. 170)).[1,2,3,4] When injected subcutaneously into fat, Kybella causes adipocytolysis, and stimulates a local tissue response consisting of macrophage infiltration (to remove cellular debris and liberated lipids), fibroblast recruitment, and collagen production (neocollagenesis).[3] The desired effect is to improve the submental contour and decrease submental fullness. The treatment process is performed as a 20-minute procedure in an office setting and usually requires 2 to 4 treatments to achieve maximal improvement in neck contour.[1] This technique has minimal downtime and can often replace submental liposuction, in addition to having off-label potential for body contouring in other areas.[5]

12.5.2 CoolSculpting

The recently developed CoolSculpting (ZELTIQ Aesthetics, Inc.) device utilizes thermogenic damage of superficial adipocytes to induce what the company has named *cryolipolysis* (see Product Index (p. 180)). For days to weeks following the treatment, the damaged adipose tissue is cleared by macrophages and neutrophils and theoretically results in a reduction of the superficial fatty tissue.[6] The length of the procedure is approximately 60 minutes on average, and effects can be apparent in weeks to months after the procedure. Most patients will have 1 to 2 treatments depending on the individual patient response and patient preference.

The CoolSculpting device is FDA-approved for use in the abdomen, thigh, flank, back, axilla, and submental areas, and it is sometimes used off-label in other areas as well.[7,8] Advantages to CoolSculpting treatments are that it is noninvasive and does not require an anesthetic or incision. There is virtually no postprocedure downtime, and there is minimal discomfort to the patient during and after the procedure. Side effects are mild and include temporary erythema and ecchymosis, paresthesia/numbness, and mild pain, with severe complications exceedingly rare.[7] In those patients who are surgery-averse, CoolSculpting offers a reasonable option for improvement in body contour. Also, because this procedure can be performed by a nurse, technician, or aesthetician, it does not require a large time commitment by the surgeon. Disadvantages to the treatment include inconsistent results and the repeated or additional treatments required by some patients. The cost averages approximately $2000 per treatment, but this amount varies geographically. From a cost perspective, a fair amount of the charges are composed of relatively high-cost consumables, particularly the applicators. As far as the durability of results, long-term data has not yet been published. This makes it difficult to communicate the predictability of the treatment to patients. Anecdotally, practitioners find that if the patient gains body weight during the postprocedure period, the results are somewhat truncated.

12.5.3 Ultherapy

Ultherapy (Ulthera, Inc.) is designed as a skin-tightening device that uses ultrasonic energy to induce collagen production and deposition in the subcutaneous tissues (see Product Index (p. 185)). Using a combined imaging and treatment ultrasound probe, the Ultherapist provides pulses of ultrasound at various depths of the subdermis and superficial fat.[9] Treatments average approximately 60 minutes depending on the number of area(s) treated. Ultherapy is FDA-approved for use in the neck, upper chest, and brow, and its off-label uses include the midface and other areas of the body.[10]

Advantages of the Ultherapy procedure include another nonsurgical and scarless approach to induce facial rejuvenation, with little to no downtime and postprocedure healing (▶ Fig. 12.1). Also, the Ultherapist does not have to be an MD or nurse in most U.S. states, thus providing an opportunity cost-benefit in freeing the surgeon for other productivity. The therapy has also been shown to be safe with relatively few complications.

The major disadvantages of Ultherapy is the variability of results and some patients may even report worsening of their skin laxity. Also, the procedure itself can be somewhat uncomfortable and even painful, sometimes requiring oral analgesics or anxiolytics.[9] The device is quite expensive to purchase, and the consumables have similarly high prices, which often translates into bigger charges to the patients, averaging $2,000 to $3,000 with additional charges for added subsites.

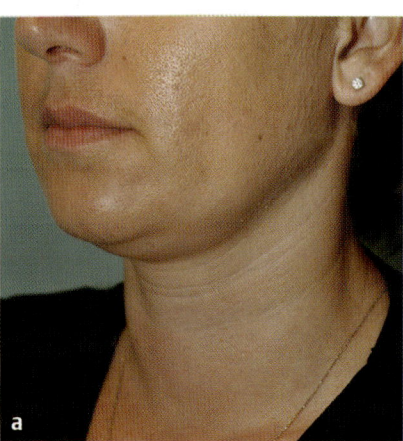 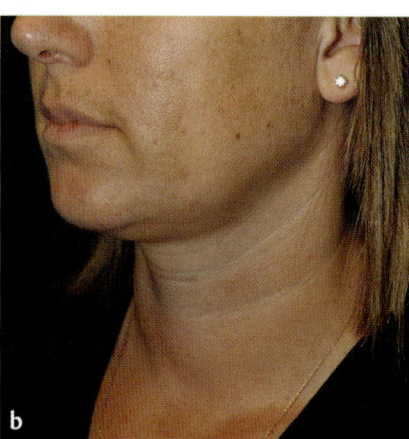

Fig. 12.1 (a) Before and (b) after Ultherapy treatment.

Integrating Technology in Facial Plastic Surgery

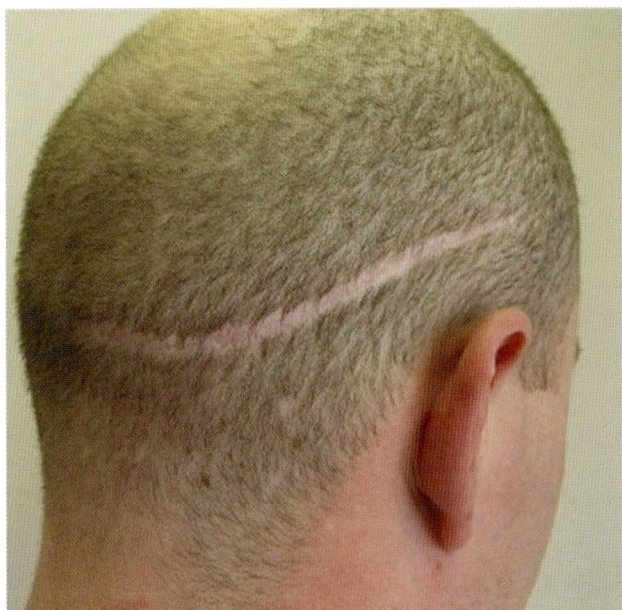

Fig. 12.2 Poorly scarred strip harvest site.

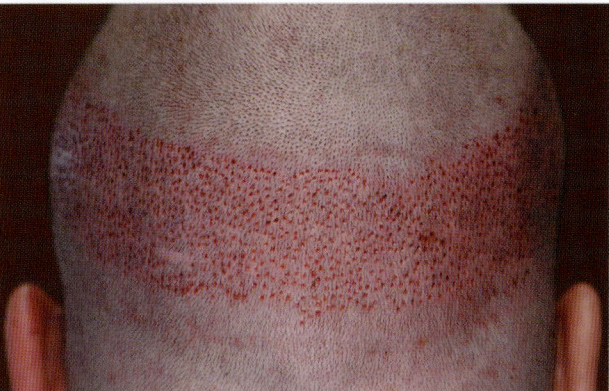

Fig. 12.3 Immediate postoperative following follicular unit extraction (FUE).

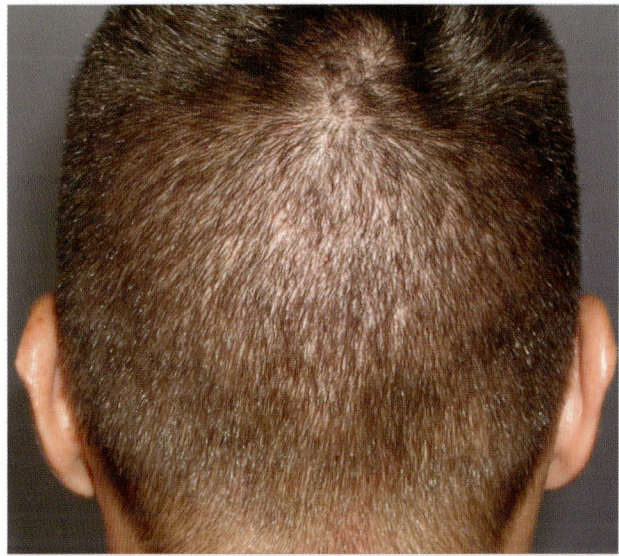

Fig. 12.4 One-week postoperative following follicular unit extraction (FUE).

12.5.4 New Devices for Microfollicular Hair Transplantation

The most utilized method of surgical hair restoration is follicular unit transplantation (FUT).[11] The most common mode of donor harvest of hair follicle units has been this strip technique. In this procedure, a midoccipital transverse strip of scalp is excised (approximately 1 cm wide × 10 to 30 cm long) at a level just below the hair follicles within the subcutaneous fat layer. This strip is then cut into microfollicular units, and the individual transplant units are reimplanted using a "stab-and-stick" method. The disadvantage of this technique is that an occipitoparietal scar is made, which is often noticeable in patients with short, dark hair.[11,12] (▶ Fig. 12.2).

Many new devices have been designed to extract individual follicular units that are ready for reimplantation immediately after harvest and do not require sectioning into follicular units (as do the hair grafts from FUT). This technique is called *follicular unit extraction* (FUE). The most popular of the devices that perform FUE is the NeoGraft (NeoGraft Solutions, Inc.), which allows individual follicular units to be harvested from the parietooccipital region of the scalp in a random pattern (▶ Fig. 12.3). More expensive robotic models perform both donor harvest and recipient implantation.[13] With this device, not only are the grafts harvested, but also precise cuts are made in the recipient region followed by graft implantation. The primary advantage of FUE is prevention of an occipital donor scar. This is a valuable selling point for prospective hair transplant patients. The rapid hair regrowth in the donor area allows patients to return to daily activity fairly soon after the procedure[13] (▶ Fig. 12.4).

12.5.5 Lasers in Facial Plastic Surgery

Laser technology has become a common tool for addressing various needs in facial skin care and rejuvenation (see Product Index (p. 176)). Laser stands for "light amplification by the stimulated emission of radiation," and energy emitted by a laser has specific properties. These include monochromaticity, allowing the energy to be focused to a certain frequency/wavelength and thus targeting specific chromophores; collimation, causing laser light to travel in parallel beams and resisting diffraction, thus allowing for a specific area of treatment; coherence, meaning the light beams travel in phases so that there is consistent delivery of the energy. As a result of these properties, each individual laser is specific to target a single chromophore. Some chromophores are as ubiquitous as water or hemoglobin, whereas some are less prevalent such as tattoo ink or melanin.

The use of lasers in a facial plastic surgery practice can be a successful nonsurgical adjunctive set of procedures that can supplement the surgical offerings. For uses such as laser hair removal, tattoo removal, and cutaneous lesion depigmentation, the surgical alternative is an onerous and often unreasonable option. Patients who seek these treatments would otherwise not visit a surgical practice. This can be advantageous in the direct sense of providing the laser procedure itself, and also it could provide exposure to any practice's array of services and provide an opportunity for pull marketing.

However, in some applications of lasers, there are common and acceptable surgical alternatives such as facial skin resurfacing and eyelid skin treatment (in lieu of blepharoplasty). Although these can be useful to offer as an alternative for surgical treatments, the surgeon must take care to supplement but not cannibalize his or her surgical practice.

12.6 Device Decision-making

The decision to integrate any given technology into an aesthetic surgery or medicine practice is a complex one involving many factors. Considerations include the resources required to make a technology successful, the cost of the device and associated consumables, and the practitioner's thought as to whether the treatments will be efficacious and safe. Because most devices are costly, the business plan for each device is an important factor.

The business model for aesthetic devices is significantly different than the model for most injectables, such as botulinum toxins or facial fillers. The cost of a vial of botulinum toxin or a syringe of a facial filler is relatively small, and this allows the practitioner to create a profit and recover this expense relatively quickly. Additionally, if the practitioner decides that they do not want to continue providing the service (e.g., injectable facial fillers), there is not a large capital expense that needs to be recuperated after the service is discontinued (**see Video 1.1**).

The financial model for a large device such as a laser, Ultherapy, or an FUE hair device is much different. For example, a typical skin resurfacing laser may cost $100,000 to $150,000. After adding the nursing or technician and consumable costs to the original laser cost, it may require approximately $200,000 of patient revenue before a financial break-even point occurs. Although practitioners would often rather think about the effectiveness of treatment rather than financial models, it is very important to consider the costs of a given device before deciding on including it in the practice.

The efficacy and safety of any given device are also important considerations. In order to determine if a given device/procedure is effective, it is necessary to analyze patient results and adverse event data. The burden for FDA approval for devices is less than the burden for drug approval. Because of this, less efficacy and safety data are available. In that device companies desire to sell products, the information available is jaded, and the buyer must be careful in considering the effectiveness of any device and scrutinize any potential purchase with these factors in mind.

12.7 Conclusion

Integrating technology into plastic surgery practice is an important component to offering a complete range of services. Most patients request new procedures and technologies, because these services are heavily marketed on the Internet. It is the job of the aesthetic practitioner to carefully consider each device and the associated technology in order to provide efficacy and safety, and to predict honest results. It is this combination that will allow each patient to make an informed decision regarding the technology and procedure.

12.8 Commentary

Julius W. Few Jr.

The authors present a perspective of a past president for the Facial Plastic Surgery Society and a hybrid practice model, with strong academic and private practice perspectives. I asked Dr. Sykes to produce a chapter that gives a dynamic perspective to the topic of nonsurgical strategies and how to incorporate them from his perspective. He has presented a present-day assessment of strategies to consider globally, and this can apply to anyone seriously considering cosmetic medicine. This chapter brings to bear, in pure economic and marketing terms, concepts at work but not described in the world of aesthetics.

We are presented with a dynamic that illustrates how one application can beget a second, a third, and so on. The patient that presents for nonsurgical, focused ultrasound, tissue tightening, and lifting may also be the patient who wants resurfacing and then hair restoration. It then becomes a delicate balance of awareness vs. "selling" offerings. We know, through a variety of well-established business models, that businesses with related offerings have the scale to grow, because their consumer only needs to go to one location for related services. These businesses with related offerings are similar to the hair salon that offers hair styling, cutting, coloring, and product support.

It is increasingly more difficult to be a "pure surgical" practice today, and this chapter helps to explain in very technical detail why this is reality.

This chapter also shows how rapidly technology is evolving in this space, given that now cryolipolysis can be done in approximately half the time with the newly available applicators coming onto the market. In addition, the cost–benefit discussion, for the patient and treating practice alike, is very real. I think the descriptions and considerations are fair, but it is easy to see the glass as "half full" or "half empty" depending on the reader's bias.

Ultimately, one cannot deny the overwhelming desire of our patients to pursue nonsurgical face and body options for enhancement. For the facial plastic surgeon, the use of nonsurgical body contouring may be a new frontier, and the relevant expectation for the given patient must be seriously considered and understood by the plastic surgeon to avoid patient dissatisfaction. The ability to combine applications that have no disposable cost, such as external radiofrequency, can give a significant buffer to allow for results in patients who obtain less than the ideal enhancement and can effectively salvage an unhappy relationship between the surgeon and the patient.[14]

In addition, one must be careful to not fall into a practice solution that leads to an uncharted space. In particular, the use of nonsurgical body contouring should not be seriously considered in a more severe case in which surgery is clearly indicated. Pushing the limits in severe cases only leads to disappointment, and the treating practice is often expected to offer an alternative or a refund of the patient's money. If the surgeon does not specialize in body contouring surgery, this can create a significant dilemma and lead to potential loss of a patient and/or a nonspecialist feeling pressured into a more involved treatment option with a very different risk profile.

Ultimately, it is well described that it is much more satisfying and financially beneficial to obtain patients by internal practice base than externally based marketing efforts. If one offers treatment options that do not match the patient expectation, that patient will leave the given practice and search for a new one. When this occurs, it is more than just a loss of the patient, because it is also the loss of a revenue source and the associated referral source. The bottom line is that the nonsurgical solutions not only work and produce happy patients, but also they must be used in the right setting, and combinations can help expand the given potential for a practice model.

References

[1] Humphrey S, Sykes J, Kantor J, et al. ATX-101 for reduction of submental fat: A phase III randomized controlled trial. J Am Acad Dermatol. 2016; 75(4):788–797.e7

[2] Jones DH, Carruthers J, Joseph JH, et al. REFINE-1, a multicenter, randomized, double-blind, placebo-controlled, phase 3 trial with ATX-101, an injectable drug for submental fat reduction. Dermatol Surg. 2016; 42(1):38–49

[3] Ascher B, Hoffmann K, Walker P, Lippert S, Wollina U, Havlickova B. Efficacy, patient-reported outcomes and safety profile of ATX-101 (deoxycholic acid), an injectable drug for the reduction of unwanted submental fat: results from a phase III, randomized, placebo-controlled study. J Eur Acad Dermatol Venereol. 2014; 28(12):1707–1715

[4] Rotunda AM, Weiss SR, Rivkin LS. Randomized double-blind clinical trial of subcutaneously injected deoxycholate versus a phosphatidylcholine-deoxycholate combination for the reduction of submental fat. Dermatol Surg. 2009; 35(5):792–803

[5] Sykes JM, Allak A, Klink B. Future applications of deoxycholic acid (Kybella) in body contouring. J Drugs Dermatol. 2017; 16(1):43–46

[6] Manstein D, Laubach H, Watanabe K, Farinelli W, Zurakowski D, Anderson RR. Selective cryolysis: a novel method of non-invasive fat removal. Lasers Surg Med. 2008; 40(9):595–604

[7] Dierickx CC, Mazer JM, Sand M, Koenig S, Arigon V. Safety, tolerance, and patient satisfaction with noninvasive cryolipolysis. Dermatol Surg. 2013; 39(8):1209–1216

[8] Ingargiola MJ, Motakef S, Chung MT, Vasconez HC, Sasaki GH. Cryolipolysis for fat reduction and body contouring: safety and efficacy of current treatment paradigms. Plast Reconstr Surg. 2015; 135(6):1581–1590

[9] Sklar LR, El Tal AK, Kerwin LY. Use of transcutaneous ultrasound for lipolysis and skin tightening: a review. Aesthetic Plast Surg. 2014; 38(2):429–441

[10] Gadsden E, Aguilar MT, Smoller BR, Jewell ML. Evaluation of a novel high-intensity focused ultrasound device for ablating subcutaneous adipose tissue for noninvasive body contouring: safety studies in human volunteers. Aesthet Surg J. 2011; 31(4):401–410

[11] Rassman WR, Bernstein RM, McClellan R, Jones R, Worton E, Uyttendaele H. Follicular unit extraction: minimally invasive surgery for hair transplantation. Dermatol Surg. 2002; 28(8):720–728

[12] Onda M, Igawa HH, Inoue K, Tanino R. Novel technique of follicular unit extraction hair transplantation with a powered punching device. Dermatol Surg. 2008; 34(12):1683–1688

[13] Ors S, Ozkose M, Ors S. Follicular unit extraction hair transplantation with micromotor: eight years experience. Aesthetic Plast Surg. 2015; 39(4):589–596

[14] Few J. Continuum of beauty: blending of surgical and nonsurgical cosmetic medicine. Treatment Strateg Dermatol. 2012; 2(1):29–31

13 Cryolipolysis

W. Grant Stevens, Michelle Manning Eagan, Cory Felber, Deniz Sarhaddi, and Marc Vincent Orlando

Summary

Cryolipolysis, a controlled cooling treatment to reduce fat deposits, induces apoptosis in fat cells without damaging the surrounding tissues, muscles, nerves, or blood vessels. One of the most popular cryolipolysis patented technologies is CoolSculpting®.

Keywords: apoptosis, comprehensive contouring, CoolSculpting®, cryodermadstringo, cryolipolysis, debulking, DualSculpting®, liposuction, thermal injury

Key Points

- Fat cells are more susceptible to cold injury than surrounding tissues. Cryolipolysis extracts energy to cool fat cells and selectively trigger their natural cell death (apoptosis), while leaving surrounding cells and tissues unharmed.
- Patients tolerate the procedure well without the need for pain medication during treatment.
- Cryolipolysis requires little staff time for greater profitability. Once the treatment has started, little to no additional staff time is required until the end of the treatment.
- Body assessment is different for women and men: the goal for women is to have an hourglass shape, whereas the goal for men is to have a V-shaped back.
- Results are operator-dependent. The proper applicator choice and placement are key for optimal results.
- The first important step in patient evaluation is assessing skin laxity and the thickness of the adipose tissue.
- Locating the peaks of fat, the orientation of the fat deposit, and where the fat tapers are crucial to choosing the correct applicator and proper placement.
- CoolMax® (ZELTIQ Aesthetics, Inc.) is the most commonly used applicator for debulking. For comprehensive contouring, it is important to overlap the treatment areas.
- Patients should be weighed and photographed to clearly demonstrate pretreatment asymmetries and to document posttreatment results.
- Overall reduction in subcutaneous fat after treatment is approximately 20% to 25%. This is not a treatment for obesity.
- Immediate posttreatment massage can dramatically improve results, increasing results by up to 68% more fat reduction. The senior author (Dr. Stevens) recommends a 3-minute massage after every treatment. The first minute consists of vigorous massage and the second and third minutes consist of circular motions. Hand massage or a 2.5-minute Zimmer percussion (2500 pulses, 16hz, 120mJ) for 3 minutes to the treatment area can be used.
- Suction settings vary based on the applicator and the location of treatment. Increasing suction can improve applicator adherence. The cupped applicators, such as the CoolMini® (ZELTIQ Aesthetics, Inc.) and CoolAdvantage® (ZELTIQ Aesthetics, Inc.), require less suction than the flat-plated, vacuum-assisted applicators.
- Most areas will require two treatments to see the desired optimal results. The inner thighs can be very responsive and may only need one application.
- Patients should return for follow-up in 4 to 8 weeks.
- Temporary side effects may include ecchymosis, neuropraxia, swelling, and pain.
- Rare complications can occur and include contour irregularities and paradoxical adipocyte hyperplasia.
- Contraindications include cryoglobulinemia or paroxysmal cold hemoglobinuria. The effects on hernias have not been studied, but caution is advised adjacent to areas with possible hernia or previous surgical scarring. Applicator placement over hernias is not advised. Placement over enlarged thyroids is also not advised.

13.1 Introduction

Cosmetic surgical and nonsurgical procedures are on the rise, according to the Cosmetic Surgery National Data Bank Statistics by The American Society of Aesthetic Plastic Surgery (ASAPS) in 2016.[1] Nearly 12.8 million procedures were performed in 2015. More than 1.9 million surgical and 10.8 million nonsurgical procedures were performed in 2015, with nonsurgical cosmetic procedures accounting for 42% of the total expenditures. Liposuction was the number one procedure performed on both men and women, with 396,048 procedures completed. In 2015, nonsurgical fat reduction procedures increased by 18.7%.[1]

The majority of patients undergoing both surgical and nonsurgical fat reduction is between 35 and 50 years of age. Nonsurgical techniques in fat reduction offer patients an opportunity to decrease fat deposits without recovery, downtime, pain, or the risks associated with surgery and anesthesia.[1,2]

The most popular nonsurgical fat reduction system, which accounts for approximately 99% of nonsurgical body contouring performed at Marina Plastic Surgery, is CoolSculpting® (ZELTIQ Aesthetics, Inc.). We have used 10 other nonsurgical devices, and none of them compare to this system with regard to effectiveness, tolerability, efficient use of staff time, and patient satisfaction.

CoolSculpting employs controlled cooling to reduce fat deposits using a mechanism known as cryolipolysis. Fat cells are uniquely sensitive to cold and crystallize at a warmer temperature than water in surrounding tissues.[3] Consequently, cryolipolysis induces apoptosis in fat cells and an inflammatory response in the treated tissue, without damage to overlying skin and surrounding muscles, nerves, and blood vessels. The CoolSculpting patented technology protects the skin from freezing while the adipose cells are exposed to therapeutic levels of cooling[4] (▶ Fig. 13.1). Over the course of 2 to 4 months, the damaged fat cells are metabolized, resulting in gradual, permanent fat reduction in the treated region. The results have been shown to be long-term[5] (▶ Fig. 13.2).

Fat reduction related to cold exposure was first described in 1970, with the observation of inflammatory nodules followed

Cryolipolysis

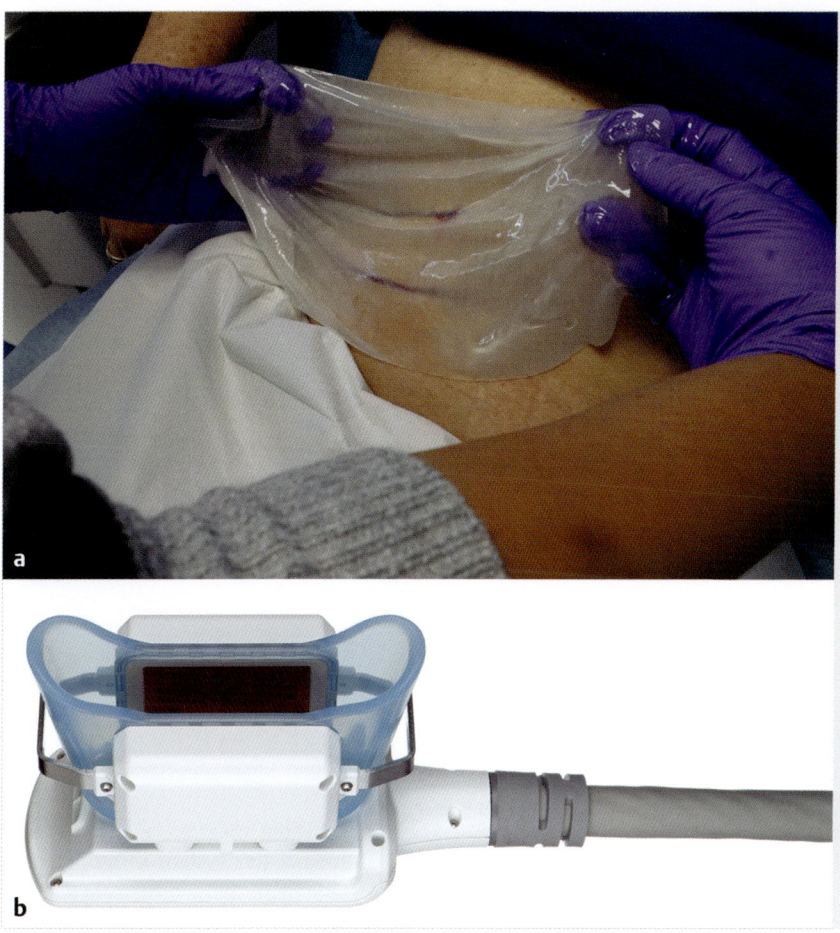

Fig. 13.1 (a) Safety measures to prevent thermal injury include the thermal coupling gel pad. Applied before placement of the applicator, it ensures consistent thermal contact and insulates the skin during the treatment. (b) Freeze Detect® (ZELTIQ Aesthetics, Inc.) sensors and software are patented technology that detect changes in skin temperature and will stop the treatment if a freeze is detected. (Courtesy of ZELTIQ Aesthetics, Inc)

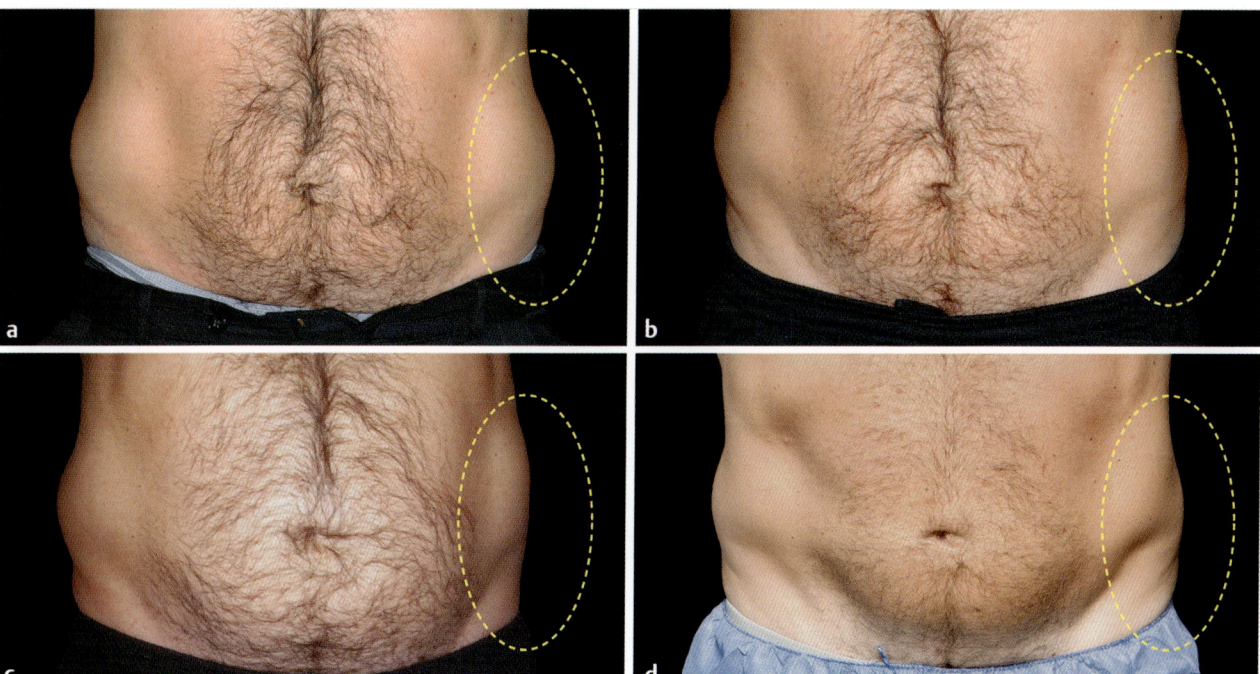

Fig. 13.2 Long-term results of cryolipolysis. (a) Flanks before treatment. (b) Left flank treated after 8 weeks. (c) 2 years after and (d) 6 years after the left flank treatment with weight gain of +10 pounds. Procedure by Dr. Eric Bernstein. (Reproduced with permission from Bernstein EF. Long-term efficacy follow-up on two cryolipolysis case studies: 6 and 9 years post-treatment. J Cosmet Dermatol. 2016 Dec;15(4):561-564.)

Cryolipolysis

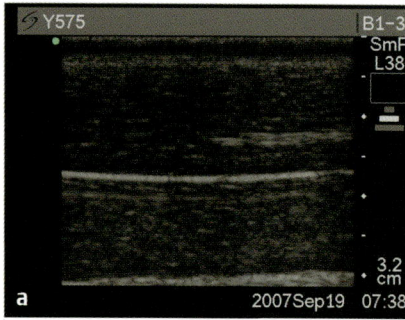
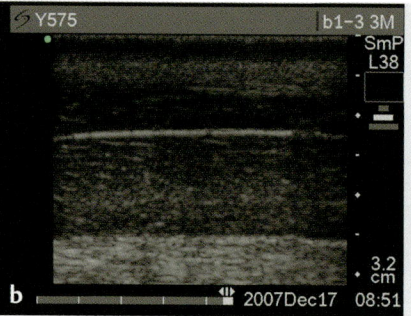
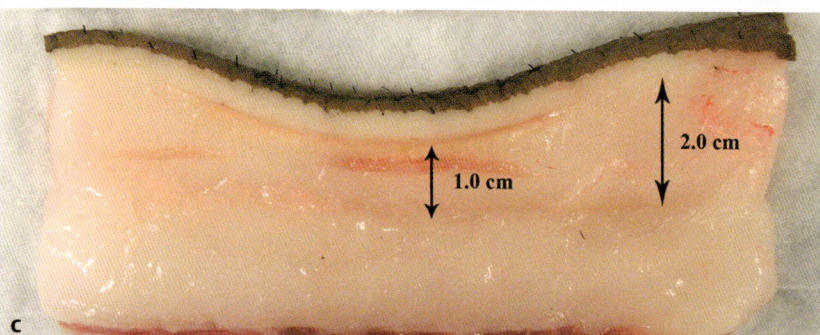

Fig. 13.3 Porcine abdominal specimen showing the effectiveness in fat reduction after cryolipolysis. **(a)** Ultrasound image showing pretreated subcutaneous fat. **(b)** Ultrasound at 3 months shows a 0.7-cm, or greater than 40% decrease, in the thickness of the fat layer. **(c)** Gross pathology from the same treatment side shows the superficial fat layer at the center of the treatment site reduced 1 cm, or 50%, at 90 days posttreatment compared to the untreated region. (Reproduced with permission from Zelickson B, Egbert BM, Preciado J et al. Cryolipolysis for noninvasive fat cell destruction: initial results from a pig model. Dermatol Surg 2009;35:1462–1470, 2009)

by fat necrosis and change in cheek contour of an infant who had been sucking on a popsicle.[6] In 1980, the term *equestrian cold panniculitis* was coined to describe the inflammation of the inner thighs of female equestrians who rode horses in cold temperatures for at least 2 hours a day without insulated pants. A decrease in thigh fat was noted after resolution of the inflammation.[7] Cryolipolysis was performed on abdominal porcine tissue, showing the clinical reduction of fat 90 days after the treatment[8] (▶ Fig. 13.3). Several studies on various areas of the body and its effects on peripheral nerves and lipid levels have validated cryolipolysis as a safe and effective procedure for reducing subcutaneous fat.[3,9,10,11,12]

CoolSculpting is the only cryolipolysis machine in the United States approved by the Food and Drug Administration (FDA). In 2010, it was approved for use on the abdomen. Since then, the FDA has approved its use on the flanks (2012), thighs (2014), and chin (2015).[13] Other areas can be treated at the discretion of physicians and with consent disclosing non-FDA-approved use. These areas include "bra-fat" rolls, inner thighs, knees, arms, axillary fat pads, and the male chest.

In addition to safety and efficacy, cryolipolysis has high tolerability, excellent patient satisfaction, and offers the potential for tremendous growth of a plastic surgery practice. From a business perspective, offering an alternative to surgical fat reduction with CoolSculpting has increased the number of new patients to the practice by attracting people who are interested in body contouring but who are reluctant to undergo invasive procedures. CoolSculpting has increased the number of male patients in our practice more than any other technology. Of the 66% new patients seen within 2 years, 62% had never had any aesthetic procedure. Forty percent of those who underwent CoolSculpting became established patients, undergoing additional aesthetic procedures within the next 3 years.[14] Multiple concomitant procedures can be performed while a patient is undergoing cryolipolysis, such as hair transplantation, neuromodulator injections, filler injections, laser treatments and so on (**see Video 1.1**).[14]

Cryolipolysis has been successfully integrated into the Marina Plastic Surgery practice. Unique to this system is the potential to use multiple devices simultaneously, a term called *DualSculpting®* (Seattle Aesthetics), to reduce overall treatment times (▶ Fig. 13.4) Currently, there are nine devices available at the main office in Marina del Rey, California, and eight devices at the satellite offices in the Orange County offices. An average of 80 cycles are delivered each week in Marina Del Rey and 70 cycles in Orange County, totaling over 240,000 CoolSculpting procedures. Patients can reduce overall treatment time if multiple machines are being used simultaneously. Also, it is possible for multiple concomitant procedures to be performed while a patient is undergoing cryolipolysis, such as hair transplantation, neuromodulator injections, filler injections, laser treatments, and so on (▶ Fig. 13.5). CoolSculpting is convenient and efficient for both the patient and the clinician.[14]

Dr. W. Grant Stevens (author) has been a pioneer in unlocking the potential of this technology. The treatment plans have ranged from one to two cycles per treatment area, with optimal results attained after at least two cycles per area. *Comprehensive contouring* is a term coined by Dr. Stevens that describes a strategy to debulk fat and sculpt the body.

Comprehensive contouring can produce liposuction-like results and has even proved useful in softening contour irregularities from previous liposuction procedures[14] (▶ Fig. 13.6). This technique utilizes multiple, varying applicators, a variable number of cycles depending on the treatment area, and overlapping treatment sites. With the addition of the nonsuction flat panel and the mini-cupped applicators, clinicians are able to target nearly any desired area. As the technology continues to advance, more applicator variations will assist the clinician and patient in achieving the desired nonsurgical fat reduction in more regions.

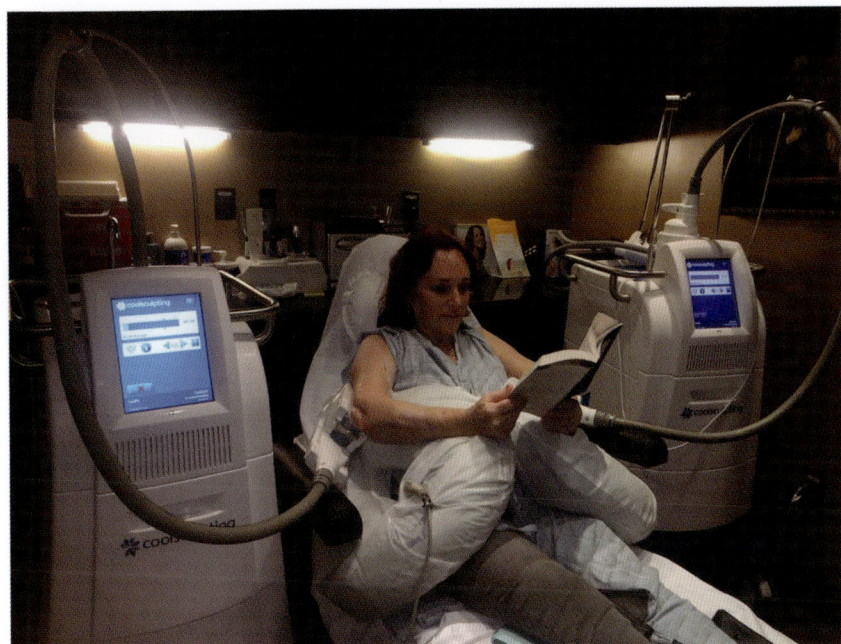

Fig. 13.4 DualSculpting. Multiple cycles can be performed, saving time and money for both the patient and clinician.

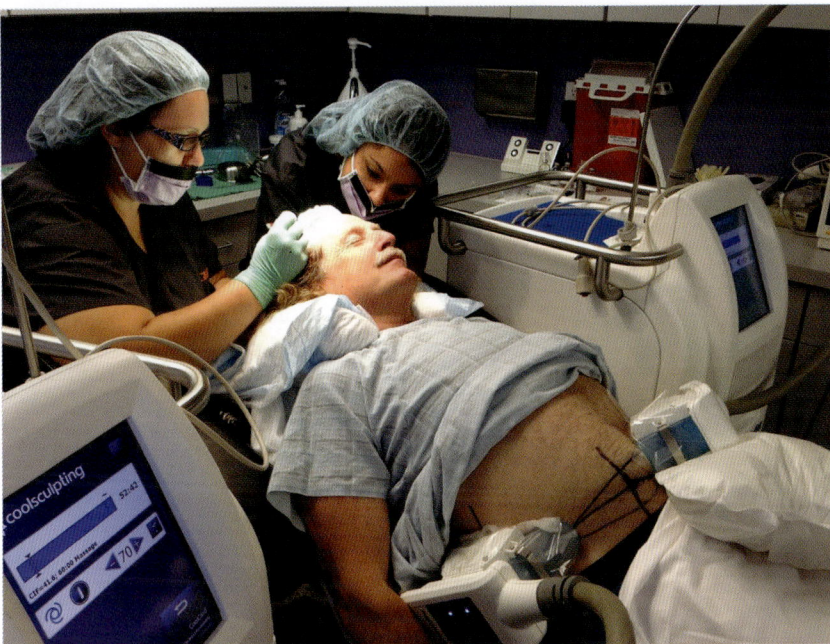

Fig. 13.5 Multiple procedures can be done concomitantly. This patient is undergoing cryolipolysis of the right flank and left abdomen as well as hair transplantation. Procedure by Dr. W. Grant Stevens.

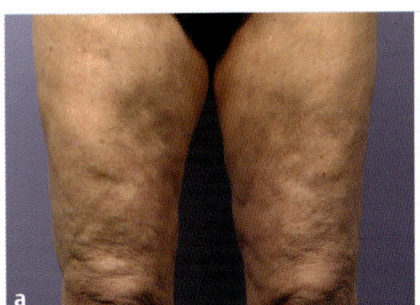
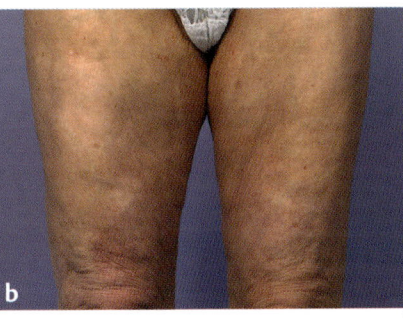

Fig. 13.6 Cryolipolysis can be used to smooth the contour irregularities. CoolSmoothPro used circumferentially around thighs in (a) a 66-year-old woman, who presented for treatment of her anterior thighs. (b) 2 years after circumferential treatment of the thighs with CoolSmooth Pro. Procedure by Dr. W. Grant Stevens. (Reproduced with permission from Stevens WG, Pietrzak LK, Spring MA. Broad overview of a clinical and commercial experience with CoolSculpting®. Aesthet Surg J. 2013 Aug 1;33(6):835-46.)

Consequently, cryolipolysis can freeze fat cells without inducing damage to overlying skin and surrounding muscles, nerves, and blood vessels. The exposure to cold induces apoptosis in the fat cells and an inflammatory response in the treated tissue. Over the course of 2 to 4 months, the damaged fat cells are cleared by the body, resulting in gradual, permanent fat reduction in the treated region. Several studies on various areas of the body, cholesterol, and peripheral nerve effects have shown cryolipolysis to be a very safe and effective procedure for the nonsurgical reduction of subcutaneous fat.[3,9,10,11,12]

In addition to safety and efficacy, cryolipolysis has high tolerability, excellent patient satisfaction, and brings potential for tremendous business growth to a plastic surgery practice. Cryolipolysis has been successfully integrated into the Marina Plastic Surgery practice, attracting new patients who are interested in body contouring but not yet ready for invasive procedures. Of the 66% new patients, 62% had never had any aesthetic procedure. Forty percent of those who underwent CoolSculpting became established patients, undergoing other aesthetic procedures. CoolSculpting has increased the number of male patients to the practice greater than any other technology.[14] Unique to this practice is the multiple machines available for each patient to improve treatment times.

The idea of cryolipolysis stems from two papers that describe fat reduction related to cold temperatures.[6,7] The first was fat reduction of the cheeks in infants after prolonged sucking on popsicles.[6] There was an altered cheek structure noted after the resolution of the inflammation. The second study referred to a group of female equestrians who were noted to ride horses in the near freezing temperatures for at least 2 hours without insulated pants. Beacham, et al.[7] described the resulting inflammation of the inner thighs as "equestrian cold panniculitis." A decrease in fat was noted in these areas. The technology of controlled-cooling therapy to reduce fat was a huge undertaking. The most difficult part was to freeze the fat without affecting the skin.

With the addition of the nonsuction, flat-panel, and mini applicators, clinicians are able to target nearly any desired area. Comprehensive contouring results in liposuction-like results (▶ Fig. 13.6).

From a business perspective, offering an alternative to surgical fat reduction with CoolSculpting has increased the number of new patients to the practice, specifically men who are normally averse to cosmetic treatments, and neophytes reluctant to undergo invasive procedures. These patients often will undergo other procedures, because they have seen good results with CoolSculpting. Multiple procedures can also be done while the patient is undergoing cryolipolysis, such as hair transplantation, neuromodulator injections, filler injections, laser treatments, and so on.[14] Cryolipolysis is an excellent nonsurgical body contouring procedure because of its high safety, tolerability, efficacy, and business growth potential.

This chapter will cover the patient selection, technique, post-procedural care, typical results, and possible complications related to cryolipolysis.

13.2 Patient Selection

Proper patient selection is essential to achieving an optimal result. Cryolipolysis has been proven to be safe and effective, but it is not the fat-reduction strategy of choice for all patients.

All patients should be counseled for a treatment-to-transformation. Comprehensive contouring is the ideal treatment plan for total body contouring (▶ Fig. 13.7). The patient should be aware of the optimal number of cycles required for desired fat reduction. Patients who elect to undergo suboptimal treatment, whether because of personal desire or financial constraints, should be informed of the likely suboptimal results. One should consider avoiding treatment in such a scenario, because both the patient and the clinician may be disappointed with the fat-reduction outcome.

Two crucial factors to assess during the patient examination are (1) local skin laxity and (2) thickness of adipose tissue. Gender and ethnic background do not affect outcomes. To use the vacuum-assisted application heads, tissue laxity should allow for adequate draw into the applicator. Areas with dense cutaneous attachments near bony prominences, such as the iliac crest and ribs, may have less mobility. For areas with less skin laxity, the nonsuction, flat-panel applicators are suitable. The nonsuction applicators can also be used to help smooth severe liposuction irregularities, because the prominent fat peaks are cooled more than the depressions. This management, however, is only attempting to improve irregular contours.

Patients with moderate to severe skin laxity often demonstrate the phenomenon of cryodermadstringo, or skin tightening[14,15,16] (▶ Fig. 13.8).

Patients with thick adipose tissue will require debulking in addition to sculpting, and patients should be made aware that debulking necessitates more than one treatment cycle. Furthermore, treatment of one area may give the illusion of increased adiposity in an adjacent, untreated area; therefore, the comprehensive plan should include treatment of an entire region to avoid deformities or irregularities.[17] For patients who only want or only can afford less than ideal treatment, it may be best to avoid treatment altogether, because both the patient and the clinician will be unsatisfied with the results.

Potential treatment areas should be examined for the presence of open wounds or infection. These areas should be avoided, because tissue injury with cooling can worsen the condition. Patients with prior abdominal surgeries should be evaluated for abdominal hernias, which would present a contraindication to treatment in that area. Any large skin incisions or scars should be noted, because they can draw into the vacuum-assisted device, or they can cause diffusion of the cooling through the flat-panel applicators, which may enhance scar depression. Treatment should be altogether avoided in patients with cryoglobulinemia or paroxysmal cold hemoglubinuria; although the effects of CoolSculpting in patients with these disorders has not been studied or reported, it is reasonable to assume that induced cooling will exacerbate these conditions. Also, when using the CoolMini® (ZELTIQ Aesthetics, Inc.) to treat the submental region, an enlarged thyroid should be avoided.

13.3 Technique

The CoolSculpting system is an FDA-approved device for cryolipolysis on the abdomen, flank, thighs, submental area, and other flexible treatment parameters[4] (▶ Fig. 13.9). The control console contains a thermoelectric cooling element that modulates the temperature of two cooling plates, which are housed

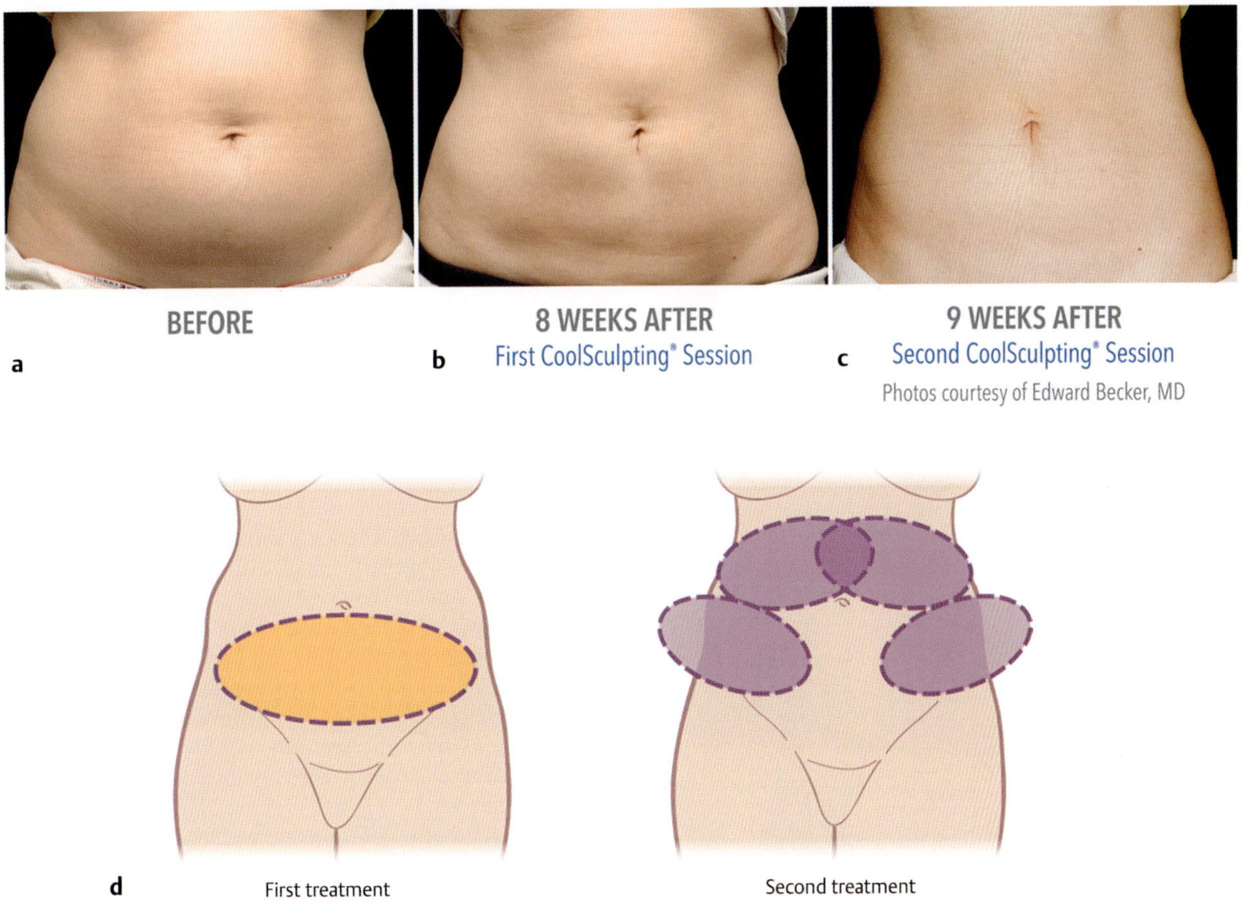

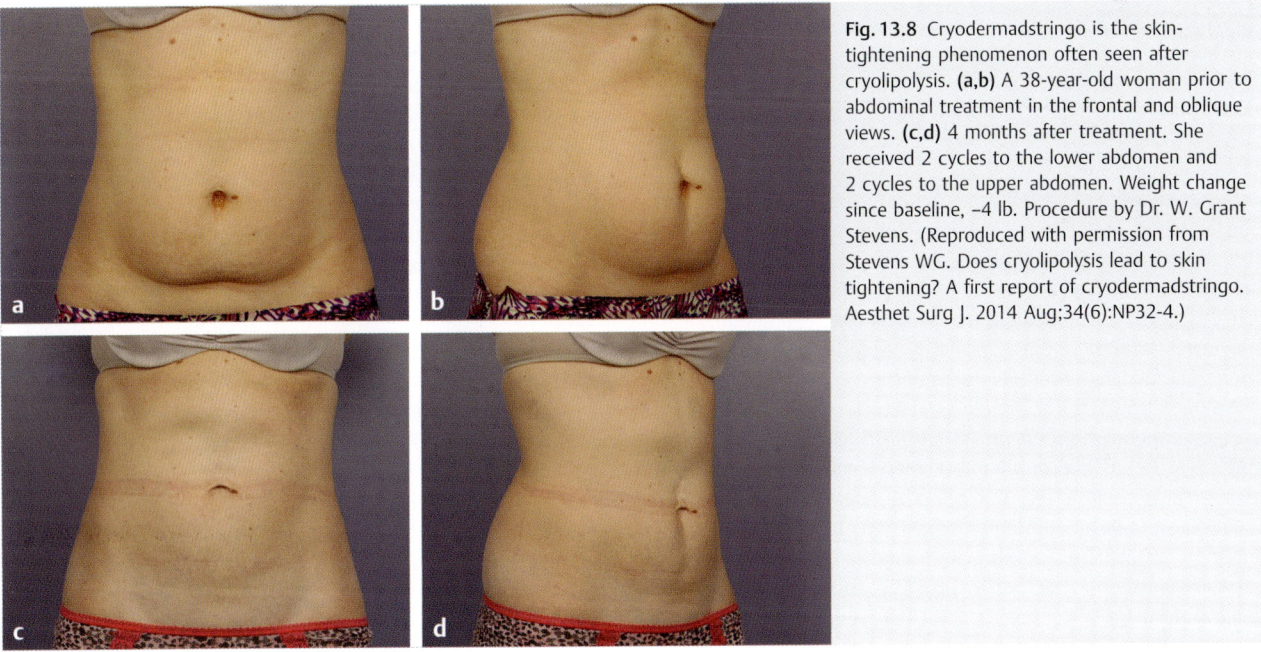

Fig. 13.7 Comprehensive Contouring utilizes the various cryolipolysis applicators to shape the body using the aesthetic shapes of the male and female body as a guide. Multiple cycles per area are often required, and debulking and sculpting applicators are used to achieve optimal results. **(a)** Patient before cryolipolysis. **(b)** 8 weeks after debulking. **(c)** 9 weeks after the second treatment using sculpting applicators. No weight change was noted. Procedure by Dr. Edward Becker. **(d)** Applicator placements used in the first and second treatments. ((d) (Courtesy of ZELTIQ™ Aesthetics, Inc))

Fig. 13.8 Cryodermadstringo is the skin-tightening phenomenon often seen after cryolipolysis. **(a,b)** A 38-year-old woman prior to abdominal treatment in the frontal and oblique views. **(c,d)** 4 months after treatment. She received 2 cycles to the lower abdomen and 2 cycles to the upper abdomen. Weight change since baseline, –4 lb. Procedure by Dr. W. Grant Stevens. (Reproduced with permission from Stevens WG. Does cryolipolysis lead to skin tightening? A first report of cryodermadstringo. Aesthet Surg J. 2014 Aug;34(6):NP32-4.)

Cryolipolysis

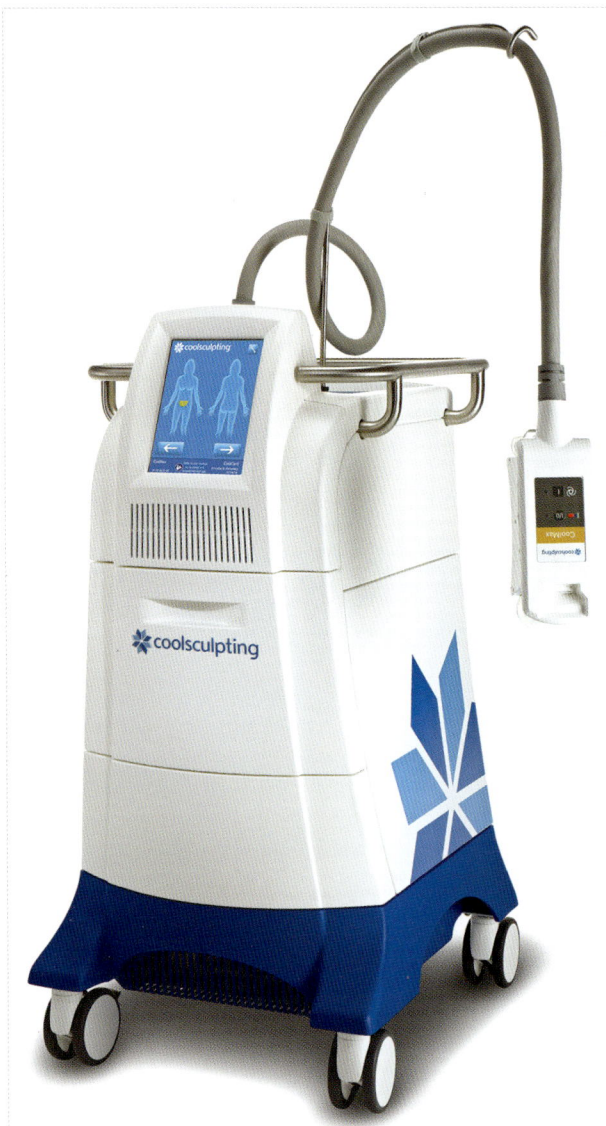

Fig. 13.9 CoolSculpting machine that performs cryolipolysis. There is a console, beeper, patient push button (not shown), and umbilical cord with applicator attached. (Courtesy of ZELTIQ™ Aesthetics, Inc. CoolSculpting® Available from: http://www.coolsculpting.com/for-physicians/coolsculpting-technology.)

within a cup-shaped applicator of variable size and configuration attached to the console by an umbilical[18] (▶ Table 13.1). The control unit also regulates the rate of energy extraction (mW/cm^2), which is expressed as the cooling intensity factor (CIF). In most clinical studies, the CIF falls between 0 and 5 °Celsius. The vacuum applicators apply negative pressure when applied across the specified treatment area. The adipose tissue is drawn between the cooling plates, which maintain a variable, preset temperature between -10 and -13 °Celsius.[19] The negative pressure of the applicator limits local cutaneous blood flow; this, in conjunction with selective energy extraction from the adipose tissue, eliminates convective heat exchange and leads to therapeutic cooling and cryolipolysis. The nonvacuumed applicators lack draw into the applicator and utilize cooling alone for fat reduction; thus, they require slightly longer treatment times.

Applicators, of which there are seven currently, vary in size and shape to improve adherence to various anatomic treatment areas. There are (1) vacuumed-assisted, flat-plated applicators with flanges, (2) vacuum-assisted, cupped-plated applicators, and (3) non-suctioning, contoured, flat-plated applicators. The most common treatment areas include

- Abdomen.
- Arms.
- Brassiere rolls.
- Lumbar rolls.
- Hip rolls/flanks.
- Peritrochanteric areas.
- Inner and outer thighs.
- Medial knee.

The applicators that generate vacuum suction do not require additional measures to maintain applicator fixation to the skin. These include the CoolCurve+®, CoolCore®, CoolFit® and CoolMax® (all ZELTIQ Aesthetics, Inc.). Both the CoolCurve+ and CoolCore share similar cooling plate footprints, but differ in the flange configuration. The CoolMax applicator has a larger surface area than the others listed, and is ideal for debulking. To treat the medial thigh, CoolCore can treat horizontally oriented fat bulges, and CoolFit, a flat vacuum applicator with longer cooling plates, can be used for more vertically oriented fat bulges. The CoolMini uses less negative pressure and is designed for small areas of adiposity including submental, axillary, and knee fat.

Applicators that do not provide vacuum suction or use less suction usually require straps to maintain the device-to-skin interface and may require longer treatment times. The CoolSmooth Pro® (ZELTIQ Aesthetics, Inc.) is a flat applicator that may be used for FDA-approved areas of the lateral thighs, abdomen, or off-labeled use for the banana rolls.[18]

The previously mentioned applicators all use flat cooling plates. The other two applicators use cupped cooling plates that increase contact with the tissue, therefore cooling tissues faster and to cooler temperatures with less suction needed. The two available cupped applicators are the CoolMini and the newer CoolAdvantage® (ZELTIQ Aesthetics, Inc.). The CoolMini is smaller and designed to fit little areas of adiposity including submental, axillary, and knee fat. The CoolAdvantage, released in March 2016, has the surface area of the CoolFit with interchangeable flanges to help fit different contours. The 3-in-1 applicator offers three different flanges that create three different applicators: CoolFit Advantage®, CoolCore Advantage®, and CoolCurve+Advantage® (all ZELTIQ Aesthetics, Inc.). These each treat similar areas to the corresponding CoolFit, CoolCore, and CoolCurve+. Due to the specialized cooling cupped-plates, the time required is nearly half the treatment time, 35 minutes, with nearly 45% increased comfort.[20]

Typical settings for the vacuum suction may vary as the applicators are changed. For the CoolCurve+, CoolCore, CoolFit, and CoolMax, the vacuum suction is set to 60 to 70 mmHg, and the massage suction is set between 60 and 75 mmHg. The recommended maximum massage suction setting is 15 mmHg above the minimum suction setting. The cupped applicators will require less suction. The CoolMini is set to 50 mmHg. While the nonsuction, flat-panel applicators do not have suction settings to set, some do have length of time and temperature settings to select.

Cryolipolysis

Table 13.1 CoolSculpting Applicators

Vacuum Applicators	Image	Description	Treatment Area
CoolCurve+®		Sculpting applicator; ideal for curves	Flanks
CoolCore®		Sculpting applicator; same footprint as CoolCurve+ but a different flange that is more ideal for bulges with more gentle curves	Abdomen
CoolFit®		Sculpting applicator; ideal for longer, vertical areas of fat	Abdomen; off-labeled use for arms; occasionally inner thighs
CoolMax®		Debulking applicator for larger surface areas	Abdomen and flanks
CoolMini®		Sculpting applicator; ideal for smaller, pliable tissue	Abdomen; off-labeled use for arms; occasionally inner thighs
CoolAdvantage®		Sculpting applicator; interchangeable flanges	Outer thighs and abdomen; off-labeled use for posterior thighs
Non-vacuum Applicators			
CoolSmooth Pro®		Sculpting applicator; ideal for larger surface areas with less tissue pliability and pinchability; requires 75 minutes of treatment	Outer thighs and abdomen; off-labeled use for posterior thighs

From CoolSculpting®. Available from: http://www.coolsculpting.com/for-physicians/coolsculpting-technology. Accessed Nov. 18, 2015

Patient assessment and marking should be performed with the patient standing. The operator begins by outlining the area of interest with a pen, encircling the borders of excess adiposity, and drawing a midsagittal line or "X" through its apex to assist with CoolSculpting applicator placement. By grasping fat between both hands, it is easier to see which type of applicator is needed and which direction the applicator should be placed. Using the templates provided by CoolSculpt® (ZELTIQ Aesthetics, Inc.) is helpful with this process.

When marking, all patients should be assessed for comprehensive contouring so that the ideal number and types of cycles can be recommended, and the patient's expectations can be addressed. Once all areas are marked out, the decision for dual treatments can be made. For example, if both the arms and flanks are to be treated, then four machines can be used to shorten a treatment from 4 hours to 1 hour. There are many variations in machine use to increase efficiency and decrease the patient's overall treatment time and number of visits.

It is beneficial to both the patient and clinician to be efficient. Discussing with the patient other procedures they are interested in is also recommended during consultation. If the patient desires other cosmetic procedures, they can be scheduled simultaneously during the cryolipolysis. For example, if a male patient desires hair transplants or fillers, all treatments and procedures can usually be performed simultaneously.

Once the patient is marked and the areas to be treated simultaneously are determined, the treating clinician positions the patient on an exam table or a reclined chair for the duration of treatment. Most CoolSculpt® applicators currently recommend treatments that last 60 minutes (75 minutes when using the CoolSmooth Pro).[18,20] Soon, there will be newer applicators that will decrease the treatment time to 35 minutes.

Applicator placement differs for nonsuction versus suction applicators. For each applicator, a specific card is placed into the console before initiating a treatment cycle. If the applicator is the nonsuction, flat-panel applicator, the Pretreatment Skin Wipe® (ZELTIQ Aesthetics, Inc.) is used to clean the skin with firm pressure to remove skin oils. Only for the flat-plated applicators, adhesive foam liners are placed around the treatment areas. Next, a skin-protective Gelpad® (ZELTIQ Aesthetics, Inc.) is placed on the skin and gently tucked into the corners of the foam borders. Because the gel prevents the skin from freezing, if this gel pad tears, it could lead to skin injury or the cycle canceling. Using the back of the clinician's finger is recommended to prevent tearing the gel pad. A clear liner is placed on top of the gel pad. The applicator is aligned with previous markings placed in the midline of the adiposity, with care to ensure that the peak of the fat deposit lies within the center of the applicator. The straps are connected to the applicator, securing it in place. After positioning the patient and umbilical in the securement arm, the applicator is checked to ensure that it did not move out of position. The cycle is then started.

For suction applicators, the patient should be sitting in a reclining chair to assist with enhancement of the bulges and to prevent the applicator from detaching when the patient finds a comfortable position on the chair. A gel liner is placed directly on the skin (▶ Fig. 13.10**a**). The clear liner is attached to the applicator cup prior to placing the applicator on the patient. The vacuum-suction is started and then the treatment applicator is placed over the markings. The tissue should be checked to ensure that it is above the side bars on the flanges. For better tissue draw, it is recommended that the applicator is applied starting at the bottom of the treatment area, and rolled upward into place. Using the patient's body posture can help enhance the roll of fat to assist with better tissue draw. If the tissue is not above the side bars, remove the applicator and try again (▶ Fig. 13.10). For the abdomen, if tissue draw is inadequate, the patient can sit up and flex at the waist to increase skin laxity and provide the quality tissue draw needed.

The vacuum-assisted cupped-applicator, CoolAdvantage, uses the largest gel liner, which is placed on the skin. There is a foam gasket that is used as the "liner" to protect the device and encircles the edge of the metal plates. This is changed between cycles. The gel trap is placed within the base of the cup and removed between patients only. The flange is chosen and held in place with locking clips on the sides of the applicator. Because of the use of less suction with this applicator, a unique strap is used to hold the applicator onto the patient. The vacuum is turned on and then the cycle is started once the patient is in position. After the cycle, the gel trap and liner are removed. The applicator's plates and crevasses are thoroughly cleaned with rubbing alcohol with a soft cloth or cotton-tipped applicator.[8]

Use of the CoolMini applicator can be tricky, because it is slightly different. The patient should be marked while standing, as described above. For off-label use on axillary fat pads, for example, the patient must lay supine with arms down by his or her side. The patient is then positioned in a reclining chair. The Pretreatment Skin Wipe is used to clean the skin with firm pressure to remove skin oils. Care is taken to clean the metal plates and its crevasses using rubbing alcohol. A transparent tape dressing, such as Tegaderm® (chlorhexidine gluconate topical, 3 M Medical), is used as the liner and placed over the metal cupped-plate (▶ Fig. 13.11). The vacuum is turned on to a preset 50 mmHg of negative pressure. The film dressing is then drawn into the applicator. The vacuum must be maintained for skin protection from the plates. Once the tape remains adherent to the plate, the gel trap is placed in the middle of the cupped device. Apply the entire CoolGel Mini® (ZELTIQ Aesthetics, Inc.) syringe on the skin, extending 1 cm beyond the treatment area. If the syringe is being used in the submental area, place the patient's head between a head-stabilizing pillow. The applicator is placed over the marked area. A strap is then used to hold the applicator in place if it is being used in the submental region. The patient should be comfortable, without having any pressure on the thyroid cartilage. The umbilical is placed in the securement arm using a c-clamp. It is helpful to remove any slack in the umbilical to prevent it from pulling the applicator out of position.

Pillows and blankets are strategically placed to hold the applicators in place and to increase patient comfort. ▶ Fig. 13.12 shows examples of patient positioning and the importance of pillows. The use of hospital-grade boppy pillows, and pillows that are easily wiped clean or have disposable covers, are ideal for this. Finally, once the cooling plates are activated and the patient is in a comfortable position, the cycle is allowed to proceed without any additional operator intervention. Patients may feel some discomfort until the tissue becomes numb.

For all CoolSculpting procedures, a pager is carried by the clinician that is triggered by the call button given to the patient. The pager notifies if something is needed by the patient or if an issue with the machines arises. Periodic assessment of patient comfort during the treatment cycle continues as needed as he or she relaxes. Small details of using the restroom before treatment, having a television with a remote, and having a magazine or glass of water nearby may add to the overall positive experience (▶ Fig. 13.13).

Occasionally, an error message will occur. The clinician will be alerted through the pager. Errors may include an applicator detachment or loss of suction, tissue not cooling to temperature, or possible breach in skin protection.

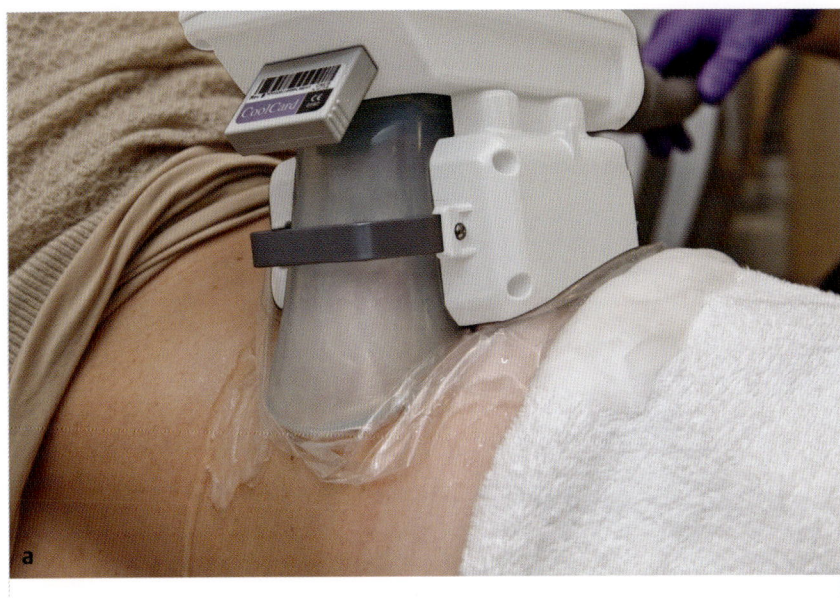
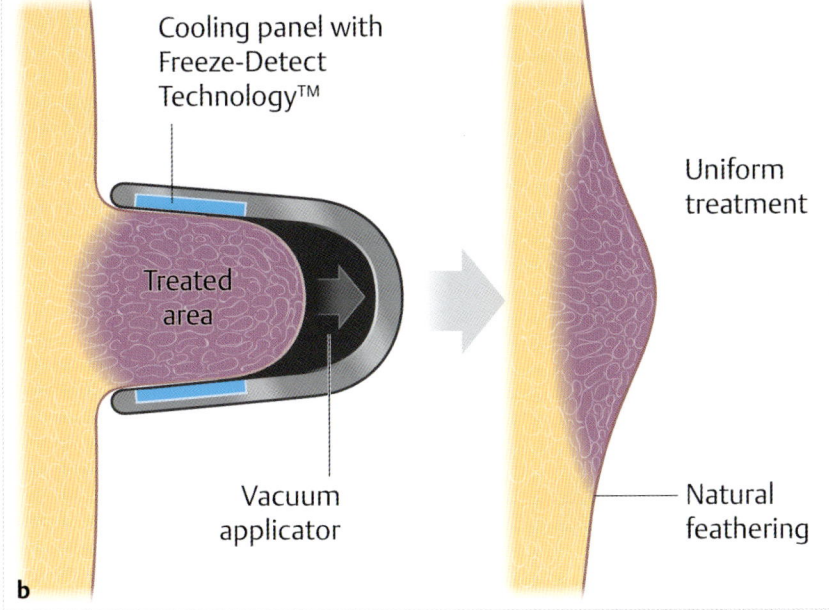

Fig. 13.10 (a) CoolSculpting vacuum applicator placed on the right flank. (b) Illustration of how the tissue is drawn into applicator with vacuum-suction. The plates are in full contact with the tissue and lead to a natural feathering of fat reduction with maximum uniform treatment at the apex. (Courtesy of ZELTIQ™ Aesthetics, Inc. CoolSculpting Available from: http://www.coolsculpting.com/for-physicians/coolsculpting-technology)

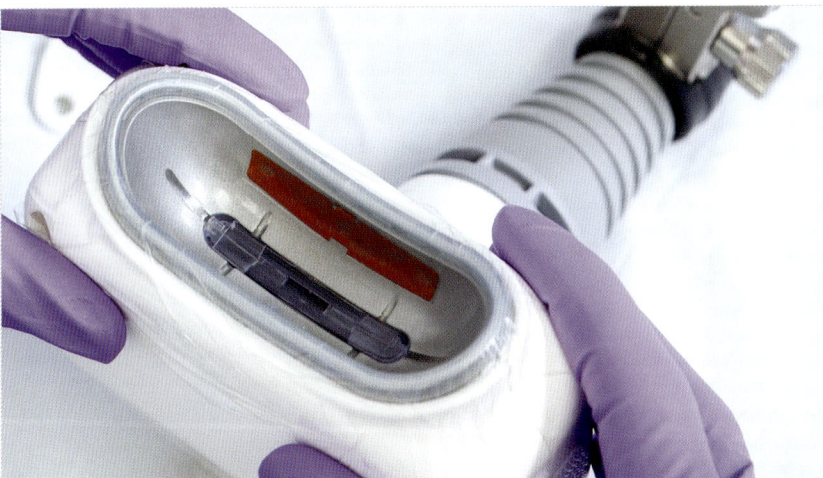

Fig. 13.11 CoolMini uses tape adhesive in place of the protective gel pad. This tape adhesive must be secured around the end. Suction is applied and then a gel trap is placed in the middle of the cupped applicator. (Courtesy of ZELTIQ™ Aesthetics, Inc. CoolSculpting Available from: http://www.coolsculpting.com/for-physicians/coolsculpting-technology)

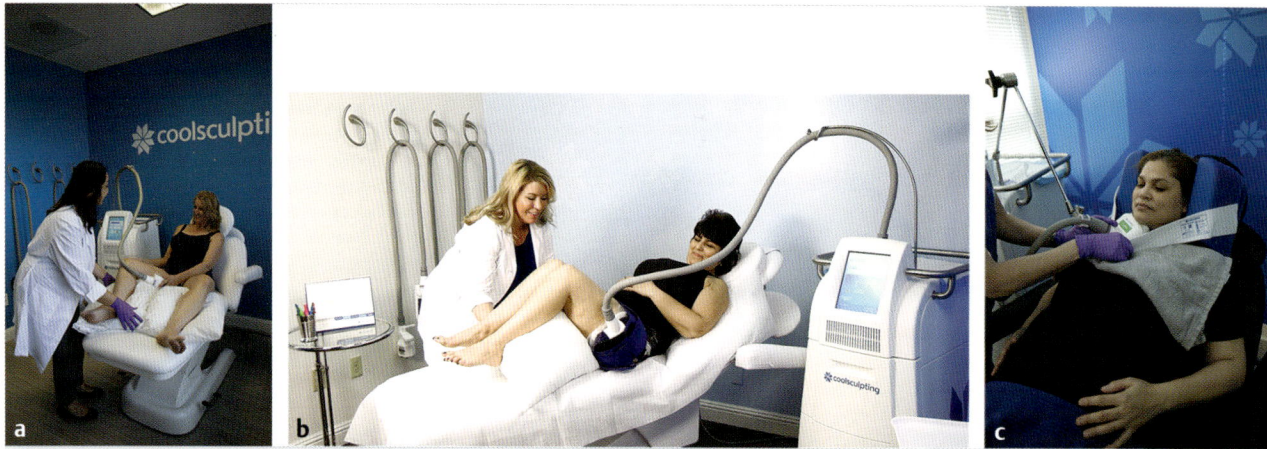

Fig. 13.12 Examples of positioning the applicator and pillows to assist with maintaining contact for the procedure. (a) CoolFit is placed with the patient in a frog-legged position with supportive pillows. (b) CoolSmoothPro is placed on the outer thigh and held in place with straps and pillows. (c) CoolMini is held in place with the special securing arm, headrest pillow, and straps. (Courtesy of ZELTIQ™ Aesthetics, Inc. CoolSculpting Available from: http://www.coolsculpting.com/for-physicians/coolsculpting-technology)

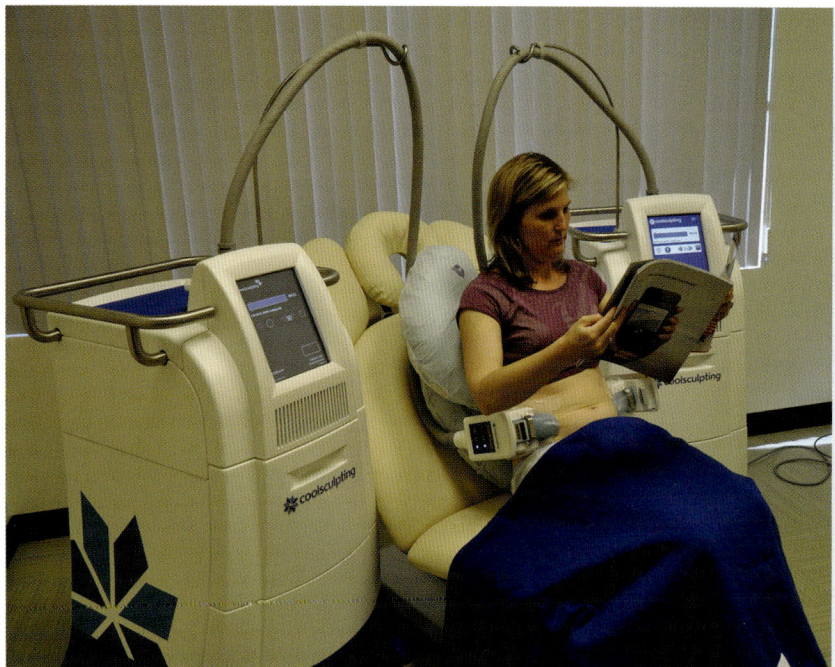

Fig. 13.13 CoolSculpting allows patients to have a comfortable experience of fat reduction while saving time. (Courtesy of ZELTIQ™ Aesthetics, Inc. CoolSculpting Available from: http://www.coolsculpting.com/for-physicians/coolsculpting-technology)

13.4 Posttreatment Care

Once the treatment concludes, the applicator is removed, and a 3-minute firm massage of the treated tissue ensues. At our institution, we prefer a 3-minute application of Zimmer percussion (2500 pulses, 16 Hz, 120 mJ) in all areas except the submental area, where hand massage is preferred. This posttreatment massage results in an increase in fat reduction.[21] Boey and Wasilenchuk[21] demonstrated a 68% increase in mean fat-layer reduction of the abdomen ($p < 0.0007$) at 2-month follow-up in patients who received manual massage for 2 minutes following a 60-minute treatment with the CoolCore applicator at CIF 42 (72.9mW/cm^2). At the 4-month follow-up, the massaged sites maintained 44% greater mean fat-layer reduction when compared to nonmassaged treatment sites ($p < 0.01$).[21] This additional fat-layer reduction may be attributable to ischemic perfusion injury from rewarming the cooled adipose tissue with massage. Reperfusion is thought to lead to increased reactive oxygen species and cytosolic calcium concentrations, activation of several calcium-dependent and calcium-independent proteolytic enzymes, and subsequent apoptosis of a large number of adipocytes that were only sublethally injured after cryolipolysis.[22] Sasaki et al[23] demonstrated a faster return to pretreatment skin temperature and significant additional fat reduction in patients who received massage at 0, 15, 30, and 45 minutes after cryolipolysis. However, the importance of re-establishing pretreatment temperatures and indirectly increasing the return of blood flow to the treated site has yet to be defined.[23]

Multiple treatments (2 to 3) may lead to further contour improvement, although the efficacy of cryolipolysis may be attenuated with successive treatments. Additional cryolipolysis is recommended for most areas 8 weeks after initial treatment to allow the resolution of inflammation. Bernstein et al[24] sequentially administered two 60-minute cycles at a CIF of 41.6 with a 50% treatment area overlap, followed by 5 minutes of vigorous manual massage. This resulted in an average appearance of flank fat reduction by 44.3%. On average, excess adipose tissue may be reduced by 20 to 25% per treatment cycle.[24]

13.5 Results

There have been more than 23 million cycles of cryolipolysis completed, with efficacy and safety consistently demonstrated.[25] ▶ Fig. 13.14, ▶ Fig. 13.15, ▶ Fig. 13.16, ▶ Fig. 13.17, ▶ Fig. 13.18, ▶ Fig. 13.19, ▶ Fig. 13.20, ▶ Fig. 13.21 show before and after results obtainable using cryolipolysis.[14,26]

The efficacy of this technology has been demonstrated not only by patient satisfaction and independent rater scales, but also objectively using a variety of techniques including standardized clinical photography, ultrasound evaluation of fat layer reduction, fat caliper measurements, circumferential measurements, and VECTRA 3D imaging (Canfield Scientific, Inc.). Overall, patients can expect a gradual fat layer reduction over the course of 2 to 4 months after treatment, and, as previously mentioned, results can be enhanced with immediate posttreatment massage. Without significant weight change, long-term fat reduction in the treated area remains for up to 5 years after cryolipolysis.[27]

Multiple studies using various outcomes measures have demonstrated the efficacy of a single cryolipolysis treatment to reduce abdominal and flank fat. At 6-month follow-up examinations using ultrasound, Sasaki et al[23] found a 19.6% reduction of subcutaneous fat above Scarpa's fascia after a single 1-hour cycle. Coleman et al[9] found similar reductions in fat of the flank, with 20.4% reduction at the 2-month follow-up and 25.5% reduction at the 6-month follow-up. Volumetric quantification of fat reduction was performed by Garibyan et al[27] using Vectra 3D photography. This showed an average of 40 mL loss of fat from a flank treated with a single 1-hour cycle compared to the patient's contralateral, untreated side, which served as the control. Caliper measurements revealed a 14.9% average reduction in thickness at the 2-month follow-up.[28]

Off-label use of cryolipolysis includes the inner thighs, arms, chest, knees, axillae, and "bra-fat" rolls. Research on the knees and axillae is under way but currently lacking. For treatment of the inner thighs, Zelickson et al[28] demonstrated a mean fat-layer reduction of 2.8 cm through ultrasound evaluation, and a 0.9-cm reduction in thigh circumference 16 weeks after a single-cycle, 60-minute treatment using a vacuum applicator. With this same treatment, Sasaki et al[23] measured a 0.5-cm reduction of inner thigh fat by caliper measurement, corresponding to a 17% reduction at the 6-month follow-up. The outer thighs pose a unique challenge for the cryolipolysis system due to the inability to draw this adherent tissue into a vacuum applicator. With the development of a conformable surface applicator, Stevens and Bachelor[26] demonstrated the efficacy of a single 120-minute cryolipolysis treatment of the lateral thigh, achieving a 2.6-mm mean reduction in fat thickness through ultrasound measurement at 16 weeks posttreatment.

Data results and outcomes of the arms and chest are scarce. For the upper arms, Saltz et al[17] found a 2.3-mm reduction in fat thickness through ultrasound measurement after 2 months, and a 4.4-mm reduction after 4 months. To treat the male chest, Munavalli and Panchaprateep[29] sequentially administered 2 60-minute treatments with 50% site overlap using a vacuum applicator, separated by 2 minutes of manual massage, followed 2 months later with an additional 60-minute treatment. They

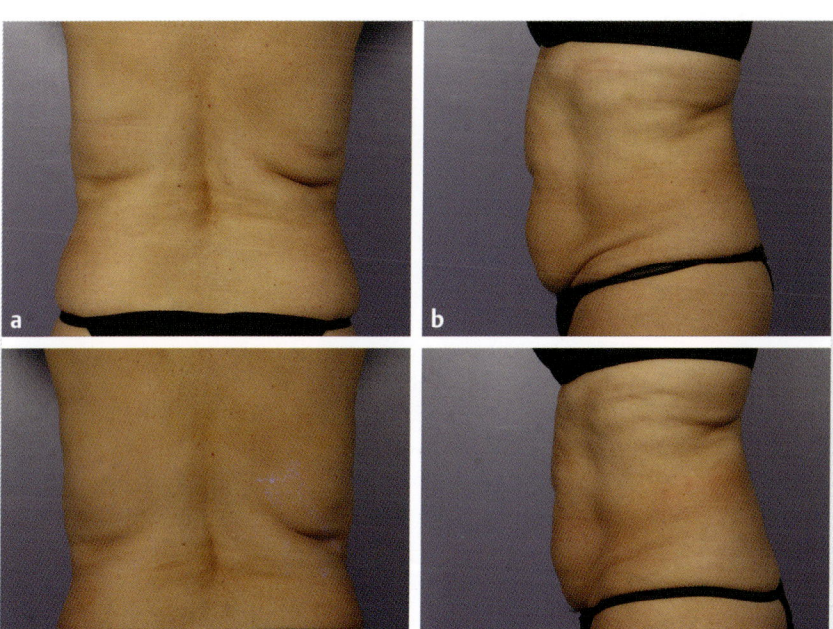

Fig. 13.14 Abdominal and "bra-fat" rolls cryolipolysis. (a,b) This 58-year-old woman was dissatisfied with subcutaneous fat in her abdomen and back: pretreatment. (c,d) 4 months after the first treatment, which consisted of 2 treatment visits spaced 2 months apart (each consisting of 4 cryolipolysis cycles to the abdomen and 2 cycles to the bra-fat area), the fat was visibly reduced and the skin noticeably tightened. Despite the appreciable fat volume loss, the skin draped well across the new body contours, rather than sagging. The weight change since baseline was −5 lbs.

Cryolipolysis

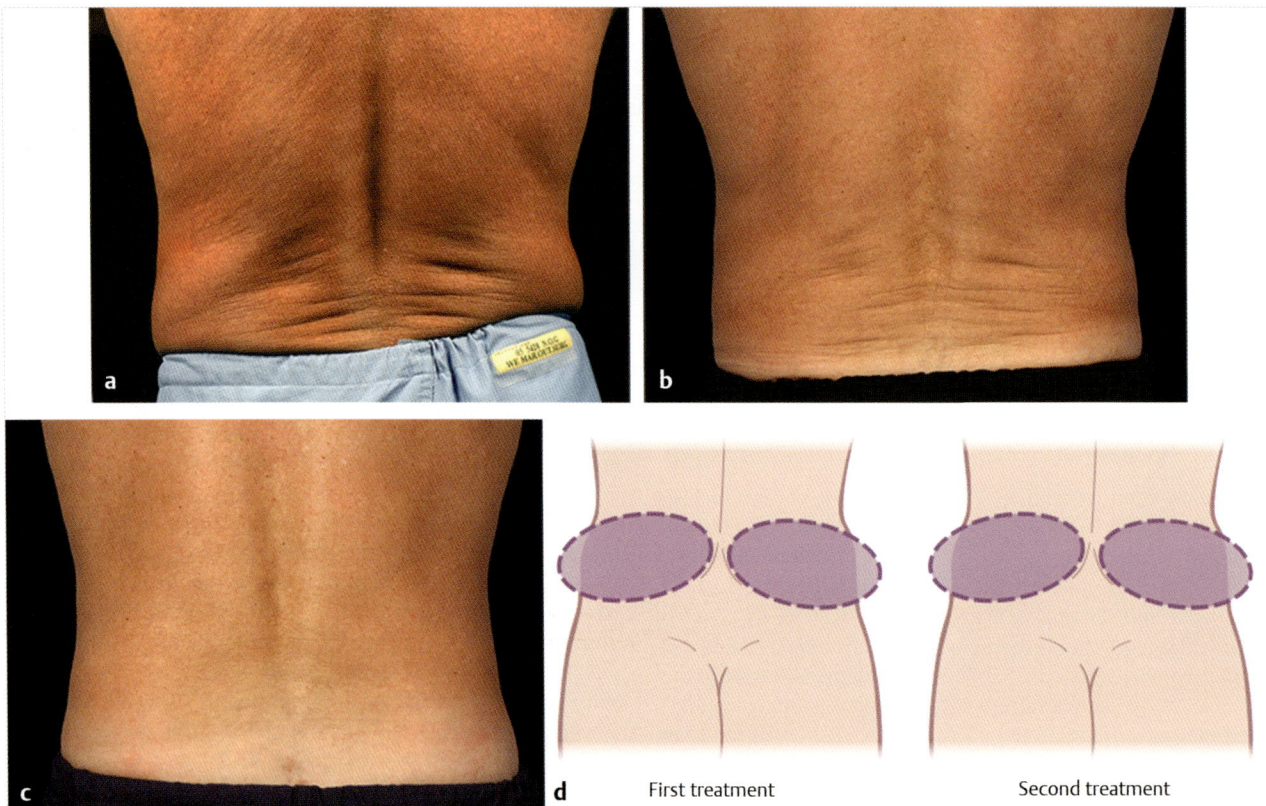

Fig. 13.15 Cryolipolysis of the flanks. (a) This 58-year-old man was fit overall but displeased about the fat in his flanks. (b) 1 year after the first treatment. (c) 1 year after the second treatment. The patient is shown with no weight change since baseline. (d) Illustration of applicator placements. Procedures performed by Dr. W. Grant Stevens. (Reproduced with permission from Stevens WG, Pietrzak LK, Spring MA. Broad overview of a clinical and commercial experience with CoolSculpting. Aesthet Surg J. 2013 Aug 1;33(6):835-46. (d) Courtesy of ZELTIQ™ Aesthetics, Inc. CoolSculpting Available from: http://www.coolsculpting.com/for-physicians/coolsculpting-technology.)

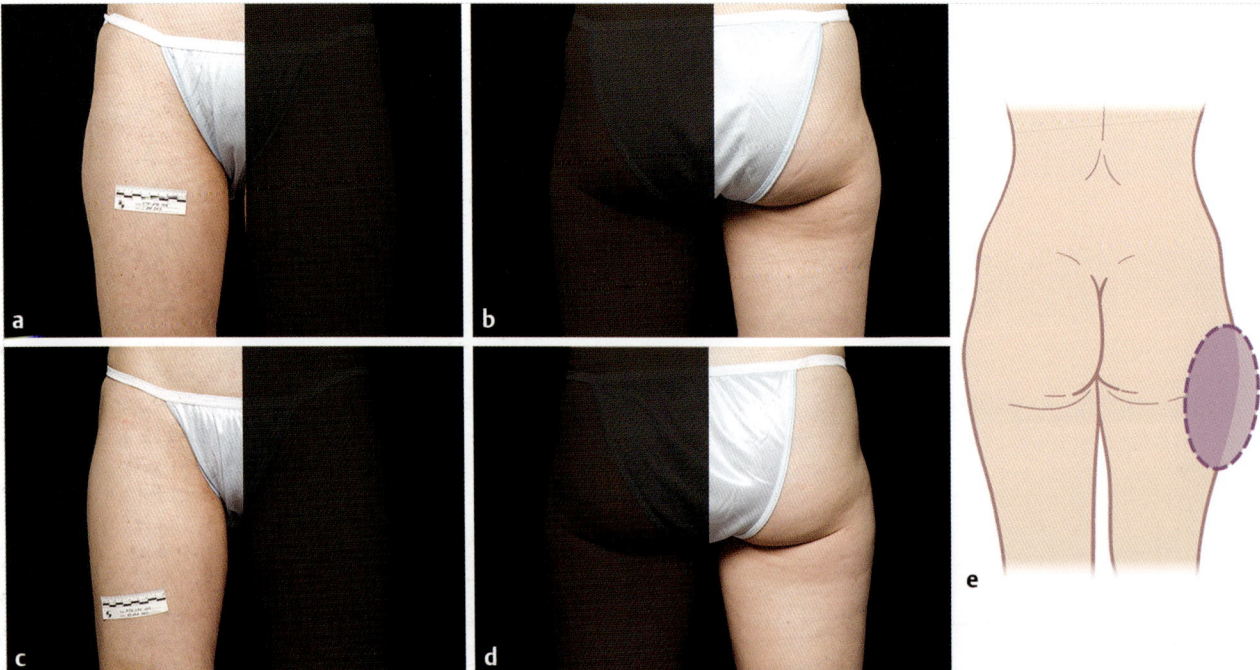

Fig. 13.16 CoolSmoothPro: lateral thighs. (a,b) Before a single-sided cryolipolysis treatment. (c,d) Four months after a single treatment. Procedure by Dr. W. Grant Stevens. (e) Illustration of applicator placement. (Reproduced with permission from Stevens WG, Bachelor EP. Cryolipolysis conformable-surface applicator for nonsurgical fat reduction in lateral thighs. Aesthet Surg J. 2015 Jan;35(1):66-71.(e) Courtesy of ZELTIQ™ Aesthetics, Inc. CoolSculpting Available from: http://www.coolsculpting.com/for-physicians/coolsculpting-technology.)

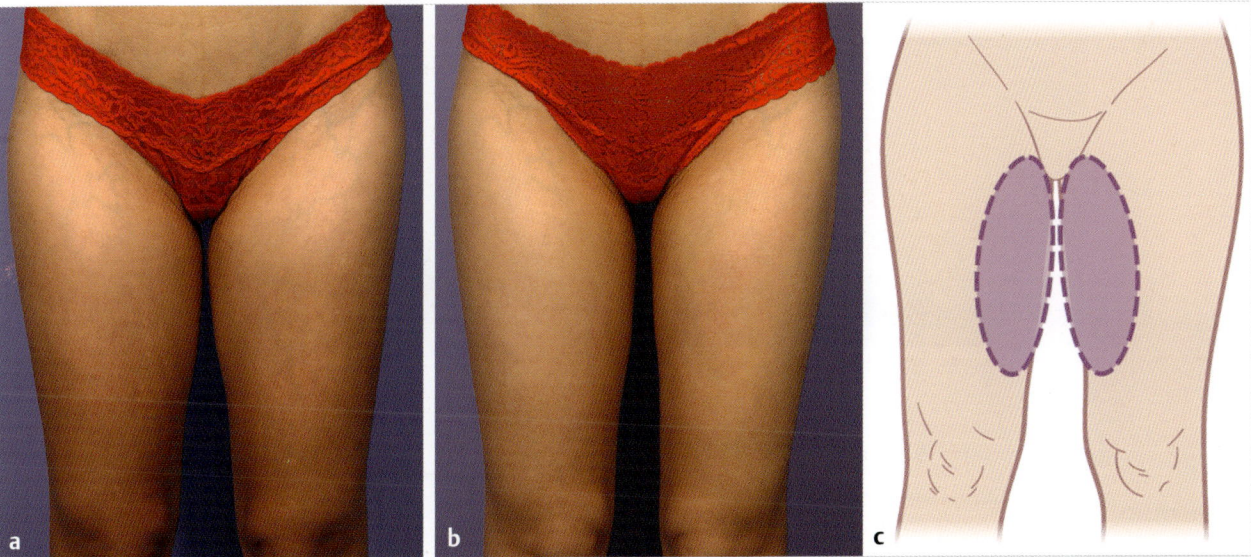

Fig. 13.17 CoolFit: medial thighs. (a) Before cryolipolysis treatment. (b) 2 months after a single treatment. (c) Illustration of applicator placements. (Reproduced with permission from Stevens WG, Pietrzak LK, Spring MA. Broad overview of a clinical and commercial experience with CoolSculpting. Aesthet Surg J. 2013 Aug 1;33(6):835-46. (c) Courtesy of ZELTIQ™ Aesthetics, Inc. CoolSculpting Available from: http://www.coolsculpting.com/for-physicians/coolsculpting-technology.)

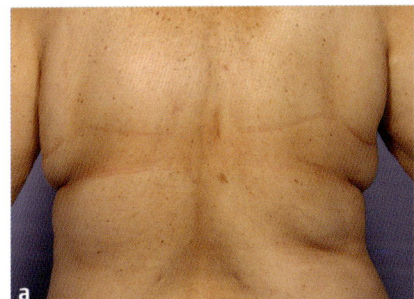 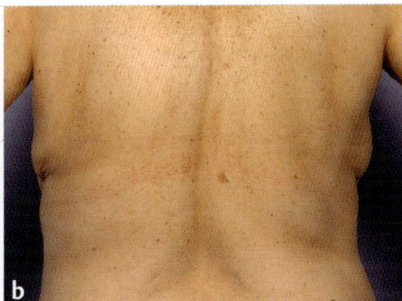

Fig. 13.18 Cryolipolysis of "bra-fat" rolls. (a) This 58-year-old woman was unhappy about her "bra-fat" rolls. (b) Three months after cryolipolysis treatment to the upper back, the patient is shown with no weight change since baseline. (Reproduced with permission from Stevens WG, Pietrzak LK, Spring MA. Broad overview of a clinical and commercial experience with CoolSculpting. Aesthet Surg J. 2013 Aug 1;33 (6):835-46.)

achieved a reduction of 1.6 mm noted 2 months after the last treatment.[29]

The use of cryolipolysis has been broadened from the treatment of discrete areas to comprehensive fat reduction using multiple treatments in overlapping sites. Saltz et al.[17] have described this methodology through a *Treatment to Transformation Protocol*, which requires thoughtful customization of applicator placement and the number of treatment cycles for individual patients and for each, often contiguous, treatment area. Patients in this study underwent up to 4 treatment cycles of overlapping target areas at the initial treatment visit, with additional treatments spaced 2 months apart. Follow-up at 2, 4, and 12 months demonstrated long-term fat reduction from cryolipolysis and excellent tolerability with no reported adverse effects.[17]

In addition to fat reduction, areas that have been treated with cryolipolysis demonstrate cryodermadstringo, or skin tightening (▶ Fig. 13.8) This has been subjectively studied after treatment of the abdomen, flanks, arms, thighs, and back, especially where skin folds often accompany excess fat. This effect has yet to be objectively evaluated in the literature, but pretreatment and posttreatment images in the literature consistently demonstrate this positive ancillary effect.[15,16]

13.6 Complications

Although side effects are rare, the most common side effects of cryolipolysis are transient, mild, and self-resolving. These may include erythema, edema, bruising, and/or soreness, which typically resolve within 1 to 2 weeks. Temporary sensory changes, such as numbness, itching, and neuralgia in the treatment area, are also to be expected, and they resolve without intervention within a few days to months. Zelickson et al[28] reported neuralgia of the inner thighs after a single treatment that did not fully resolve for 132 days. In similar cases, short-term treatment with gabapentin has proved helpful for patients.[30] There have been no reports of ulcerations, scarring, hematomas, blistering, or bleeding after the use of FDA-approved cryolipolysis systems, but these outcomes have been reported after the use of counterfeit, non-FDA-approved cryolipolysis systems, which

Cryolipolysis

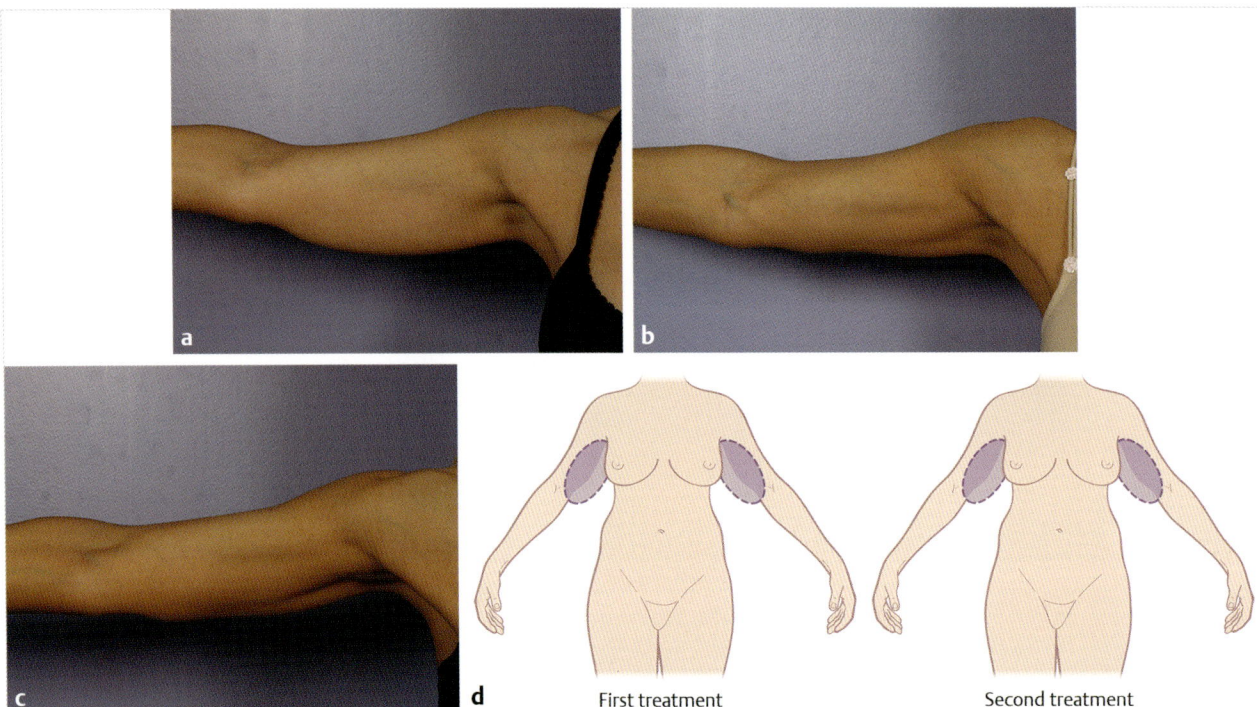

Fig. 13.19 (a) This 48-year-old woman presented for treatment of her upper arms. (b) Two months after one treatment cycle. (c) 4 months after the first treatment, by which time she had undergone 1 additional cycle at the 2-month visit. The patient is shown with a weight change of −4 lbs. under baseline. (d) Illustration of applicator placements. (Reproduced with permission from Stevens WG, Pietrzak LK, Spring MA. Broad overview of a clinical and commercial experience with CoolSculpting. Aesthet Surg J. 2013 Aug 1;33(6):835-46. (d) Courtesy of ZELTIQ™ Aesthetics, Inc. CoolSculpting Available from: http://www.coolsculpting.com/for-physicians/coolsculpting-technology.)

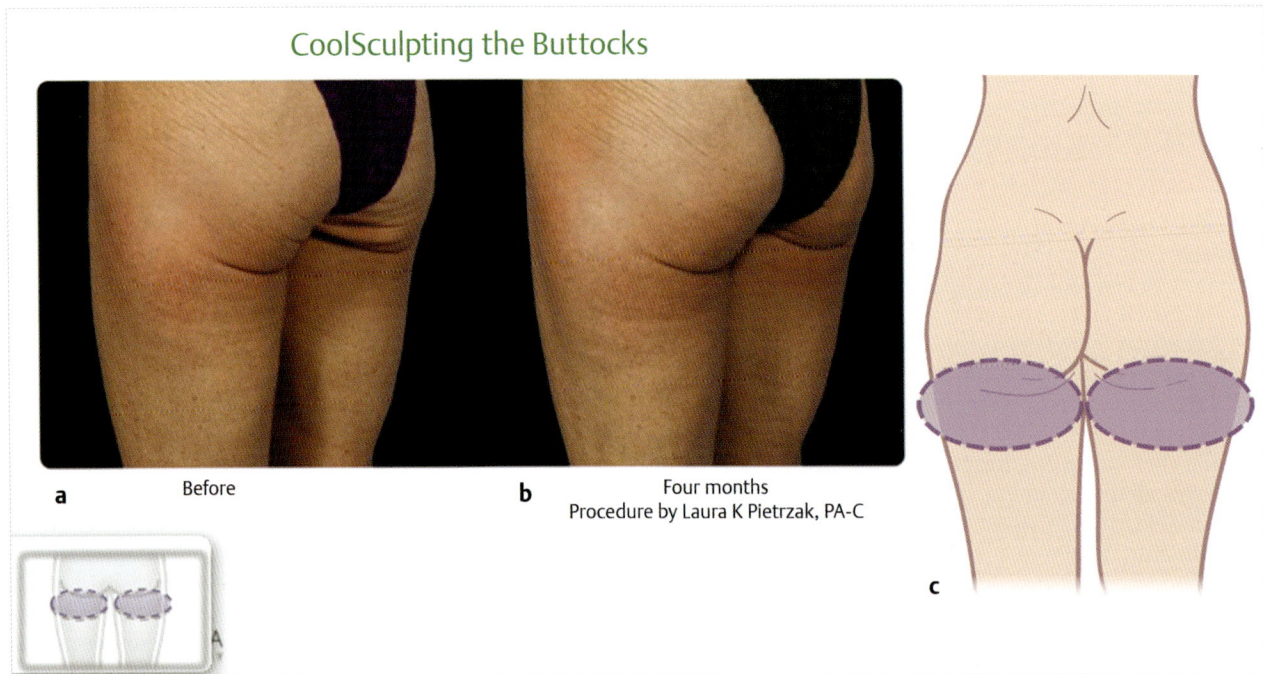

Fig. 13.20 CoolCore: "banana rolls." (a) Before cryolipolysis treatment. (b) 4 months after a single treatment. (c) Illustration of the placement of applicators. ((c) Courtesy of ZELTIQ Aesthetics, Inc.)

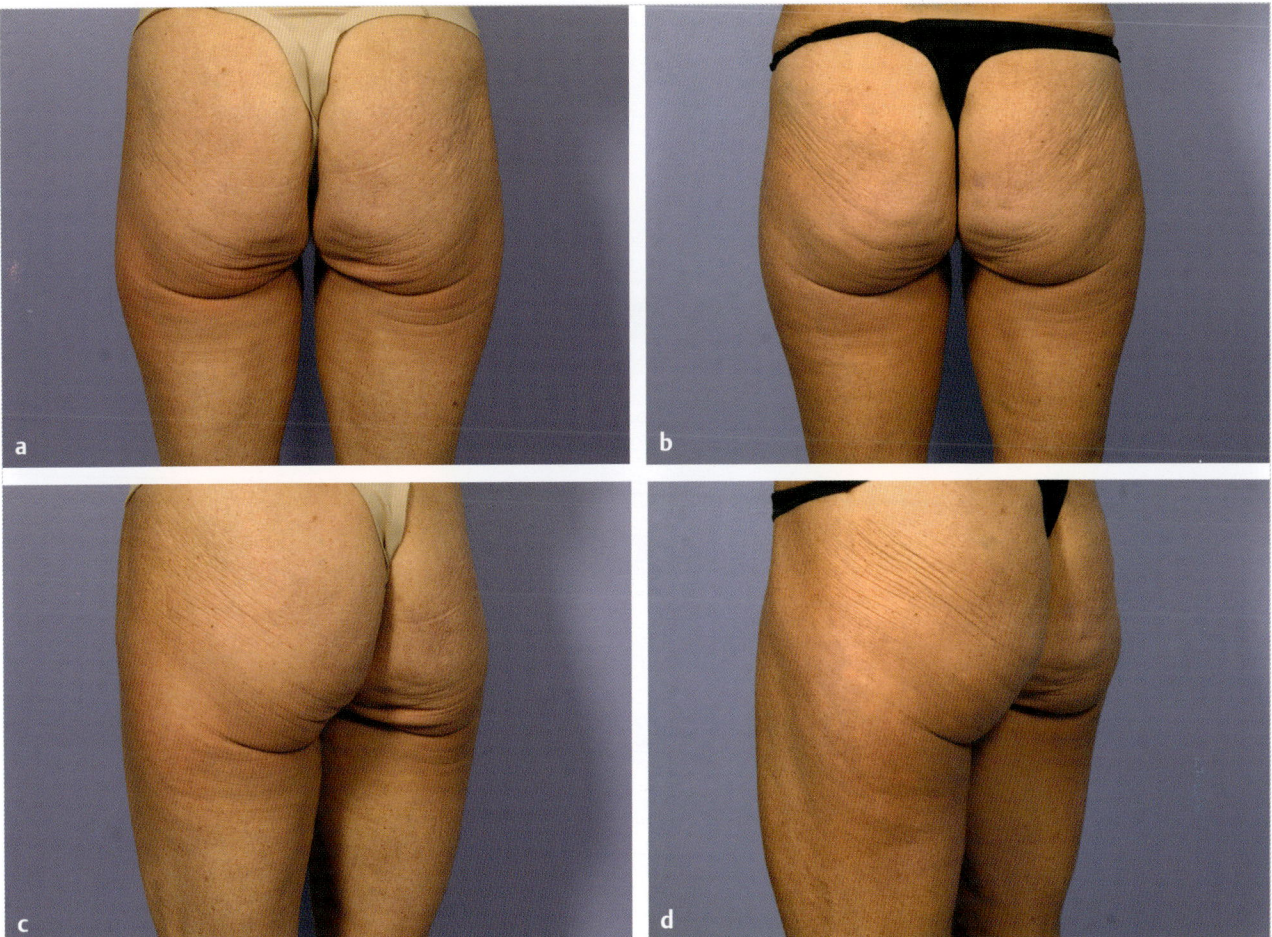

Fig. 13.21 Cryolipolysis of "banana rolls." **(a,b)** This 57-year-old woman presented for treatment of "banana rolls" under her buttocks. **(c,d)** Five months after two cryolipolysis cycles on each side, the patient is shown with a weight change of +4 lbs. over baseline. (Reproduced with permission from Stevens WG, Pietrzak LK, Spring MA. Broad overview of a clinical and commercial experience with CoolSculpting. Aesthet Surg J. 2013 Aug 1;33 (6):835-46.)

are available commercially and online[31] (▶ Fig. 13.22). A rare adverse effect of cryolipolysis, which does not resolve spontaneously, is paradoxical adipose hyperplasia. This has been reported in approximately 33 patients to date and has been estimated to occur in 1 in 20,000 cycles.[32,33] A painless, firm, well-demarcated tissue mass, usually occurring 3 to 6 months posttreatment, characterizes the treated area.[32,33] The treatment for paradoxical adipose hyperplasia is liposuction.[34] Because cryolipolysis is an effective fat-reduction technique, contour irregularities and indentations can occur. As with all fat reduction interventions, fluctuations in the patient's weight will significantly affect the long-term results of cryolipolysis, and are outside of the practitioner's control. Current studies that demonstrate long-term fat-reduction after cryolipolysis qualify these findings with the stipulation that patients' weight did not fluctuate significantly, and in fact, was often maintained within 5 lbs of the baseline weight.

13.7 The Future

New applicators are being developed with different contours and different shaped-plates, which are new ways to decrease treatment time and increase comfort. New cooling cupped surfaces, including more cupped-shaped applicators like the CoolMini and CoolAdvantage, are being developed that may have less required treatment times with colder tissue temperatures. Because less suction is needed, there is less bruising and increased comfort. Applicators with exchangeable flanges will be available soon with more development and may lead to less storage space needed. The current technology may also lead to an improvement in skin quality, such as less dimples or cellulite. Further research is needed.

13.8 Conclusion

Cryolipolysis with the only FDA-approved device, CoolSculpting, uses a controlled-cooling method to nonsurgically reduce adiposity through apoptosis. Several studies have shown that it is effective and safe with high patient satisfaction. As one of the best alternatives to nonsurgical fat reduction, CoolSculpting is an excellent tool for a surgeon to offer his or her patients. This technology has been shown to help grow neophyte and male patient populations. Increasing the available devices has increased the number of treatment cycles and treated patients.

Cryolipolysis

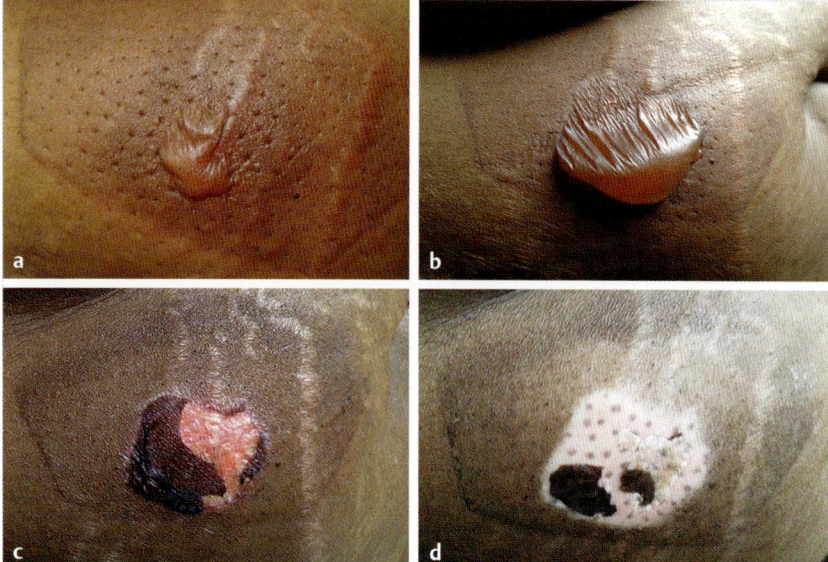

Fig. 13.22 The non-FDA-approved Cryolipolysis system has led to skin injuries. This abdominal injury in a 50-year-old woman was caused by a counterfeit Cryolipolysis system that was not cleared by the FDA. Appearance of the injury on **(a)** day 1, **(b)** day 2, **(c)** day 7, and **(d)** day 13 following treatment with the counterfeit system. (Reproduced with permission from Stevens WG, Spring MA, Macias LH. Counterfeit medical devices: the money you save up front will cost you big in the end. Aesthet Surg J. 2014 Jul;34(5):786-8.)

The staff requirements and posttreatment care is minimal for the results that can be achieved. CoolSculpting does work and is operator-dependent; therefore, excellent results can be achieved with proper application.

13.9 Commentary

Julius W. Few Jr.

Cryolipolysis is the current gold standard in nonsurgical body contouring by lipolysis, and the authors of this chapter have more experience than anyone in the world for treatment of and research on cryolipolysis. I have been an investigator for this technology as well. This chapter helps to present a versatile technology that has been reinvented several times to the benefit of the patient and physician alike. The reader is able to quickly understand how such a technology can be scaled and focused to an individual practice, and this is presented in a clear and concise manner. I strongly agree with the business model presented and the translation to our practice as a dual-sculpting center.

I applaud the authors for emphasizing how to avoid potential complications with the technology, and we have found the suboptimal response rate to be acceptably low, at approximately 10%. In those individuals who have not responded ideally, we have provided the option for the patient to undergo liposuction vs. supplemental radiofrequency treatment, after at least 6 months of postcryolipolysis recovery, at no or significantly limited financial obligation.

We readily apply body-contouring cryolipolysis with facial aesthetic nonsurgical injectable, neuromodulators, and related facial enhancements. This creates a powerful, efficient way to rejuvenate a patient using a full body model. We have found that such packaging enables us to expand our treatment base, grow our body-contouring base, and create a true continuum of beauty.

With the introduction of cryolipolysis to our practice, we have seen double-digit growth in both surgical and nonsurgical body contouring. The addition of submental fat treatment has further enhanced our offering, creating a growth center for the face as well.

My personal enthusiasm for cryolipolysis is significant, primarily due to its longevity in the marketplace and our experience, and there are also other technologies presented in this book that are very effective and powerful. I believe that the presentation in this chapter shows us how a focused application with a very good technology can deliver good results.

Although the authors show results of very good skin remodeling with lipolysis, we have found that some patients with significant skin laxity can be challenging. This was the basis of our recent study. We used a randomized, double-blind approach with separate reviewers to show the benefit of combining radiofrequency after cryolipolysis to the flanks in individuals with lax skin. There was a significant benefit to this combination, and it helps to power the concept of stackable treatments.

References

[1] The American Society for Aesthetic Plastic Surgery. 2016 Cosmetic Surgery National Data Bank Statistics. 19th Annual Multi-Specialty Statistical Data. http://www.surgery.org/media/statistics. Accessed 11/2016

[2] The American Society for Aesthetic Plastic Surgery. 2014 Cosmetic Surgery National Data Bank Statistics. 18th Annual Multi-Specialty Statistical Data. Accessed 11/2016

[3] Manstein D, Laubach H, Watanabe K, Farinelli W, Zurakowski D, Anderson RR. Selective cryolysis: a novel method of non-invasive fat removal. Lasers Surg Med. 2008; 40(9):595–604

[4] ZELTIQ™ Aesthetics, Inc. http://www.coolsculpting.com/

[5] Bernstein EF. Long-term efficacy follow-up on two cryolipolysis case studies: 6 and 9 years post-treatment. J Cosmet Dermatol. 2016; 15(4):561–564

[6] Epstein EH, Jr, Oren ME. Popsicle panniculitis. N Engl J Med. 1970; 282(17):966–967

[7] Beacham BE, Cooper PH, Buchanan CS, Weary PE. Equestrian cold panniculitis in women. Arch Dermatol. 1980; 116(9):1025–1027

[8] Zelickson B, Egbert BM, Preciado J, et al. Cryolipolysis for noninvasive fat cell destruction: initial results from a pig model. Dermatol Surg. 2009; 35(10):1462–1470

[9] Coleman SR, Sachdeva K, Egbert BM, Preciado J, Allison J. Clinical efficacy of noninvasive cryolipolysis and its effects on peripheral nerves. Aesthetic Plast Surg. 2009; 33(4):482–488

[10] Klein KB, Zelickson B, Riopelle JG, et al. Non-invasive cryolipolysis for subcutaneous fat reduction does not affect serum lipid levels or liver function tests. Lasers Surg Med. 2009; 41(10):785–790

[11] Dierickx CC, Mazer JM, Sand M, Koenig S, Arigon V. Safety, tolerance, and patient satisfaction with noninvasive cryolipolysis. Dermatol Surg. 2013; 39(8):1209–1216

[12] Derrick CD, Shridharani SM, Broyles JM. The safety and efficacy of cryolipolysis: a systematic review of available literature. Aesthet Surg J. 2015; 35(7):830–836

[13] US Food and Drug Administration. 510(k) clearance K151179: CoolSculpting System. 2015. Available from: http://www.accessdata.fda.gov/cdrh_docs/pdf15/K151179.pdf. Accessed 18 Nov, 2015

[14] Stevens WG, Pietrzak LK, Spring MA. Broad overview of a clinical and commercial experience with CoolSculpting. Aesthet Surg J. 2013; 33(6):835–846

[15] Stevens WG. Does cryolipolysis lead to skin tightening? A first report of cryodermadstringo. Aesthet Surg J. 2014; 34(6):NP32–NP34

[16] Carruthers J, Stevens WG, Carruthers A, Humphrey S. Cryolipolysis and skin tightening. Dermatol Surg. 2014; 40 Suppl 12:S184–S189

[17] Saltz R, Burns J, Stevens G, Kilmer S. Abstract: Cryolipolysis treatment to transformation: one year safety and efficacy follow-up. The Aesthetic Meeting. 2014

[18] CoolSculpting® Available from: http://www.coolsculpting.com/for-physicians/coolsculpting-technology

[19] Wanitphakdeedecha R, Sathaworawong A, Manuskiatti W. The efficacy of cryolipolysis treatment on arms and inner thighs. Lasers Med Sci. 2015; 30(8):2165–2169

[20] Coolsculpting®. ZELTIQ(R) launches 3-in-1 CoolAdvantage® applicator for the CoolSculpting® system at American Academy of Dermatology Annual Meeting. http://investor.coolsculpting.com/releasedetail.cfm?releaseid=958687. March 3, 2016

[21] Boey GE, Wasilenchuk JL. Enhanced clinical outcome with manual massage following cryolipolysis treatment: a 4-month study of safety and efficacy. Lasers Surg Med. 2014; 46(1):20–26

[22] Ingargiola MJ, Motakef S, Chung MT, Vasconez HC, Sasaki GH. Cryolipolysis for fat reduction and body contouring: safety and efficacy of current treatment paradigms. Plast Reconstr Surg. 2015; 135(6):1581–1590

[23] Sasaki GH, Abelev N, Tevez-Ortiz A. Noninvasive selective cryolipolysis and reperfusion recovery for localized natural fat reduction and contouring. Aesthet Surg J. 2014; 34(3):420–431

[24] Bernstein EF, Bloom JD, Basilavecchio LD, Plugis JM. Non-invasive fat reduction of the flanks using a new cryolipolysis applicator and overlapping, two-cycle treatments. Lasers Surg Med. 2014; 46(10):731–735

[25] Bernstein EF. Longitudinal evaluation of cryolipolysis efficacy: two case studies. J Cosmet Dermatol. 2013; 12(2):149–152

[26] Stevens WG, Bachelor EP. Cryolipolysis conformable-surface applicator for nonsurgical fat reduction in lateral thighs. Aesthet Surg J. 2015; 35(1):66–71

[27] Garibyan L, Sipprell WH, III, Jalian HR, Sakamoto FH, Avram M, Anderson RR. Three-dimensional volumetric quantification of fat loss following cryolipolysis. Lasers Surg Med. 2014; 46(2):75–80

[28] Zelickson BD, Burns AJ, Kilmer SL. Cryolipolysis for safe and effective inner thigh fat reduction. Lasers Surg Med. 2015; 47(2):120–127

[29] Munavalli GS, Panchaprateep R. Cryolipolysis for targeted fat reduction and improved appearance of the enlarged male breast. Dermatol Surg. 2015; 41(9):1043–1051

[30] Keaney TC, Gudas AT, Alster TS. Delayed onset pain associated with cryolipolysis treatment: a retrospective study with treatment recommendations. Dermatol Surg. 2015; 41(11):1296–1299

[31] Stevens WG, Spring MA, Macias LH. Counterfeit medical devices: the money you save up front will cost you big in the end. Aesthet Surg J. 2014; 34(5):786–788

[32] Seaman SA, Tannan SC, Cao Y, Peirce SM, Gampper TJ. Paradoxical adipose hyperplasia and cellular effects after cryolipolysis: a case report. Aesthet Surg J. 2015; •••:sjv105

[33] Jalian HR, Avram MM, Garibyan L, Mihm MC, Anderson RR. Paradoxical adipose hyperplasia after cryolipolysis. JAMA Dermatol. 2014; 150(3):317–319

[34] Stefani WA. Adipose hypertrophy following cryolipolysis. Aesthet Surg J. 2015; 35(7):NP218–NP220

14 Minimally Invasive Techniques: Preventing and Managing Adverse Events

Mark S. Nestor, Paige Paparone, and Mitchell Manway

Summary

Preventing adverse events in minimally invasive blended aesthetic treatments begins with appropriate patient selection. It is critical to understand patient anatomy, the risks and benefits of the procedure, and to understand and master the techniques associated with optimal patient outcome. Managing adverse events requires recognizing them when they occur and understanding how to treat them. Complications include the inherent risk of bleeding, damage to important tissues and structures, wound closure difficulties, poor healing, and infection.

Keywords: complications, deoxycholic acid, dermal filler, infection, intense pulsed light (IPL), laser resurfacing, microfocused ultrasound, neurotoxin injection

> **Key Points**
>
> - Always take a comprehensive medical and cosmetic procedure history and speak to the patient about other potential lifestyle factors that may impact the aesthetic outcome.
> - Many complications can be avoided by making sure to only select appropriate patients.
> - When performing any procedure, it is critical to understand patient anatomy, the risks and benefits of the procedure, and to understand and master the techniques associated with optimal patient outcome.
> - Adverse events can occur with any procedure and at the hands of any clinician. It is critical, therefore, to prevent them whenever possible, recognize them when they occur, and understand how to treat them.
> - Informing the patient of every potential risk and complication inherent to a product or procedure is the moral and ethical duty of the provider.

14.1 Introduction

Blended aesthetic medicine is a sophisticated and personalized cosmetic approach that, by definition, uses a combination of procedures incorporating neurotoxin injections, injectable fillers, and devices, including both ablative and nonablative lasers, radiofrequency and microfocused ultrasound, chemical peels, absorbable lifting sutures, and/or surgery. The ideal blending of procedures combines the benefits of multiple modalities and result in a cumulative effect that no one method can accomplish alone. However, with the increased potential afforded in blended aesthetic medicine also comes the increased complexity of safety considerations and the increased risk of complications.[1,2]

A variety of complications can arise from aesthetic medical procedures. Well-known surgical complications include the inherent risk of bleeding, damage to important tissues and structures, wound closure difficulties, poor healing, and infection. Less frequently, secondary events due to an adverse reaction to anesthetics or sedatives can even be life-threatening. Although less invasive, even the modern nonsurgical cosmetic techniques that many patients actively seek and prefer are also certainly not without the risk of very minor or even rarely severe complications.[2]

If and when complications and adverse events occur while employing blended aesthetic medicine, a physician with a deeper understanding of each product, each technique, and the contributing factors involved will be more able to effectively prevent, perceive, and manage complications.[3]

In this chapter, we will discuss a variety of minimally invasive procedures that are commonly used in blended aesthetic medicine, such as neurotoxin injection, dermal filler, laser resurfacing, deoxycholic acid, and microfocused ultrasound. First, appropriate patient selection and common indications and contraindications will be listed, followed by the potential complications of each method and how one can effectively prevent, treat, and manage such adverse events.

14.2 Patient Selection

The selection of suitable patients and the exclusion of inappropriate patients is the first and perhaps the most important step in avoiding complications. For any cosmetic procedure, a thorough and comprehensive medical and cosmetic history must be elicited in order to avoid treating patients with preexisting conditions that are contraindicated to treatment. Obviously, it is also critically important to discuss realistic expectations of the aesthetic outcome, as well as the number of treatments required to reach personalized goals. Patients will undoubtedly be unsatisfied with the results if they are not sufficiently informed of the limitations of these minimally invasive techniques.

14.2.1 Dermal Fillers

Dermal fillers of all types are frequently used to replace lost volume, decrease the appearance of wrinkles, and improve the overall contour of the skin on the face. In addition, off-label use for the correction of facial depressions caused by prior surgery, as well as administration to other areas of the body to help treat volume loss, is also common.[4] When considering any dermal filler injection, patients with evidence of active skin infection in the proposed treatment area should force a delay of the treatment, because the infecting organism can spread to deeper tissues with trauma induced through the needle. Examples of such cases include viral infections such as herpes simplex virus (HSV) and human papilloma virus (HPV), molluscum contagiosum, bacterial infections such as streptococci or staphylococci, and rarely fungal and yeast infections[5] (▶ Fig. 14.1). With

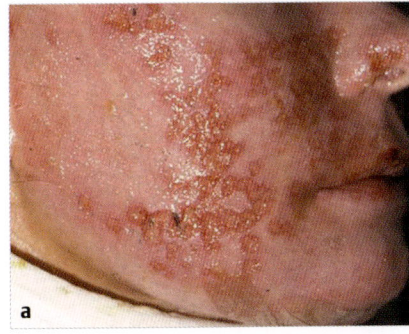
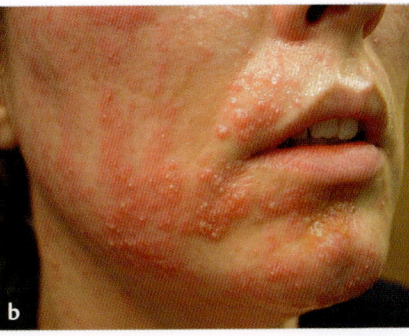

Fig. 14.1 (a) Lesions of the treated areas often indicate infection. Punched-out circular lesions are typical of herpetic infection. (b) Posttreatment appearance of common fungal infection.[5] (Reproduced with permission from Bass L and Pozner J: Laser Facial Resurfacing. In Cohen M and Thaller S: The Unfavorable Result in Plastic Surgery: Avoidance and Treatment, Thieme Medical Publishers, St. Louis, 2017)

evidence of any of these organisms, cultures should be obtained, treatment with an appropriate medication should be administered, and resolution should be confirmed before any injections are performed.

Likewise, dermal fillers can exacerbate chronic preexisting skin conditions such as autoimmune and connective tissue diseases. Poor candidates for dermal fillers may include patients with history of hypertrophic and keloid scarring, discoid lupus erythematosus, active scleroderma or psoriasis, Marfan syndrome, and Ehlers-Danlos syndrome. In patients with systemic disease such as human immunodeficiency virus (HIV), diabetes mellitus, or scleroderma, treatment can cautiously be performed if the patient has displayed a history of normal wound healing. Therefore, immunosuppressed patients should be screened carefully to determine if they are good candidates for treatment.[6,7]

Indications for Dermal Fillers

- Lipoatrophy
- Rhytides and folds
- Depressed facial defects
- Cosmesis

Relative Contraindications for Dermal Fillers

- History of multiple or severe allergies or anaphylaxis
- Active skin infection in the treatment area
- Isotretinoin for 6 months before or after treatment (controversial)
- Autoimmune and connective tissue diseases
- Pregnant or lactating women
- Certain psychiatric conditions such as body dysmorphia

14.2.2 Botulinum Toxin

Patients with dynamic rhytides and no static component will show the most impressive improvement from injection with botulinum toxin. Patients who have rhytides visible at rest will also benefit from this type of treatment, although peak improvement is likely to require numerous administrations. These deeper wrinkles may become softened over time, but combination treatment with dermal fillers or resurfacing procedures may be required to achieve the desired results. The most notable contraindications to botulinum toxin injection include patients with neuromuscular disorders such as myasthenia gravis, amyotrophic lateral sclerosis, Labert-Eaton myasthenic syndrome, and other myopathies that involve neuromuscular transmission. Relative contraindications include patients with impaired healing, bleeding abnormalities, a history of hypertrophic or keloidal scarring, and those with significant skin atrophy. A very unique contraindication to neurotoxin administration is the need for uncompromised facial expression. This can be found frequently in patients with occupations in the show business. As with any procedure, the clinician and the patient should discuss end treatment goals and realistic expectations.[8,9]

Indications for Botulinum Toxin

- Rhytides
- Hyperhidrosis
- Blepharospasm
- Strabismus
- Migraines
- Platysma neck muscle bands
- Dystonias (cervical, cranial, facial, oromandibular, laryngeal)

Relative Contraindications for Botulinum Toxin

- History of allergy or sensitivity
- Pregnant or nursing women
- Active infection or dermatoses in the treatment area
- Bleeding abnormalities
- Impaired healing
- Hypertrophic or keloidal scarring
- Skin atrophy
- Body dysmorphic disorder
- Dependence on uncompromised facial expression
- Myasthenia gravis
- Amyotrophic lateral sclerosis
- Eaton-Lambert syndrome
- Other neuromuscular disorders

14.2.3 Deoxycholic Acid

Recently, the FDA has approved deoxycholate treatment designed to reduce submental fat (SMF). Traditionally, SMF reduction can effectively be treated by liposuction and lower facelift and neck lift, with or without submentoplasty. However, patients continue to seek less invasive methods. A recent set of studies investigating injectable deoxycholic acid has met with very encouraging results (**see Video 2.11**).[10,11] Deoxycholic acid is thought to act by disrupting the membranes of adipocytes through solubilization of the membrane lipids, causing the targeted destruction of fat cells.[12] Future studies will hopefully look to explore a deeper understanding of this attractive modality (**see Video 1.1**).

Indications for Deoxycholic Acid

- Moderate or severe convexity associated with SMF
- History of dysphagia
- Facial neurapraxia
- Loose skin or previous trauma in the submental area
- Prominent platysma bands
- Any localized swelling in the submental area

Relative Contraindication for Deoxycholic Acid

- Infection in submental area

14.2.4 Laser Resurfacing

Ablative laser resurfacing utilizing CO_2 or erbium lasers can either be fractional or nonfractional. Proper patient selection is particularly important when considering any laser resurfacing. Most notably, it is critical to appreciate the patient's Fitzpatrick skin type, because there exists significant risk for dyspigmentation with this methodology. For example, patients with higher Fitzpatrick skin types (darker skin types) are at increased risk for postinflammatory hyperpigmentation (PIH), which can prove extremely difficult to remedy. In addition, patients with a history of poor wound healing, hypertrophic scarring, or keloids are not candidates for aggressive treatment, and thus lower fluences should be utilized on these patients. As always, a detailed history should be obtained during cosmetic consultation to accurately predict the risk of known side effects.[13]

Among others, common indications for both fractional ablative and nonablative laser treatment include mild to moderate facial and periorbital wrinkles, acne scarring, dyschromias, and postburn and surgical scars. More dramatic improvement has been shown with fine rhytides as opposed to deeper creases, and again realistic expectations should be conveyed to these patients.[14]

Indications for Ablative Laser Resurfacing

- Perioral vertical furrows
- Periorbital dynamic lines (crow's-feet)
- Mild dermatochalasis
- Glabellar dynamic lines
- Actinic damage
- Facial elastosis
- Scars, including acne scars
- Epidermal lesions
- Dyschromias
- Mild photodamaged skin
- Superficial and deep rhytides

Indications for Nonablative Laser Resurfacing

- Mild rhytides, photodamage
- Acne scar
- Postsurgical scar
- Skin texture improvement

Relative Contraindications for Laser Resurfacing

- Reduced adnexal structures
- Unrealistic patient expectations
- History of keloid scars
- Active acne
- Deep acne pits
- Isotretinoin treatment in the last 6 months
- Recent radiation therapy

14.2.5 Microfocused Ultrasound

Microfocused ultrasound is a recently developed technology used for noninvasive skin tightening and lifting. Microfocused ultrasound uses different frequencies of acoustic sound that converge and exert their effect below the epidermis, bypassing the need for invasive surgery. This modality focuses ultrasound waves to specific areas in both the dermal and subcutaneous tissues, creating tiny thermal coagulation points. Browlifting, improvement in wrinkles, and skin tightening can all be achieved by adjusting the energy and depth of the emitted sound. In addition to the potential benefits to the face and neck, microfocused ultrasound can also be used on regions including the thighs, upper arms, and knees. Microfocused ultrasound combined with imaging has also been shown to be beneficial in the removal of hyperactive sweat glands in patients with hyperhidrosis, the effects of which were shown to last more than 12 months.[15,16]

The ideal microfocused ultrasound patient has mild to moderate skin and soft tissue laxity. Because microfocused ultrasound patients have increased wound healing capacity, younger patients are favored. Similarly, patients with extensive photodamage, severe skin laxity, and dramatic platysma banding are poorer candidates and, comparatively, will require a more aggressive approach.

Relative contraindications of microfocused ultrasound include infections/wounds, severe acne, or the possession of metallic objects within the treatment area such as cardiac pacemakers and defibrillators. Relative contraindications also include treatment areas containing keloids, permanent dermal fillers, or patients with risk factors that inhibit proper wound healing such as uncontrolled diabetes or chronic tobacco smokers.[15]

Indications for Microfocused Ultrasound

- Axillary hyperhidrosis
- Soft tissue laxity
- Mild to moderate rhytides
- Photodamage
- Platysmal banding

Contraindications for Microfocused Ultrasound

- Infections
- Open skin lesions
- Severe acne
- Metallic implants

14.2.6 Intense Pulsed Light

Intense pulsed light (IPL) uses a broad wavelength of noncoherent light to exert nonablative effects on many cell types. The photobiology is not as well understood, but the procedure appears to affect many more chromophores and cell types due to a wider spectrum. In theory, this may have a greater and more thorough potential for exerting a regenerative effect.

IPL is ideal for photodamage-associated dyschromia and telangiectasia as well as mild rhytides and the improvement of large pores. IPL has many advantages compared to laser-based technologies. There is minimal downtime when undertaking an IPL procedure. It can be performed during the patient's lunch break with the patient returning directly back to work after completion of a session. In addition to being used on the face, IPL can be used on the chest, neck, and hands. Moreover, IPL can penetrate deeper tissues than most laser-based technologies and yet maintains a reduced risk for purpura and hyperpigmentation. The benefit for using IPL to treat rhytides is modest when compared to laser-based therapies, but the relative safety profile of IPL is unmatched.

More often, however, IPL is used to remove hair, treat telangiectasias, improve skin texture, and correct irregular pigmentation.[17] The contraindications to IPL are fairly limited.

Indications for Intense Pulsed Light

- Hair removal
- Vascular lesions
- Spider angiomas
- Port-wine stains
- Broken facial veins
- Rosacea
- Pigmented lesions
- Age spots
- Melasma
- Photoaging
- Acne
- Rhytides

Contraindications for Intense Pulsed Light

- Tanned or sunburned skin
- Depilatory cream in the past 6 months
- History of hypertrophic or keloid scarring

14.3 Avoidance and Management of Complications

An experienced physician with knowledge of anatomy, appropriate technique, and aftercare is the single most important factor to decrease the incidence of complications and adverse events. However, despite flawless administration and proper patient instruction, complications can and do still occur, and it is again the knowledge of how to properly manage these undesirable results that will be vital to maximize the aesthetic outcome. A list of potential complications inherent to each modality, as well as steps for proper treatment and management therein, will be detailed in the following sections.

14.3.1 Dermal Fillers

In addition to basic aseptic injection technique, the safe and proper injection of dermal fillers requires the provider to possess detailed knowledge of facial anatomy, specifically the distribution of facial nerves and arteries.[18] Unfortunately, subtle individual variations in anatomy are prevalent, and even the most educated injectors will still have to exercise continuous caution. Accordingly, aspiration should be done prior to injection, especially in high-risk areas such as the glabella and nose.[2] Slow injection gives the clinician time to rapidly react to impending complications. Immediate evidence of such problems can manifest as acute changes in skin color or disproportionate or excessive pain.[6] That being said, a patient may paradoxically report no pain if the dermal filler is combined with a local anesthetic or if a nerve block has been utilized.[2] Small-gauge needles are preferred to slow the injection rate, and although there is no data confirming decreased incidence of adverse events, blunt cannulas are recommended to reduce the risk of vessel injury. Postinjection massage is an important practice to prevent the uneven dispersal of product, which can manifest as lumps or beading; however, massage by the patient at home is to be avoided. The patient should not massage the injected area for 2 weeks and should avoid extremes of temperature. Finally, proper depth placement inherent to each type of filler is not to be adjusted. Overcorrection and erroneous placement of filler is much more common than other serious adverse events. For instance, a very superficial injection of a filler meant for deeper placement, or even too much volume given to very thin skin, can result in a displeasing outcome.[19] Likewise, synthetic fillers should not be injected into muscle, because contraction will dislodge the filler and may result in asymmetry and/or lumps.[20]

Both short-term and long-term complications are associated with all types of fillers. Early complications arising in days to weeks include swelling, erythema, bruising, pain, pruritus, infection, allergic reaction, and the rare risk of vascular compromise or embolism. The related side effects of local injections are transient and can be minimized by standard ice and compression. Although rare, infection from filler implantation can occur and may appear as erythematous nodules. There is speculation that such nodules are caused by a mild bacterial infection such as *Staphylococcus epidermidis* or *Propionibacterium acnes*, which festers within a biofilm in the area adjacent to filler placement. The biofilm itself consists of waste, bacteria, and nutrient material.[21] Mild infections can be treated with empirical oral antibiotics such as a macrolide or tetracycline.[6]

The most feared and serious complications of dermal fillers involve vascular compromise or embolization. Vascular occlusion may occur if the filler is placed within a blood vessel, or if a significant amount of the filler is placed next to a vessel causing compression. Immediate venous occlusion will display a bluish discoloration of the surrounding skin. Arterial blockage is a serious complication and can result in severe tissue damage and necrosis. The most vulnerable site is the glabellar region, which is supplied by an artery that lacks strong collateral circulation.[6,21] Indeed, there have been case reports of embolization to the central retinal artery resulting in blindness of the affected eye.[22] This is possible due to the retrograde flow of filler through the blood vessels exiting the supraorbital area.

Fortunately, this is an extremely rare occurrence, but it is important to note.[2]

With any suspicion of vascular occlusion, the injection must be stopped and treatment must be administered immediately. Massage, warm compresses, and/or 2% nitropaste to promote vasodilation can be given. If occlusion results from hyaluronic acid fillers, an injection of hyaluronidase is administered. Conversely, saline may be injected for hydroxyapatite fillers. Therefore, hyaluronidase has been proposed as treatment in all cases of vascular occlusion regardless of the filler type, because it has been shown to decrease swelling and vascular pressure.[23]

Later and long-term complications of dermal fillers occurring within weeks to years include incorrect placement or migration of the implanted filler, overcorrection or undercorrection, scarring, implant visibility, nodules, or granulomatous inflammation. Overcorrection is an avoidable complication commonly caused by injecting dermal filler too quickly or inappropriately. Similarly, when hyaluronic acid fillers are implanted too superficially, a bluish hue may result because of the scattering of light by particles in suspension, which is known as the *Tyndall effect*. One major advantage of hyaluronic acid fillers is that overambitious administration can be corrected with the injection of hyaluronidase.

Nodule formation can result from the incorrect placement of dermal filler or the asymmetric dispersal of product. This complication is especially common when product is injected too superficially and can develop as soon as 1-month postinjection. Luckily, nodules are usually invisible and asymptomatic. Nodules detected early can be effectively treated using massage or a 25-gauge needle to break up the product. Conversely, late-appearing nodules are best treated more aggressively and may require the injection of triamcinolone, 5-flourouracil, or methylprednisolone. If nodules are large and resistant to conservative management, excision may be necessary.[7,21]

Granulomatous foreign-body reactions are another late complication, with incidence of roughly 0.1% to 0.2%, forming months to years after treatment. Again, patients may be asymptomatic or the symptoms can be vague with mild erythema or swelling. As in any granuloma, the histological appearance will be a group of macrophages accompanied by multinucleated giant cells and scattered lymphocytes. Concerning treatment, granulomas can be unpredictable, because they may increase in size or resolve spontaneously. If treatment is needed, the gold standard is corticosteroid injection with dosages of 5 to10 mg/cc. Repeat treatment, if necessary, can be performed in 4 to 6 weeks. Unfortunately, excision is contraindicated, because granulomas have obscure borders, thus attempts at removal may cause abscesses, fistulas, or scarring.[7,24]

Complications of Dermal Filler (Early)

- Erythema
- Swelling
- Pain/tenderness
- Ecchymosis
- Itching
- Infection/inflammation
- Allergic reaction/hypersensitivity
- Vascular compromise/necrosis
- Retinal embolus

Complications of Dermal Filler (Late)

- Overcorrection/undercorrection
- Misplacement
- Implant visibility (Tyndall effect)
- Granulomatous inflammation/foreign-body reaction
- Nodules
- Migration of implanted filler
- Scarring

14.3.2 Botulinum Toxin

Once injection of a neurotoxin to the appropriate muscle is successfully completed, patients should be instructed to not lay supine for a period of 4 hours. In addition, recipients should also avoid applying heat or massage to the area to prevent the spread of the neurotoxin to unwanted locations. Likewise, activities that cause flushing, such as consumption of alcohol and exercise, should also be discouraged.

Expected complications with any injection include transient swelling, bruising, mild erythema, and tenderness over the injection sites.[8,9] These can be mitigated through the use of very small-gauge needles, ice, and compression.[25] Infection is always a risk when compromising the skin barrier, but performing an alcohol swab of the skin before injection is usually sufficient.

Complications of Botulinum Toxin (Injection-related)

- Bruising
- Swelling
- Tenderness
- Mild erythema
- Pain
- Infection

Less common than injection-related adverse events are those related to the neurotoxin itself, the most common of which are eyelid ptosis (blepharoptosis) and eyebrow ptosis. Blepharoptosis is caused by inadvertent diffusion of the toxin through the orbital septum, resulting in paralysis the levator palpebrae superioris. The risk of this complication can be decreased by using the proper technique of maintaining the injection at least 1 cm above the supraorbital ridge at the midpupillary line.[26] Noticeable within 48 hours to seven days, this particularly distressing problem can last up to 2 to 4 weeks and is most often unilaterally witnessed. Fortunately, this condition can be treated with alpha-adrenergic agonist ophthalmic drops such as naphazoline 0.025%/pheniramine 0.3% or apraclonidine 0.5%. Both of these medications act by causing the Müller's muscle to contract, which elevates the upper eyelid. Apraclonidine should be used in refractory cases if over-the-counter methods prove noncurative, because exacerbation of underlying glaucoma is a potential side effect. Quite similarly, inadvertent or excessive paralysis of portions of the frontalis muscle can cause eyebrow ptosis or asymmetry. Injection at a minimum distance of 4 to 5 cm away from the orbital rim is advised to decrease the incidence of eyebrow ptosis for those less experienced in this area. Concerning other vulnerable areas and muscle groups, recommended and established guidelines should be followed.[26]

The rarest complications in recipients of neurotoxin involve the formation of antibodies or allergic reaction. Antibody formation is observed less than 1% of the time, although it can result in resistance to treatment or render the neurotoxin ineffective. Patients with a known allergy to cow's milk are said to have a contraindication not to receive abobotulinumtoxinA (Dysport, Ipsen Biopharmaceuticals, Inc.) injections, because bovine protein is used in the manufacturing process, although reactions in even these individuals are extremely rare.[27] Serious allergic reactions are exceedingly rare but have been witnessed as well, and aggressive treatments such as systemic steroids may be necessary for cases resulting in anaphylaxis.[8]

Complications of Botulinum Toxin

- Blepharoptosis
- Eyebrow ptosis
- Antibody development
- Allergic reaction
- Facial asymmetry
- Distant neurotoxin spread

14.3.3 Deoxycholic Acid

Per the recent FDA studies, no serious or systemic adverse events have been observed in studies after deoxycholic acid injection.[10,11,12] Not surprisingly, side effects were generally related to the injection procedure, and adequate anesthetic was achieved with topical preparations and cooling with ice. However, transient mild or moderate adverse events such as pain, swelling, bruising, induration, and fibrosis were observed. One case of injection-related nerve injury was reported, but this also was only temporary and likely due to incorrect technique.[10,11,12]

Complications of Deoxycholic Acid Injection

- Pain
- Swelling
- Bruising
- Induration
- Fibrosis

14.3.4 Laser Resurfacing

Laser resurfacing perhaps allows the most dramatic improvement in aesthetic outcome next to invasive surgery. However, with greater potential comes increased complexity. The preoperative and postoperative care is just as crucial as the intraoperative technique. Some providers recommend prophylactic antibiotics, all of which should offer viral prophylaxis against herpes simplex resurgence. Likewise, wound care during the immediate postoperative period is essential to a successful outcome. Wound care promotes rapid healing and quicker resolution of minor side effects such as erythema and swelling, and there are multiple approaches of both open and closed wound dressings. The open technique requires numerous applications of bland ointments such as plain petroleum or Aquaphor (topical emollient) to the treated skin along with cold, wet compresses and ice packs. This regimen is continued for the first 72 hours. The benefit of this system affords the visualization of the treated skin, allowing the clinician to easily detect early symptoms of scar formation or infection. However, a drawback to the open technique is the requirement of significant cooperation and effort by the patient. Using the closed technique, a biosynthetic semi-occlusive dressing such as Flexzan (Mylan) or Silon-TSR (Bio Med Sciences) is applied and left on the wound for 1 or more days to promote re-epithelialization. Patient compliance is higher with the closed technique, because it requires less effort on the part of the patient, but the dressings are difficult to keep intact and the dressings do not allow wound visualization.[28]

The risk of complications from laser resurfacing is partly determined by the number of passes completed, the energy density being used, the degree of pulse or scan overlap, and the preoperative skin condition. Some degree of postoperative side effects is normal and expected. Almost all patients treated with laser resurfacing will encounter erythema, edema, crusting, or discharge. On the other hand, there are unexpected and undesired complications such as alterations in pigmentation, contact dermatitis, acne/milia formation, infection, persistent erythema, hypertrophic scarring, delayed healing, tooth and corneal damage, and ectropion formation.

PIH is the most commonly observed adverse effect of cutaneous laser surgery. It occurs in about 33% of all patients and in 100% of patients with darker Fitzpatrick skin types. No preoperative regimen has been shown to prevent PIH. Fortunately, this effect is generally transient, occurring within 1 month and resolving without treatment during the course of several months. If treatment is desired, topical products such as hydroquinone preparations, retinoic acid, azelaic acid, or glycolic acid can be used safely after 4 weeks. Additionally, the patient must be educated on the proper use of broad-spectrum sunscreen, because sun exposure will worsen hyperpigmentation. Other recent investigations have indicated that the use of orally administered *Polypodium leucotomos* may help improve PIH due to its antioxidant and photoprotective properties.[29] In contrast, hypopigmentation is a late complication, developing 6 to 12 months after laser resurfacing, and it is extremely difficult to treat. It is likely that areas near sun-damaged skin are more susceptible to hypopigmentation. Luckily, it is a rare complication and is usually seen in patients who have had aggressive dermabrasion or phenol peels.

Irritant contact dermatitis is the most common presentation of postoperative dermatitis. After laser resurfacing, the epidermal barrier is lost, causing skin to be at an increased risk of irritation from topical treatments. Topical antibiotics such as bacitracin, neomycin, and polymyxin B are common culprits of contact dermatitis after laser treatment, and as such their use should be discouraged. Diagnostic clues to irritant or allergic contact dermatitis include increased and nonresolving erythema or pruritus. Emollients such as Aquaphor or plain petroleum are recommended, and it is prudent to warn patients not to apply other lotions or creams. Contact dermatitis is treated with cessation of any topical treatments, cold compresses, and mild topical corticosteroids, if necessary.

Eruptions of acne are common following laser resurfacing secondary to occlusive ointments and wound dressings applied after treatment. In addition, the pilosebaceous apparatus can be damaged, causing acne formation even in patients without prior history of acne. This adverse event will usually resolve without treatment once ointments are discontinued. In the case of persistent acne after laser treatment, a tetracycline antibiotic can be given, and if needed topical retinoids or glycolic or azelaic acid compounds can be administered.

Infections after laser resurfacing will usually develop during the first week after treatment while the skin barrier is compromised. Opportunistic infections can include bacteria and fungi, but reactivation of the herpes simplex virus is the most common infectious complication after laser resurfacing. It is thought that the trauma induced by the laser can cause activation and shedding of the virus. It is important to note that due to the compromised epithelium, classic vesicles will not likely form, and erythematous erosions associated with pain, fever, and malaise may provide clues to a diagnosis. Because severe cases can cause systemic infection and atrophic scarring, they must be diagnosed and treated as soon as possible. Antiviral medications are commonly given 1 to 2 days before laser treatment and continued for up to 10 days until re-epithelialization has completed. Conversely, there is data that show that bacterial prophylaxis offers no significant benefit, despite many practitioners' preference. Again, the lack of complete epithelial barrier and the use of ointments postoperatively can contribute to superficial bacterial and fungal infections. Commonly witnessed species of bacteria include streptococci, staphylococci, and *Pseudomonas aeruginosa*, and if infection is suspected, empiric coverage with an oral cephalosporin is indicated. Rarely, fungal infections can occur but may be difficult to recognize, because their appearance may mimic acne and milia formation. Vulnerable patients may include those with diabetes, immunosuppression, vaginal candidiasis, or angular chelitis.[28]

Even without infection, scarring may occur. Within the first postoperative week, scars will present with erythema and are generally raised in appearance. Particularly scar-vulnerable areas include those with lesser vasculature and blood supply such as the chest, neck, mandible, and infraorbital region. As such, a decrease in the amount of energy, pulse stacking, and density in these areas is strongly advised. If scarring occurs, the type of scar will dictate the appropriate treatment. Hypertrophic scars are more likely to regress on their own, as opposed to keloids, which have shown to have a genetic component.[30] Management should include the application of steroid-impregnated tape, low-potency steroid creams or lotions, or topical silicone or silicone sheeting. If adequate improvement is not experienced, more aggressive measures like intralesional steroid injection or high-potency steroids, such as clobetasol propionate 0.5%, may be used with caution.[28] Also, pulse-dye laser treatments have also shown effectiveness in treating erythematous, hypertrophic burn scars.[31]

For reasons not entirely understood, some patients have exhibited great difficulty healing after receiving laser resurfacing. This "delayed healing" syndrome is thought to result from a combination of infection and autoimmune phenomenon that prevents normal re-epithelialization and has been documented more frequently in lighter-toned patients. Because this syndrome causes significant scarring, healing time can be prolonged up to 8 to 10 months. Management should include a comprehensive approach with oral antibiotics and antivirals in addition to topical steroids.[32]

In order to prevent ectropion formation of the lower eyelid, a "snap test" involving manual downward pull of the lower eyelid can be used to detect patients at increased risk. If the lower eyelid does not quickly return to its resting position within 3 seconds, resurfacing around the area should be avoided. Should ectropion occur, a trial of topical corticosteroid may be attempted, but most cases require surgical correction. Finally, standard protective eyewear and metal shielding should be used to avoid damage to the teeth and the cornea.[28]

Expected Short-term Side Effects of Laser Resurfacing

- Minor oozing
- Minor bleeding
- Minor crusting
- Erythema
- Edema
- Pain
- Pruritis

Complications of Laser Resurfacing

- Hyperpigmentation
- Hypopigmentation
- Contact Dermatitis
- Acne/milia
- Viral/bacterial/fungal infection
- Hypertrophic scarring
- Delayed healing
- Tooth enamel and corneal damage
- Ectropion formation

14.3.5 Microfocused Ultrasound

Micro-focused ultrasound is a relatively new technology, and fortunately, complications are rare. The most common adverse event is discomfort during treatment, which can be minimized with oral acetaminophen or NSAIDs. Reports have shown that narcotic analgesics and topical lidocaine are no more effective than NSAIDS when using transducers at greater depth.[33,34] Other adverse events regarding microfocused ultrasound include erythema, edema, and bruising. Rarely, PIH, transient numbness, and muscle weakness have been described. One case detailed temporary perioral paralysis that lasted for 2 months.[35] As a result, caution is advised against aggressive microfocused ultrasound for areas that have superficial nerves, such as the glabella and chin. Wheal and striation can be avoided with proper technique and transducer selection.[36]

Complications of Microfocused Ultrasound

- Erythema
- Edema
- Bruising
- Wheals/striations
- PIH
- Nerve Injury

14.3.6 Intense Pulsed Light

Proper patient selection is the first step in increasing the safety of IPL. Complications are rarely observed when the procedure is performed in the right patient population with the recommended energy settings based on skin type. Because the procedure can be slightly painful, some clinicians apply a local topical anesthetic cream prior to performing the procedure. Additionally, a cooling gel can be applied to ease discomfort. Other preoperative considerations include protective eye shielding to avoid injury. Afterwards, the patient should apply a daily sunscreen and a moisturizer for 1 week and only use gentle cleansers.

Complications of IPL are rare and include erythema, bruising, scarring, alterations in skin pigmentation, and rarely nerve injury. Minimal pain, edema, and erythema are expected, but an excessive amount may indicate that cooling is insufficient or that the fluence should be lowered.

Concerning alterations in pigmentation, patients with suntanned skin and darker skin types will have increased risk. However, the incidence of dyspigmentation is lowered by close attention to overlap between pulses and using lower fluences. As mentioned in previous sections, the management of hyperpigmentation includes standard topical therapies such as hydroxyquinone or azelaic acid.

Although very rare, scarring can occur with IPL. The operator must closely inspect the tissue's response to the initial pulses to decrease the risk of burns. Likewise, treating tattoos with IPL is not recommended, because this has shown propensity to from scars. Caution should also be used with skin in certain anatomic areas covering bony landmarks. There have been reports of transient nerve injury to the temporal and facial nerves overlying the zygomatic arch, particularly in the elderly or those with thinner skin and less adipose tissue.[17,37]

Complications of Intense Pulsed Light
- Erythema
- Edema
- Bruising
- Scarring
- Hyperpigmentation
- Hypopigmentation
- Nerve Injury

14.4 Conclusion

Blended aesthetic medicine is a dynamic medical art form that requires effective communication with the patient to both define the cosmetic goals and thoroughly explain the risks associated with each individual modality. A comprehensive understanding of anatomy and cutaneous pathology, combined with proper patient selection and procedural technique, is essential to prevent and minimize adverse events while achieving the optimal cosmetic outcome. There have been major advancements in minimally invasive procedures, but not without the risk of complications. Although the treatment modalities described in this chapter are generally safe, treatment must ultimately be tailored to each individual patient.

14.5 Commentary

Julius W. Few Jr.

The pursuit of excellence in any field requires a fearless effort and pushing the natural boundaries that have been established in the past. These great innovations have happened most dramatically in the computer technology world, in which 15 years ago, one would have laughed at the idea that a mobile phone would allow the owner to listen to music, make calls, answer any question you can think of, and tell you the best way to get home after having dinner in another part of the world. Through the effort of "out of the box" thinking and a willingness to push the limits, innovation is born. Unlike the pure technology space for inanimate objects, we are dealing with the human condition in cosmetic medicine, and the desire to push the limits of established norms must be balanced against safety for the patient. This is the reason the chapter presented here is so very important. The authors have given important guidelines for the avoidance of issues using combined approaches in cosmetic medicine. In addition, one of the implied advantages of blending and combining cosmetic noninvasive techniques is the ability to lower the given volume injected and/or the energy level for the given device application to achieve a desired result with true synergy.

If there is any sort of complicating factor in the patient's history or details that remain unclear regarding treatments obtained outside your control, it is mandatory to exercise caution. I would advocate staged treatments to allow for maximum control and limited stress to the anatomy.

This was clearly illustrated by a close colleague who was providing laser resurfacing to a patient who failed to inform him of a recent radiofrequency treatment series done in another clinic. The laser treatment was at a standard fluence but the patient was still recovering from aggressive radiofrequency rejuvenation leading to increased tissue trauma and from secondary compromise leading to delayed wound healing. Fortunately, the plastic surgeon providing the laser treatment was very conscientious and complete in looking after her, and there were no long-term complications.

In general, one must assume that most patients go to multiple locations for various cosmetic treatments, and the patients often do not know exactly what has been done to them. The one detail that all patients seem to recall is timing. Therefore, it is vital for us to ask all of our patients if they went to another clinic and when, to both document and display caution in our treatment plan. If someone has had an unknown treatment, my general rule has been to not utilize any energy-based treatment over the area in question for at least 3 months. Or I have found out the nature of the treatment given by another provider and then discerned my treatment options. This is not an absolute rule; rather, it is an approach that I have adopted out of consideration for most clinically relevant results to occur with nonsurgical energy-based treatments.

References

[1] Beleznay K, Carruthers JD, Humphrey S, Jones D. Avoiding and treating blindness from fillers: a review of the world literature. Dermatol Surg. 2015; 41(10):1097–1117

[2] Rzany B, DeLorenzi C. Understanding, avoiding, and managing severe filler complications. Plast Reconstr Surg. 2015; 136(5) Suppl:196S–203S

[3] Kulichova D, Borovaya A, Ruzicka T, Thomas P, Gauglitz GG. Understanding the safety and tolerability of facial filling therapeutics. Expert Opin Drug Saf. 2014; 13(9):1215–1226

[4] Alam M, Gladstone H, Kramer EM, et al. American Society for Dermatologic Surgery. ASDS guidelines of care: injectable fillers. Dermatol Surg. 2008; 34 Suppl 1:S115–S148

[5] Bass L, Pozner J. Laser facial resurfacing. In: Cohen M, Thaller S, eds. The Unfavorable Result in Plastic Surgery: Avoidance and Treatment. St. Louis: Thieme Medical Publishers; 2017

[6] De Boulle K, Heydenrych I. Patient factors influencing dermal filler complications: prevention, assessment, and treatment. Clin Cosmet Investig Dermatol. 2015; 8:205–214

[7] Vedamurthy M, Vedamurthy A, Nischal K. Dermal fillers: do's and dont's. J Cutan Aesthet Surg. 2010; 3(1):11–15

[8] Small R. Botulinum toxin injection for facial wrinkles. Am Fam Physician. 2014; 90(3):168–175

[9] Small R, Hoang D. A practical guide to botulinum toxin procedures. Philadelphia: Wolters Kluwer/Lippincott Williams & Wilkins Health; 2012

[10] Ascher B, Hoffmann K, Walker P, Lippert S, Wollina U, Havlickova B. Efficacy, patient-reported outcomes and safety profile of ATX-101 (deoxycholic acid), an injectable drug for the reduction of unwanted submental fat: results from a phase III, randomized, placebo-controlled study. J Eur Acad Dermatol Venereol. 2014; 28(12):1707–1715

[11] Rzany B, Griffiths T, Walker P, Lippert S, McDiarmid J, Havlickova B. Reduction of unwanted submental fat with ATX-101 (deoxycholic acid), an adipocytolytic injectable treatment: results from a phase III, randomized, placebo-controlled study. Br J Dermatol. 2014; 170(2):445–453

[12] Walker P, Fellmann J, Lizzul PF. A phase I safety and pharmacokinetic study of ATX-101: injectable, synthetic deoxycholic acid for submental contouring. J Drugs Dermatol. 2015; 14(3):279–287

[13] Ramsdell WM. Fractional CO2 laser resurfacing complications. Semin Plast Surg. 2012; 26(3):137–140

[14] Goel A, Krupashankar DS, Aurangabadkar S, Nischal KC, Omprakash HM, Mysore V. Fractional lasers in dermatology–current status and recommendations. Indian J Dermatol Venereol Leprol. 2011; 77(3):369–379

[15] Fabi SG. Noninvasive skin tightening: focus on new ultrasound techniques. Clin Cosmet Investig Dermatol. 2015; 8:47–52

[16] Nestor MS, Park H. Safety and efficacy of micro-focused ultrasound plus visualization for the treatment of axillary hyperhidrosis. J Clin Aesthet Dermatol. 2014; 7(4):14–21

[17] Goldberg DJ. Current trends in intense pulsed light. J Clin Aesthet Dermatol. 2012; 5(6):45–53

[18] Funt D, Pavicic T. Dermal fillers in aesthetics: an overview of adverse events and treatment approaches. Clin Cosmet Investig Dermatol. 2013; 6:295–316

[19] Pierre A, Levy PM. Hyaluronidase offers an efficacious treatment for inaesthetic hyaluronic acid overcorrection. J Cosmet Dermatol. 2007; 6(3):159–162

[20] Lemperle G, Rullan PP, Gauthier-Hazan N. Avoiding and treating dermal filler complications. Plast Reconstr Surg. 2006; 118(3) Suppl:92S–107S

[21] Lafaille P, Benedetto A. Fillers: contraindications, side effects and precautions. J Cutan Aesthet Surg. 2010; 3(1):16–19

[22] Carruthers JD, Fagien S, Rohrich RJ, Weinkle S, Carruthers A. Blindness caused by cosmetic filler injection: a review of cause and the therapy. Plast Reconstr Surg. 2014 Dec;134(6):1197-1201. doi: 10.1097/PRS.0000000000000754.

[23] Jones GH. RNA degradation and the regulation of antibiotic synthesis in Streptomyces. Future Microbiol. 2010; 5(3):419–429

[24] Cohen SR, Born TM. Facial Rejuvenation with fillers. Elsevier Health Sciences; 2009

[25] Small R, Hoang D. A Practical Guide to Botulinum Toxin Procedures. Philadelphia, Pa.: Lippincott Williams & Wilkins; 2012

[26] Ascher B, Talarico S, Cassuto D, et al. International consensus recommendations on the aesthetic usage of botulinum toxin type A (Speywood Unit)–Part I: Upper facial wrinkles. J Eur Acad Dermatol Venereol. 2010; 24(11):1278–1284

[27] U.S. Food and Drug Administration. Information for healthcare professionals: onabotulinumtoxinA (marketed as Botox/Botox Cosmetic), abobotulinumtoxinA (marketed as Dysport) and rimabotulinumtoxinB (marketed as Myobloc). http://www.fda.gov/Drugs/DrugSafety/PostmarketDrugSafetyInformationforPatientsandProviders/DrugSafetyInformationforHeathcareProfessionals/ucm174949.htm. Accessed 20 February, 2013

[28] Alster TS, Lupton JR. Treatment of complications of laser skin resurfacing. Arch Facial Plast Surg. 2000; 2(4):279–284

[29] Nestor M, Bucay V, Callender V, Cohen JL, Sadick N, Waldorf H. Polypodium leucotomos as an Adjunct Treatment of Pigmentary Disorders. J Clin Aesthet Dermatol. 2014; 7(3):13–17

[30] Ebner J, Maytin E. Dermatologic Surgery: Requisites in Dermatology. Elsevier Health Sciences; 2008

[31] Alster TS, Nanni CA. Pulsed dye laser treatment of hypertrophic burn scars. Plast Reconstr Surg. 1998; 102(6):2190–2195

[32] Rigel DS, Weiss RA, Lim HW, Dover JS. Photoaging. 1st ed. New York: CRC Press; 2004:416

[33] Gitt S. Double-blind, randomized, controlled split-face trial to assess the efficacy and safety of a liposomal lidocaine topical for pain management during microfocused ultrasound treatment. Presented at: The Aesthetic Meeting; 2012; Vancouver, BC

[34] Sunderam H. Prospective double-blind, randomized pilot study comparing ibuprofen to a narcotic for pain management during micro-focused ultrasound treatment. Presented at: American Society for Dermatologic Surgery; 2011; Washington, DC

[35] Jeong KH, Suh DH, Shin MK, Lee SJ. Neurologic complication associated with intense focused ultrasound. J Cosmet Laser Ther. 2014; 16(1):43–44

[36] Brobst RW, Ferguson M, Perkins SW. Noninvasive treatment of the neck. Facial Plast Surg Clin North Am. 2014; 22(2):191–202

[37] Nouri K. Complications in Dermatological Surgery. Elsevier Health Sciences; 2008

15 Future Considerations

Michael P. Ogilvie and Julius W. Few Jr.

Summary

Noninvasive and minimally invasive cosmetic medicine applications are undergoing rapid innovation and development on nearly a monthly basis, with new and exciting opportunities for future development. This chapter presents several new and emerging technologies that follow the typical core principles of noninvasive cosmetic medicine.

Keywords: CoolSculpting, core principles, cosmetic medicine, imaging, innovation, Kybella, microneedling, nonsurgical skin tightening, poly lactic co-glycolic acid (PLGA), Silhouette InstaLift, skin laxity, soft tissue ptosis, Thermi, three-dimensional (3D) imaging

Key Points

- The core principles of noninvasive cosmetic medicine are to restore lost volume, remove excess, and lift and/or tighten where appropriate.
- Several new technologies (Kybella® [Allergan, Inc.], Silhouette InstaLift® [Sinclair Pharma], and Dermal Rejuvenation Enhanced by Amniotic Membrane [DREAM, Advanced Dermal Sciences, LLC]), although in their infancy, show great promise and may have far-reaching effects on the field of cosmetic medicine.
- Imaging modalities, such as Vectra (CIS), not only help with patient communication but also may help to also accurately direct therapy.
- Cosmetic medicine will likely go the way of interventional cardiology, in that technological innovation will advance the field, whereas noninvasive or minimally invasive therapies, in a stackable approach, will lead to surgical or near-surgical results.

15.1 Introduction

Noninvasive and minimally invasive cosmetic medicine applications are undergoing rapid innovation and development on nearly a monthly basis, with new and exciting opportunities for future development on the horizon.

Behind any emerging technology or modality, the core principles of noninvasive cosmetic medicine are typically followed, including the return of lost volume, the removal of excess, and lifting and/or tightening where indicated. These common themes or principles help define future innovations and allow for continued development and easy integration with existing effective platforms.

Within this chapter, we will present several new and emerging technological considerations, which we feel adhere well to the previously mentioned principles and will integrate well and help advance the field of noninvasive cosmetic medicine to help the provider gain near-surgical results. We will present several areas of interest that we believe are likely areas of future investigation based on a review of current literature, both in print and pending publication. While the following represents speculation, it is based in sound science and will allow the reader to consider how one may go about evolving a clinical practice in the ever-changing world of cosmetic medicine.

15.2 Modalities

Facial volume loss is a core component seen in every facial aging patient seeking rejuvenation. Implants, fillers, and autologous fat injection have been the aesthetic surgeons answer to the problem of facial volume loss. We are seeing a new emphasis on biocompatibility in implantable technology to better compete with the concept of autologous fat grafting. There will likely be an evolution to fast, affordable, genetically engineered filler substances that will not require a donor site, given the increasingly available ability to sequence DNA/RNA through saliva/buccal swabs (**see Video 1.1**).

The nonsurgical removal of unwanted fat is a common theme among cosmetic medicine patients. CoolSculpting® (ZELTIQ Aesthetics, Inc.) has become a mainstay modality in noninvasive fat removal (see Product Index (p.180)). One issue that remains in both surgical and nonsurgical fat removal is how to treat the patient with skin laxity that is worsened by fat reduction. The ability to use nonsurgical skin tightening provides a new frontier to enhance body contouring and is the subject of an ongoing study. As technology continues to evolve in the world of nonsurgical skin tightening and resuspension, we will continue to see more near-surgical and possibly even better-than-surgical results.

Kybella® (Allergan, Inc.) is a newly FDA-approved noninvasive injection for the treatment of moderate to severe convexity or fullness associated with submental fat in adults (see Product Index (p.170)).[1] Formulated as a nonhuman, nonanimal version of deoxycholic acid (10 mg/mL), Kybella is a cytolytic agent that destroys cell membranes. Once injected into subcutaneous fat, it causes the lysis of adipocytes, no longer allowing them to store or accumulate fat. The administration of Kybella is considered fairly straightforward. In 15 to 20 minutes, the patient's submental area is typically injected with 4 to 6 mL (2 to 3 vials) of agent divided into 0.2 mL aliquots separated by 1 cm, not to exceed 10 mL per session.[1]

In two randomized, double-blind controlled trials versus placebo ($N = 514$ vs. 508), in North America, Kybella proved to be efficacious within statistical significance ($p < 0.001$) with a 79% patient satisfaction rate[1,2] (▶ Fig. 15.1). Of those studied, nearly 60% of patients required 6 treatments (at 1-month intervals) to obtain the highest percentage of improvement, with many patients noting results within 2 to 4 treatments.

Although it appears to be safe and efficacious, side effects have been noted. Because of its cytotoxic properties, Kybella's ability to destroy cell membranes is not specific, so there exists the theoretical risk of unwanted tissue destruction (i.e., skin and muscle). Additionally, within the clinical trials, 4% of patients suffered temporary marginal mandibular injury, 2%

Future Considerations

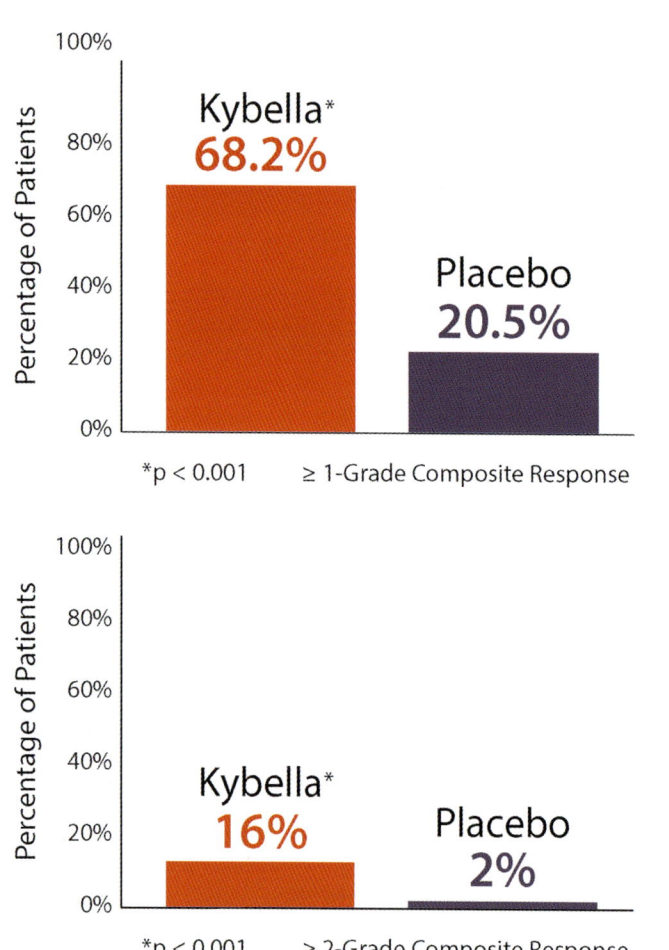

Fig. 15.1 Composite responder rates of Kybella compared to placebo. (CR, clinician reported; PR, patient reported; SMFRS, submental fat rating scale.) (Reproduced with permission from http://hcp.mykybella.com/about-kybella/clinical-results, 2015.)

suffered temporary dysphagia, and most commonly, 72% of patients suffered from various degrees of edema, bruising, pain, numbness, or redness. These findings led to the warning of not injecting within 1 to 1.5 cm of the marginal mandibular nerve and to avoid its use in patients with active or a history of dysphagia.[1]

Kybella truly is a product in its infancy, whose potential is still being unlocked and discovered. It is our opinion that it will ultimately find its utility in small areas of excess reduction, particularly when used with energy-based modalities to perform nonsurgical facial and neck rejuvenation, which will be exciting areas of research to come. This is a product of great potential excitement, not as much in its current presentation but rather as an agent to combine with focused ultrasound or radiofrequency to enhance skin tightening, skin contouring, or enhancement in skin resurfacing.

Given what we know about the inflammatory cascade and the ability of Kybella to stimulate inflammation and even targeted cell death, this could be a product that could create more permanent neurolysis and potentially replace neurotoxin use. If one allows for scientific consideration, inflammation is a necessary and key component of all things in cosmetic medicine—adipocyte lysis, thermal destruction with collagen and epithelial replacement, and longevity of surgical and nonsurgical lifting through the stimulation of collagen production in the form of what we consider scar formation. The ability to modulate these pathways is extremely exciting and will likely allow for the reduced need for traditional invasive applications.

Skin laxity and soft tissue descent are common themes in the aging face that have historically been treated through the surgical facelift. However, because younger patients have started to seek out cosmetic surgery, the need for less invasive procedures with minimal downtime have become desirable. Multiple modalities have been developed to fill this void, most of which are energy-based, namely in the form of lasers, microfocused ultrasound, or radiofrequency.

Regarding soft tissue ptosis, suture suspension systems, so-called thread lifting, have fallen in and out of favor over the years.[3] Barbed suture was once thought to be the answer for noninvasive soft tissue lift[4] (▶ Fig. 15.2). However, due to its unidirectional design, lack of absorption, and need for superficial placement to catch dermis, barbed suture was fraught with complications such as breakage, palpability, extrusion, and short-lasting results.

Silhouette InstaLift (Sinclair Pharma), is a newly FDA approved facial soft tissue suspension system. Based closely on

Future Considerations

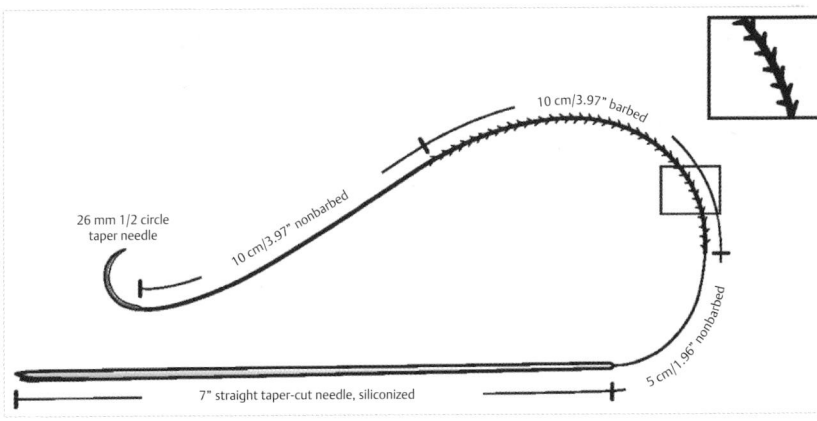

Fig. 15.2 Traditional barbed suture. (Adapted with permission from Nahai F and Saltz R. Endoscopic Plastic Surgery, ed 2, Thieme Medical Publishers, St. Louis, 2008.)

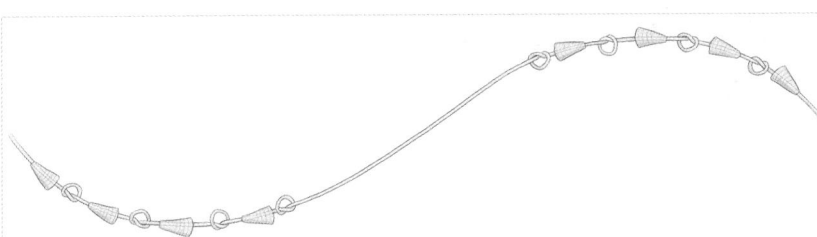

Fig. 15.3 Suture design of Silhouette InstaLift. (Adapted with permission from Sinclair Pharmaceuticals. Instruction Packet – INSTALIFT. INSTALIFT. http://www.instalift.com. Published 2015. Accessed Sept 5, 2016.)

its European counterpart, Silhouette Soft® (Sinclair Pharma), InstaLift is a fully absorbable suspension suture with 8, 12, or 16 bidirectional cones per suture, all made from poly lactic co-glycolic acid (PLGA), which is biocompatible and biodegradable[5] (▶ Fig. 15.3). The biological makeup of the material has been shown to be biostimulating when combined with injectable filler such as PLGA. This may lead to the possibility of adding volume to the lift area, thereby potentiating the result by placing injectable filler adjacent to the suspension-lifting bidirectional suture. Additionally, the resorbable cones help to provide an increased surface area to maximize suspension traction and create a strong fixation in the subcutaneous tissue, while encapsulation around the cones creates a solid support to the soft tissue, helping to mitigate the risk of migration and extrusion.[6]

Currently, the FDA indication is for midface elevation, but Silhouette Soft has been used for contouring of the entire face, neck, and jawline. The procedure is performed on an outpatient basis, under local anesthesia, in less than 1 hour.[7] Under aseptic technique, the suture is placed in the subcutaneous fat plane in a bidirectional manner and brought out of the skin through a distal site. Under slight tension, the skin and subcutaneous tissue is then contoured by hand for the desired lift effect[5,6] (▶ Fig. 15.4). Particularly for midface elevation, the majority of patients required four sutures per side to achieve the desired effect, with a maximum being six sutures per side if needed. The results evolve for up to 8 months, with the final results lasting 18 to 24 months on average, with 90% patient satisfaction at 9 months.[8]

PGLA suture has been the subject of numerous studies in the literature. In one study out of Spain ($N = 316$), the complication rate reached 13%, most of which were minor and temporary, mainly edema and bruising without any infections noted.[9] Across the literature, complications range from 2% to 10% with few reports of infection or granuloma formation. In the same study, 2 patients experienced persistent asymmetry requiring a tightening procedure at 3 months, and 1 patient required suture removal due to palpability.

Further research with this product will likely revolve around its use for other indications such as the jawline or marionette lines as well as evaluation of the maintenance of results in combination with other nonsurgical modalities, particularly energy-based and injectable adipocytic technology.

Skin laxity in the aging face has long been thought to be caused by collagen degradation over time. Several noninvasive modalities have been developed to help combat this issue, such as radiofrequency for subdermal heating (i.e., ThermiRF [THERMI]or Fractora [InMode Aesthetics Solutions, Inc.]) or subdermal suturing systems that help promote neocolagenesis (i.e., Miracu [swiss4med]).

Even less invasive, microneedling has been touted as a method of fractional rejuvenation without the pain, heat, or downtime of the previously mentioned modalities (i.e., Dermapen [Equipmed USA] or MesoPen [Bellaire Industry LLC]) (see Product Index (p.167)). Collagen induction therapy is based on the idea of creating controlled microinjuries to the skin using 6- to 12-point needles, which promote new collagen and elastin production, leading to tighter, more rejuvenated skin through the body's natural wound-healing process.

Applied Dermal Sciences, LLC has championed microneedling as a transdermal delivery system, through its production of the PRPen and delivery of platelet-rich plasma.[10] Through a new patent-pending procedure called the *DREAM*, it is using amniotic membrane to modulate collagen production and improve the epidermal recovery process. Amniotic membrane has been employed in the plastic surgery literature, for various purposes, since the 1950s.[11] Through its numerous growth factors and immune modulators, amnion has been shown to stimulate

Future Considerations

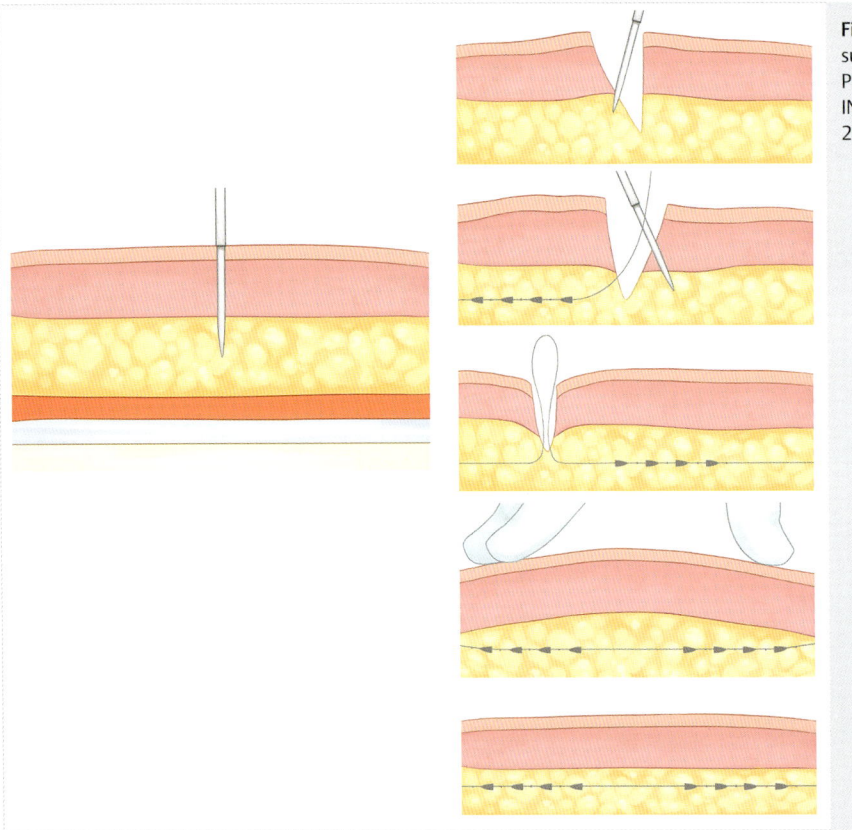

Fig. 15.4 Application of InstaLift suspension suture. (Adapted with permission from Sinclair Pharmaceuticals. Instruction Packet – INSTALIFT. INSTALIFT. http://www.instalift.com. Published 2015. Accessed Sept 5, 2016.)

multiple cell lines as well as activate and increase the productivity of dermal fibroblasts, which help explain its promotion of epithelialization while inhibiting fibrosis, scar formation, and inflammation.[12] It is with these properties in mind that Applied Dermal Sciences, LLC is looking to improve the field of facial rejuvenation through the enhancement of soft tissue healing, modulating inflammation and overall reducing scar formation.

While grounded in sound principle and research, only the application and comparison to similar techniques will tell if the use of amniotic membrane will truly improve the outcome of facial rejuvenation procedures. In addition, it needs to be determined whether this procedure can be safely integrated with other modalities to produce successful results in an established noninvasive practice.

Imaging studies have always held a significant role in the field of surgery, from the advent of the CT scan to helping identify internal pathology to the use of 2-dimensional (2D) photography to establish preoperative and postoperative outcomes.

In the visual world of cosmetic medicine, surgeons have never had a visual guide to objectively help identify and treat evidence of aging, except for the use of the naked eye. While investigators such as Val Lambros[13] have pioneered inventive ways to model and track the sequential change of aging over time (▶ Fig. 15.5; **Video 15.1**), quantifiable data particularly regarding volumetric changes, has been scarce. Hence, treatment modalities have essentially been guided by the experienced surgeons "best guess."[13] However, with the advent of three-dimensional (3D) imaging, much of this is starting to change with the use of objective, quantifiable data.

Paralleling the rapidly evolving technology seen in cosmetic medicine is the need for techniques to identify subtle pathology, evaluate the results of interventions, and communicate them with our patients. Canfield Imaging Systems, Inc. has pioneered a variety of 3D imaging platforms to help cosmetic surgeons be more objective in their analysis, more scientific with their interventions, and to help improve overall communication with the patient.[14]

Vectra is a high-resolution 3D imaging system that comes with a plethora of functionality to help the cosmetic surgeon in the previously mentioned areas[14] (▶ Fig. 15.6). Multiple studies in the literature have used Vectra in a variety of manners for research purposes. In 2007, Lowe and Lowe[15] quantified the volume effect of hyaluronic acid filler in the lips, illustrating that the volume effect could be quantifiably measured using this modality. In 2009, Meier et al[16] evaluated the long-term effects of autologous fat grafting in midface rejuvenation in 33 patients (▶ Fig. 15.6). Using Vectra, the authors were able to identify a 32% take rate at 16 months. Similarly, Donath, et al[17] analyzed the volume effects of hyaluronic acid filler for tear trough deformities in 12 patients. The authors identified an 85% volume retention rate at 14 months. In 2015, two studies evaluated midface volume changes in different scenarios.[17,18] Jacono et al[18] found a 3.2-cc volume increase in the midface after vertical vector deep-plane rhytidectomies at 1 year. The authors' conclusion was that the surgical technique could potentially obviate the need for additional volumizing interventions. In a cadaveric model, Gatherwright et al[19] identified a 3 to 5-cc volume increase with the injection of either 1.5 or 3 cc of calcium

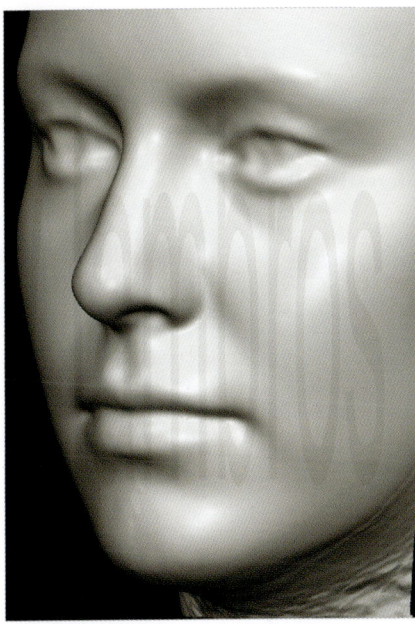 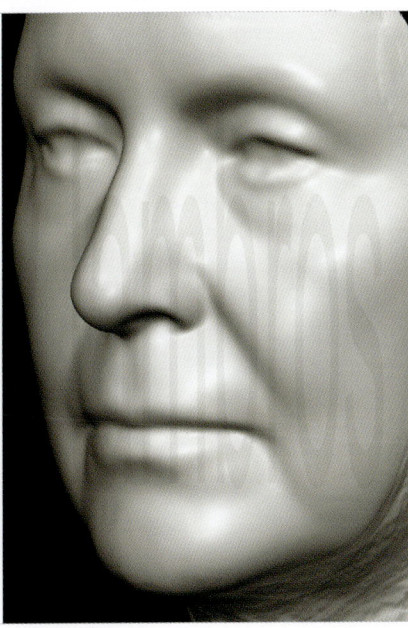

Fig. 15.5 Morph showing the average of 116 female faces from 20–30 years of age animated with 100 female faces from 68 years of age and older (average age about 76). (Courtesy Dr. Val Lambros)

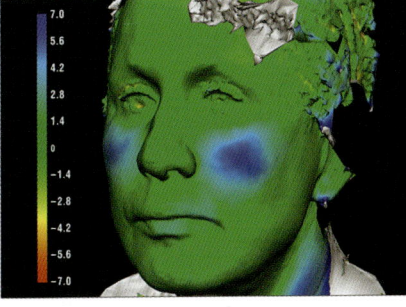 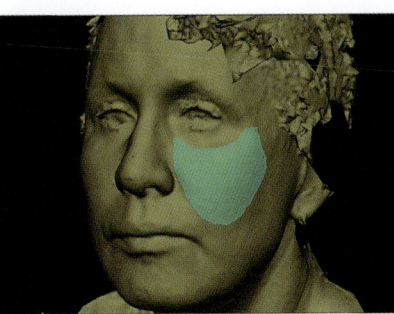

Fig. 15.6 Vectra multidimensional functionality. (Courtesy Canfield Scientific, Inc. Parsippany, NJ. www.canfieldsci.com/imaging-systems, 2016)

hydroxyapatite into the malar region of the face, illustrating the lifting effect of filler through the recruitment of ptotic tissue. Others have used the Vectra system in a true clinical setting to help guide volumization therapy with either fat or filler (▶ Fig. 15.7).

While these studies illustrate proof of concept and have given surgeons usable, quantifiable data, the next step in this exciting research is to use this data to give directed therapies for a given patient issue. As this research continues to unfold, undoubtedly a series of discoveries will ensue, which will likely change the way we look at and treat the aging face and neck. It is our belief that the future of imaging will allow for more educated predictions of facial aging, and through this better understanding, will improve treatment modalities exponentially.

15.3 Conclusion

The common objectives for the cosmetic specialist is to decrease the number of noninvasive treatments, to increase efficacy to reduce nonresponder rates, and to decrease the cost of providing a given treatment through the reduction of potential disposable costs. To this end, there will likely be a new emphasis on biocompatibility, with the end goal of taking a given patient and in 1 day treat the entire body—head to toe—nonsurgically using 3, 4, 5, or even 6 modalities to achieve efficient, minimal-downtime cosmetic enhancement. One likely example would be the idea of combining absorbable suspension sutures with microfocused ultrasound treatments, along with volume replacement and simultaneous laser resurfacing, to the aged face in order to form a single-setting construct or performed over time (▶ Fig. 15.8). Ultimately, with increased choices in applications, there will be an array of combinations to consider and choose from for a given cosmetic indication.

With increased modalities and technical enhancements, there will be a growing need to target a given cosmetic issue through imaging technology to better isolate desired end points. We will begin to see more technology aimed at objectively identifying a given point of aging and to modulate it with a given treatment to produce the most relevant clinical and aesthetic outcomes possible. Cosmetic medicine will, more and more, mirror surgery much like interventional cardiology mirrors cardiac surgery, leading to more innovation to reduce invasiveness, downtime, and cost.

Future Considerations

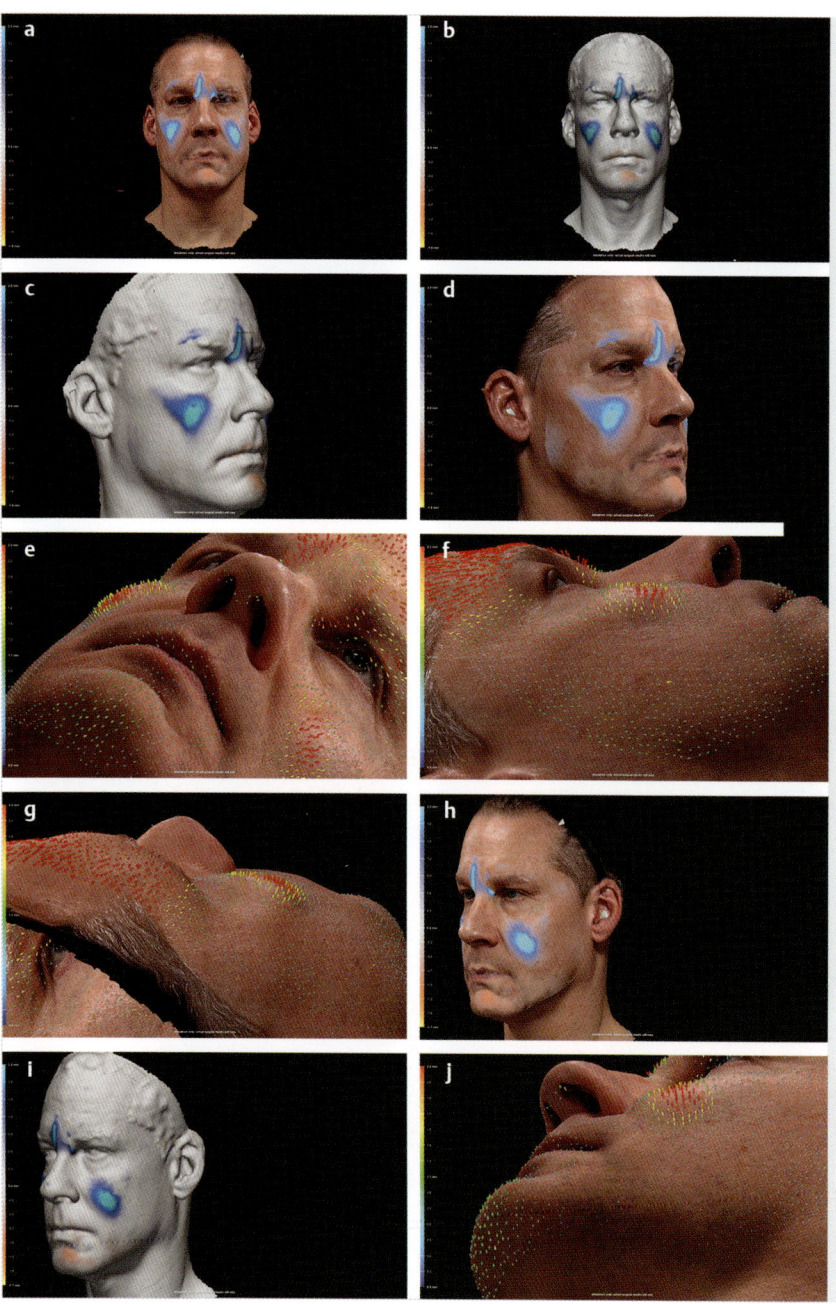

Fig. 15.7 This 52-year old man with midfacial volume deficit and glabellar frown lines was treated with hyaluronic acid filler and neuromodulator by Dr. Derek Jones. Images generated by the Vectra 3D imaging system. **(a-f)** Frontal and three-quarter views of normal and grayscale depictions with a color map illustrating the areas of change and the gross magnitude. **(g-j)** Various positions illustrating the direction and magnitude of volume change using leading-edge vector analysis.

Future Considerations

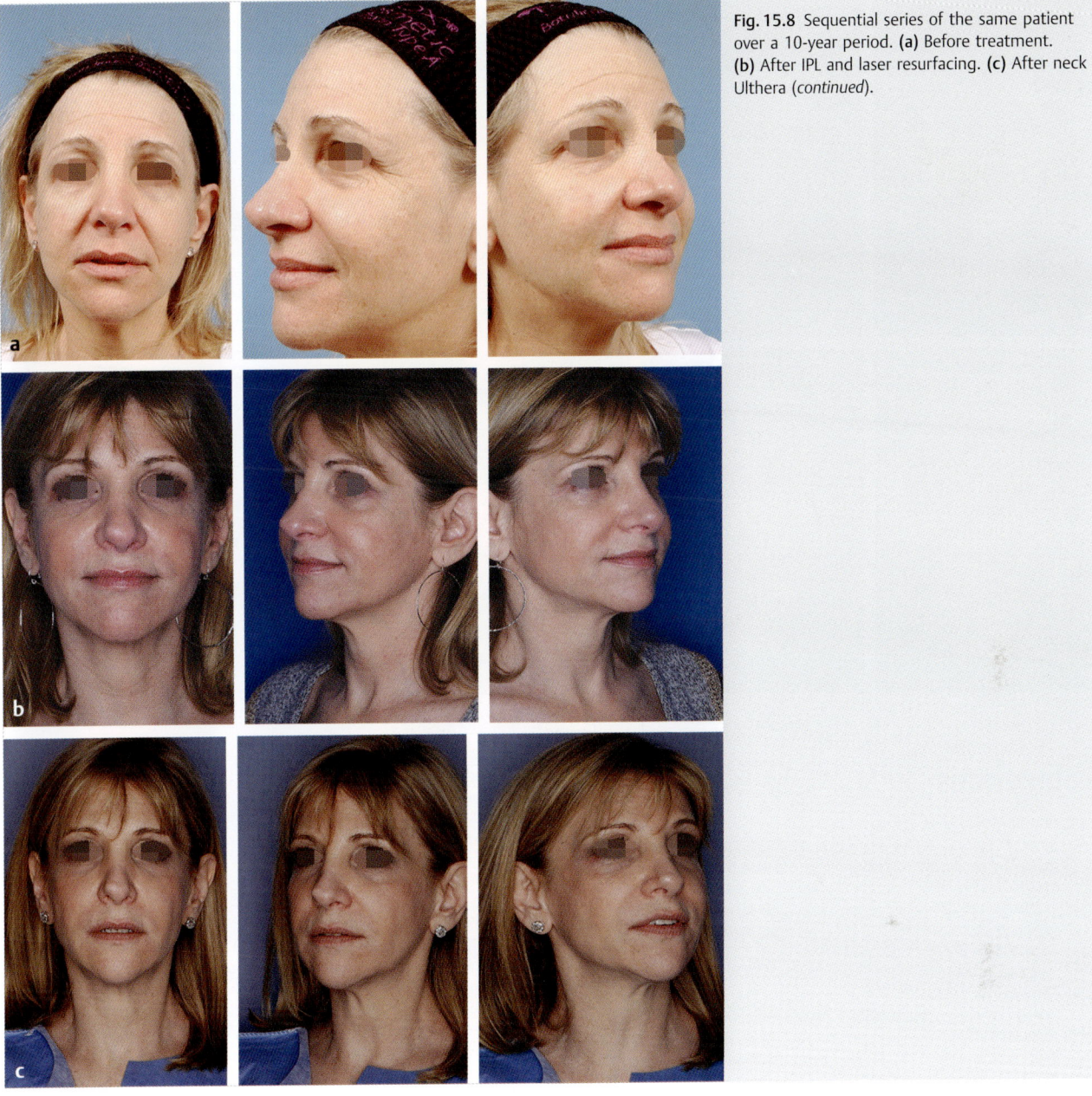

Fig. 15.8 Sequential series of the same patient over a 10-year period. (a) Before treatment. (b) After IPL and laser resurfacing. (c) After neck Ulthera (*continued*).

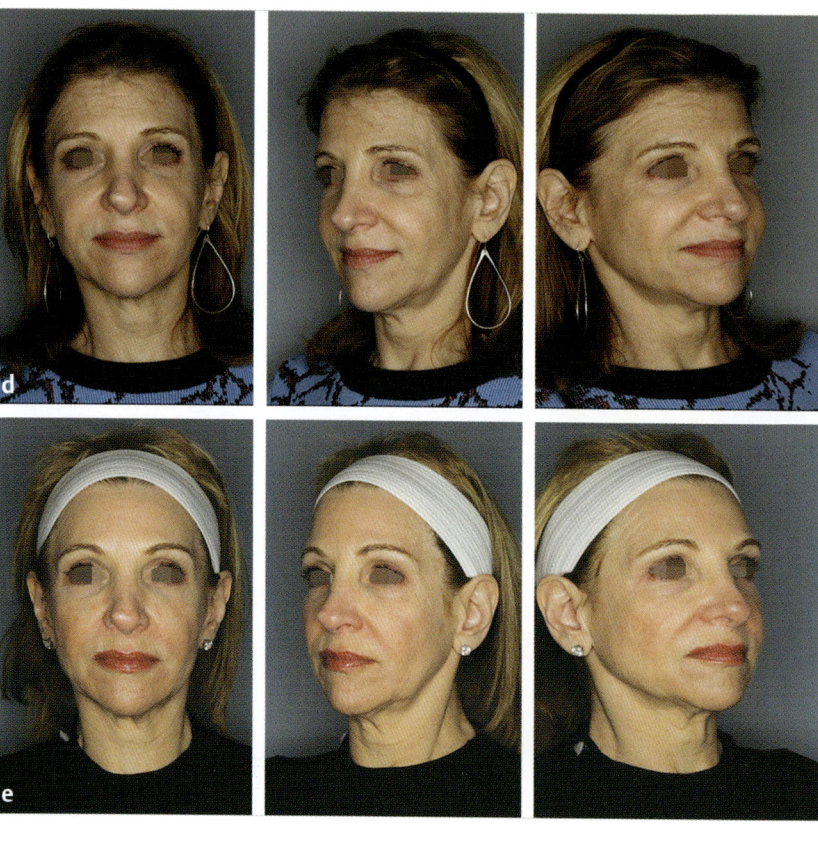

Fig. 15.8 (continued) **(d)** After upper blepharoplasty and browpexy. **(e)** After Silhouette Insta-Lift.

References

[1] http://hcp.mykybella.com

[2] Jones DH, Carruthers J, Joseph JH, et al. REFINE-1, a multicenter, randomized, double-blind, placebo-controlled, phase 3 trial with ATX-101, an injectable drug for submental fat reduction. Dermatol Surg. 2016; 42(1):38–49

[3] Nicolau PJ. Use of suspending threads in facial rejuvenation. Prime. 2014; 4(6):24–31

[4] Nahai F, Saltz R. Endoscopic plastic surgery. ed 2. St. Louis: Thieme Medical Publishers; 2008

[5] Sinclair Pharmaceuticals. Instruction Packet – INSTALIFT. INSTALIFT. http://www.instalift.com. Published 2015. Accessed 5 Sept, 2016

[6] Goldfarb, RM. Presentation at The Aesthetic Show, July 10, 2015

[7] Clark A. The aesthetic report: the non-surgical face-lift. Aesthetic & Anti-Ageing Magazine.. 2015; 2(14):28

[8] Gamboa GM, Vasconez LO. Suture suspension technique for midface and neck rejuvenation. Ann Plast Surg. 2009; 62(5):478–481

[9] de Benito J, Pizzamiglio R, Theodorou D, Arvas L. Facial rejuvenation and improvement of malar projection using sutures with absorbable cones: surgical technique and case series. Aesthetic Plast Surg. 2011; 35(2):248–253

[10] Moretti M. "Novel transdermal technologies considered next evolutionary step in aesthetic treatments". The Aesthetic Guide. Jan/Feb 2015. www.miinews.com

[11] Fairbairn NG, Randolph MA, Redmond RW. The clinical applications of human amnion in plastic surgery. J Plast Reconstr Aesthet Surg. 2014; 67(5):662–675

[12] Koob TJ, Lim JJ, Massee M, Zabek N, Denozière G. Properties of dehydrated human amnion/chorion composite grafts: Implications for wound repair and soft tissue regeneration. J Biomed Mater Res B Appl Biomater. 2014; 102(6):1353–1362

[13] Lambros V. Models of facial aging and implications for treatment. Clin Plast Surg. 2008; 35(3):319–327, discussion 317

[14] http://www.canfieldsci.com/imaging-systems

[15] Lowe P, Lowe NJ. 3D photography and lip filler: a novel assay. J Cosmet Laser Ther. 2007; 9(4):237–240

[16] Meier JD, Glasgold RA, Glasgold MJ. Autologous fat grafting: long-term evidence of its efficacy in midfacial rejuvenation. Arch Facial Plast Surg. 2009; 11(1):24–28

[17] Donath AS, Glasgold RA, Meier J, Glasgold MJ. Quantitative evaluation of volume augmentation in the tear trough with a hyaluronic Acid-based filler: a three-dimensional analysis. Plast Reconstr Surg. 2010; 125(5):1515–1522

[18] Jacono AA, Malone MH, Talei B. Three-dimensional analysis of long-term midface volume change after vertical vector deep-plane rhytidectomy. Aesthet Surg J. 2015; 35(5):491–503

[19] Gatherwright JR, Brown MS, Katira KM, Rowe DJ. Three-dimensional changes in the midface following malar calcium hydroxyapatite injection in a cadaver model. Aesthet Surg J. 2015; 35(6):NP169–NP175

16 Product Index: Fillers

16.1 Belotero Cosmetic

(see Chapter 2, Chapter 5)

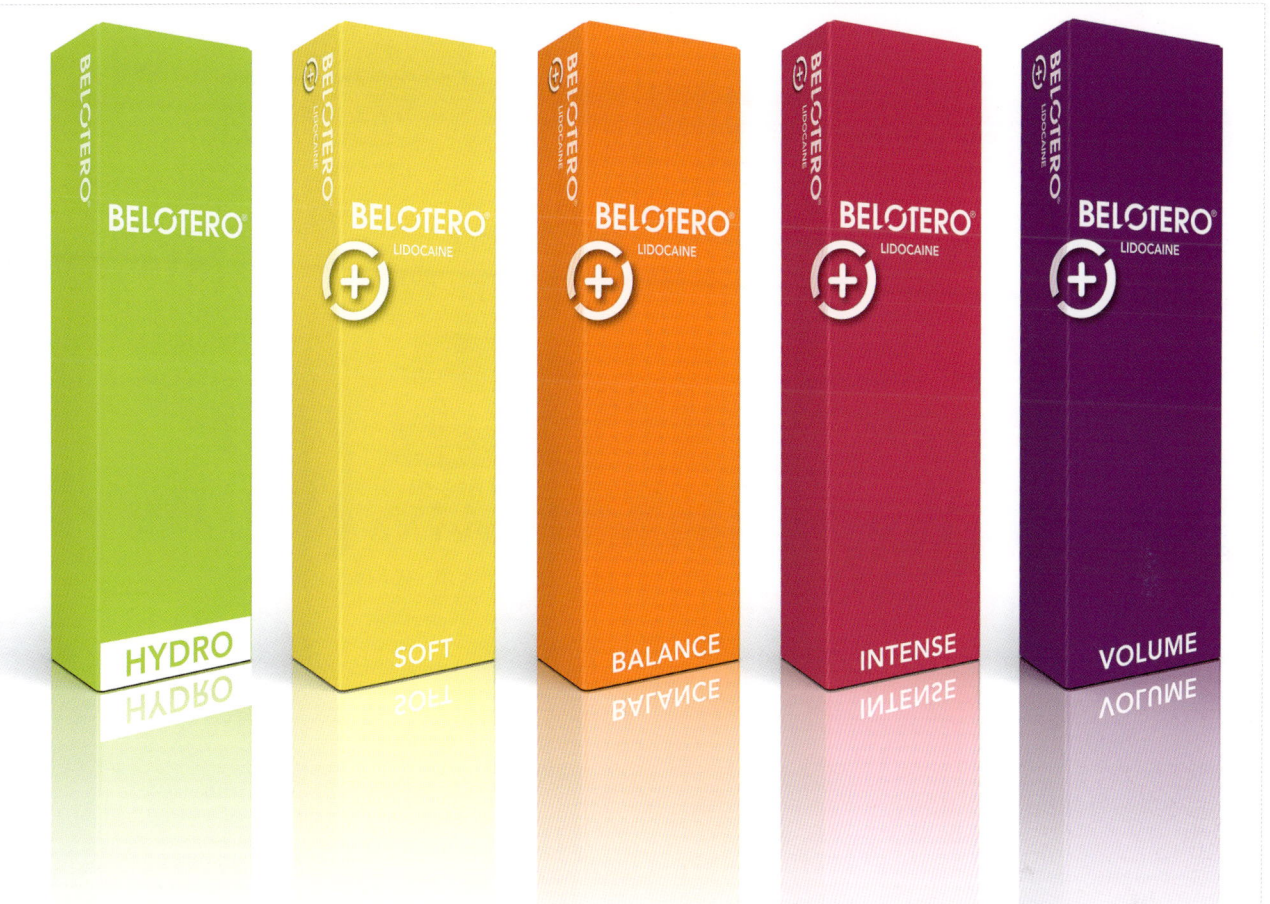

Fig. 16.1 The hyaluronic acid (HA) filler Belotero® (Belotero Volume, Belotero Hydro, Belotero Soft, Belotero Balance, Belotero Intense [Merz Aesthetics]) offers an extended portfolio for smoothing and filling wrinkles, for lip augmentation restoring facial volumes, and for rehydrating skin. Belotero integrates smoothly into an antiaging regimen that enhances confidence and self-assurance. It has an intelligent design for an advanced custom-made aesthetic solution with predictable and natural outcomes for optimal patient satisfaction and trust. The Belotero products can be used individually or in combination to tailor an aesthetic solution depending on the skin's structural and functional needs with predictable and natural outcomes. (Courtesy Merz Aesthetics)

16.2 Botox Cosmetic

(see Chapter 2, Chapter 3)

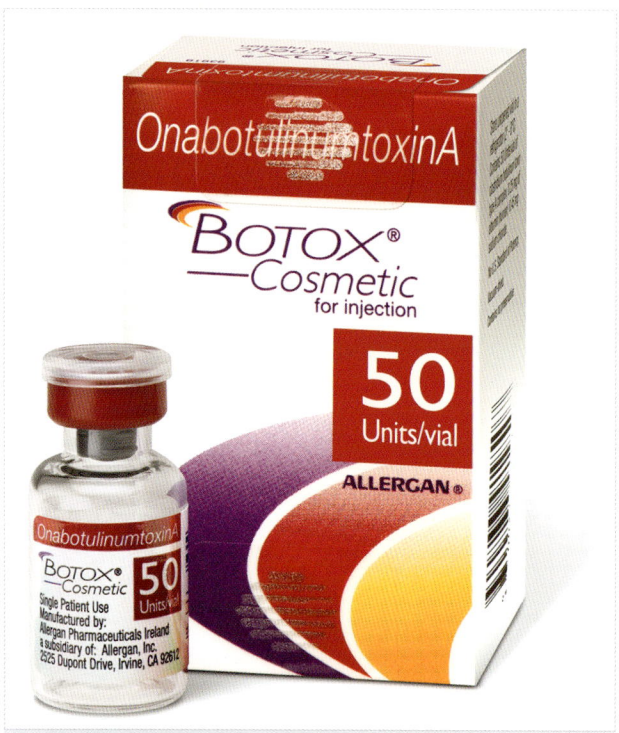

Fig. 16.2 OnabotulinumtoxinA (Botox Cosmetic, Allergan, Inc.) 50 units. (Courtesy Allergan, Inc.)

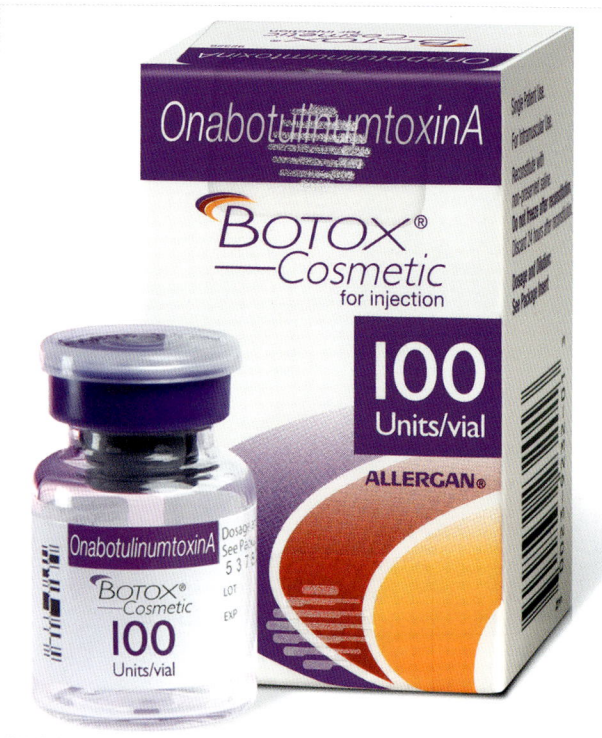

Fig. 16.3 OnabotulinumtoxinA (Botox Cosmetic, Allergan, Inc.) 100 units. (Courtesy Allergan. Inc.)

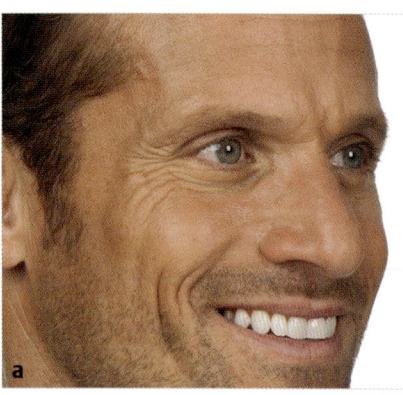
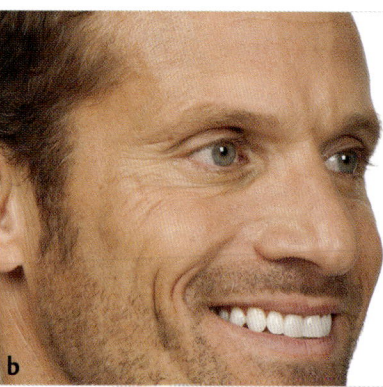

Fig. 16.4 Treatment of moderate to severe crow's-feet. **(a)** Before treatment and **(b)** 7 days after treatment. (Courtesy Allergan, Inc.)

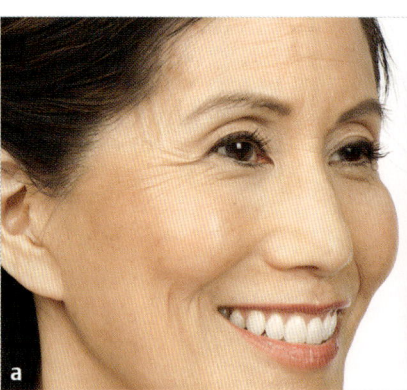
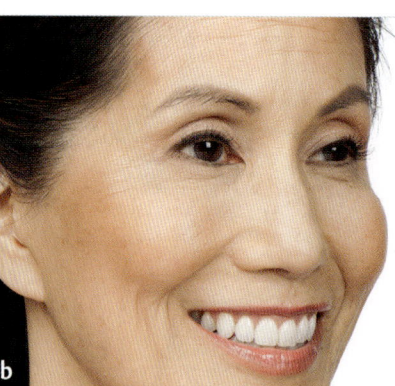

Fig. 16.5 Treatment of moderate to severe crow's-feet. **(a)** Before treatment and **(b)** 7 days after treatment. (Courtesy Allergan, Inc.)

Product Index: Fillers

16.3 Dysport

(see Chapter 2)

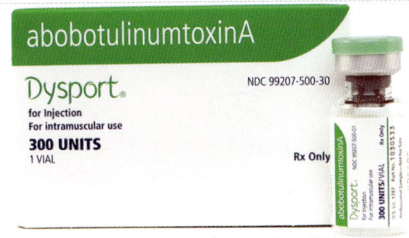

Fig. 16.6 AbabotulinumtoxinA (Dysport, Galderma, S.A.). (Courtesy Galderma)

16.4 Juvéderm

(see Chapter 2, Chapter 4)

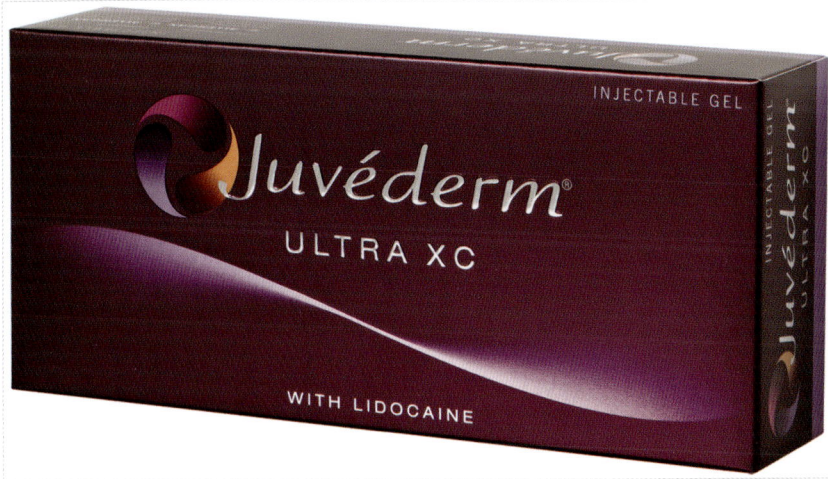

Fig. 16.7 Hyaluronic acid gel (Juvéderm Ultra XC, Allergan, Inc.). (Courtesy Allergan, Inc.)

Product Index: Fillers

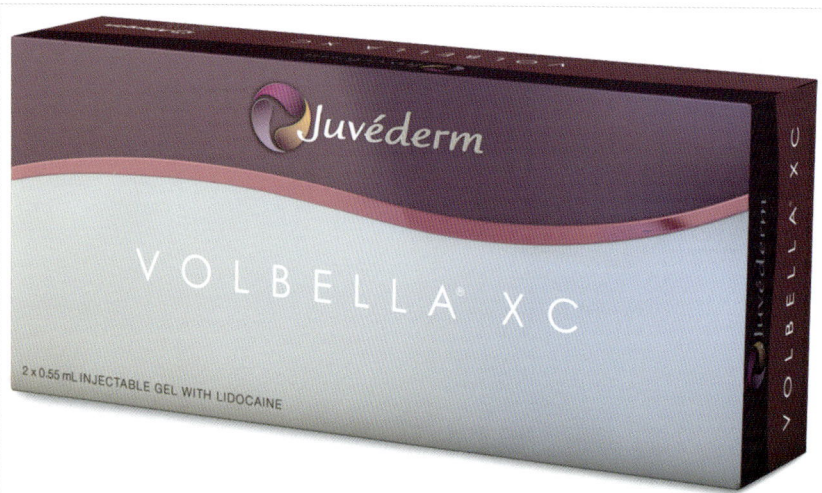

Fig. 16.8 Hyaluronic acid gel (Juvéderm Volbella XC, Allergan, Inc.). (Courtesy Allergan, Inc.)

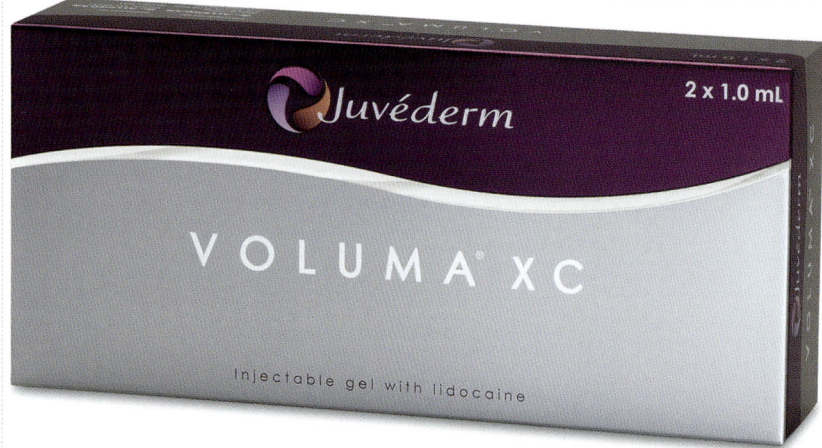

Fig. 16.9 Hyaluronic acid gel (Juvéderm Voluma XC, Allergan, Inc.). (Courtesy Allergan, Inc.)

16.5 Kybella

(see Chapter 2, Chapter 12, Chapter 15)

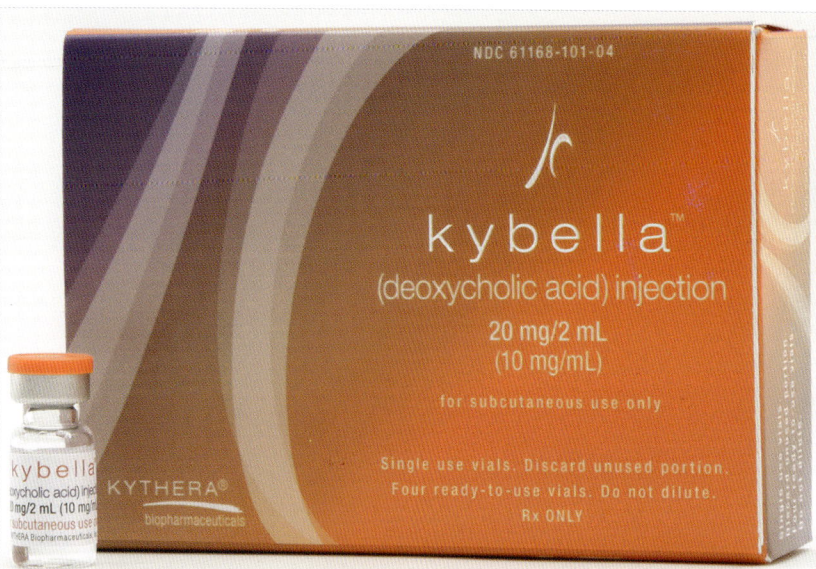

Fig. 16.10 Deoxycholic acid (Kybella, Allergan, Inc.). (Courtesy Allergan, Inc.)

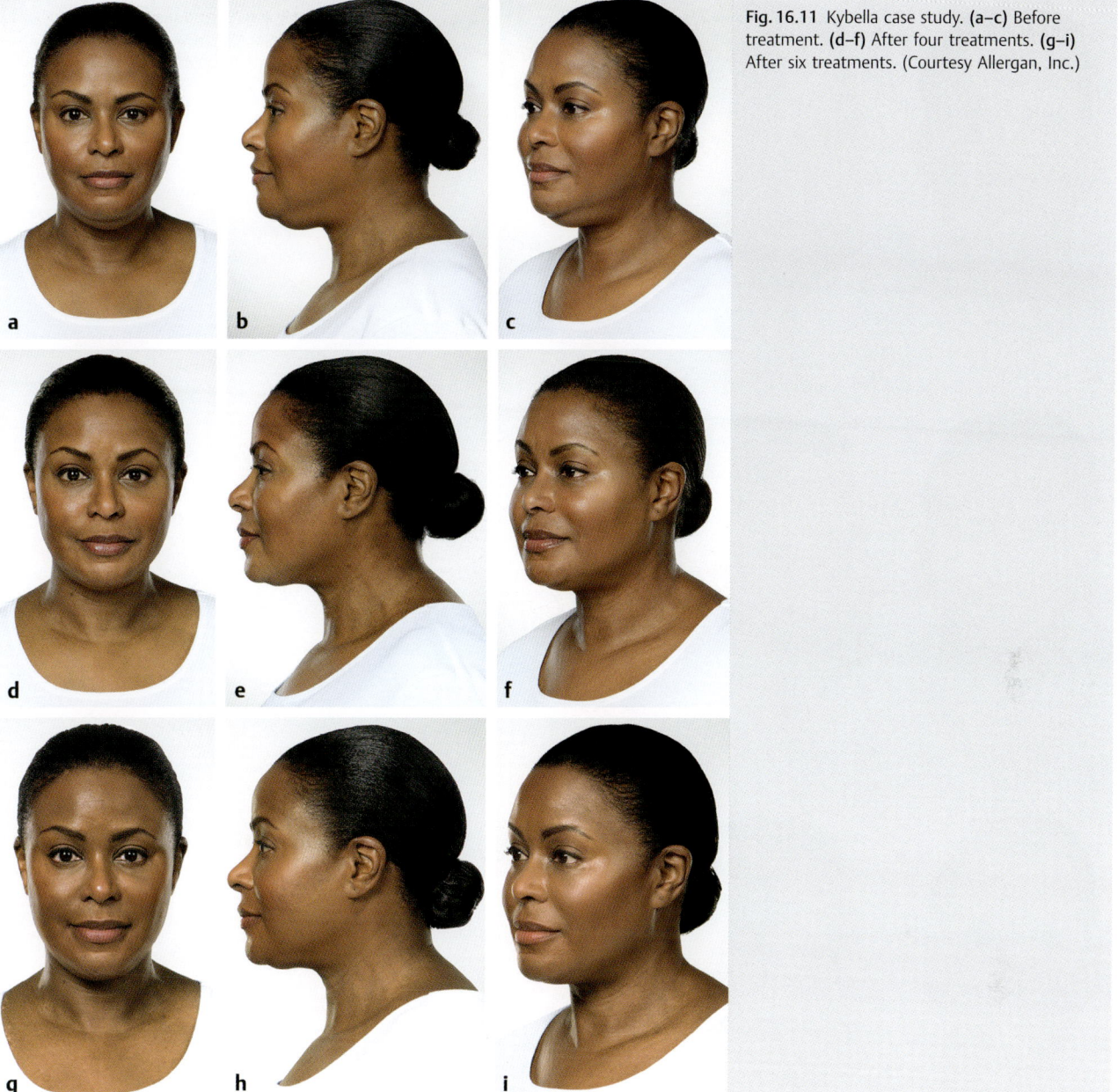

Fig. 16.11 Kybella case study. **(a–c)** Before treatment. **(d–f)** After four treatments. **(g–i)** After six treatments. (Courtesy Allergan, Inc.)

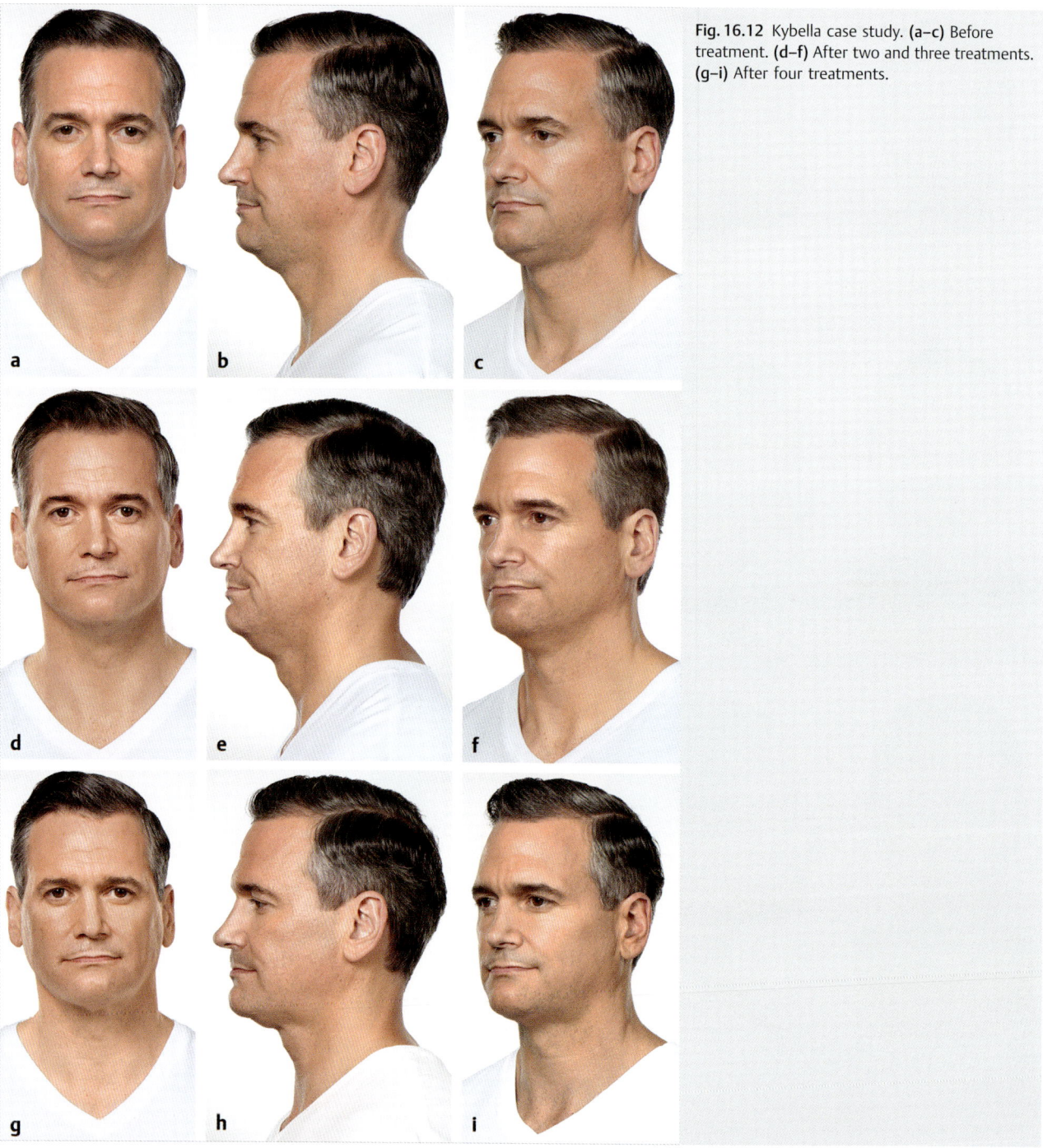

Fig. 16.12 Kybella case study. **(a–c)** Before treatment. **(d–f)** After two and three treatments. **(g–i)** After four treatments.

16.6 Sculptra

(see Chapter 2, Chapter 6)

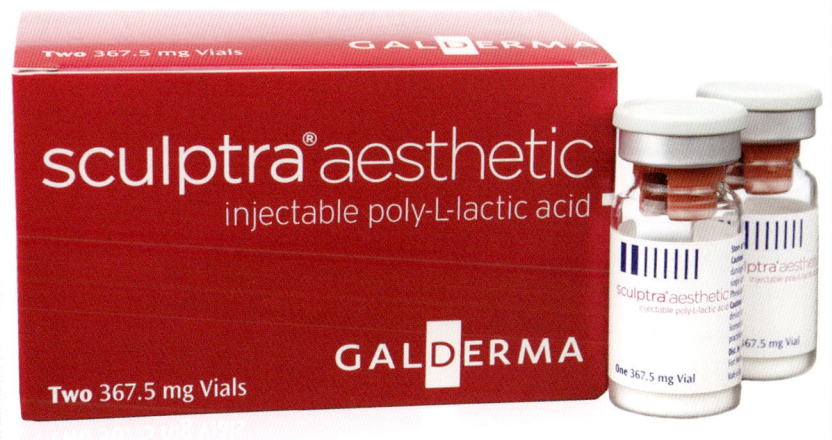

Fig. 16.13 Injectable poly-L-lactic acid (Sculptra, Galderma Inc.). (Courtesy Galderma, Inc.)

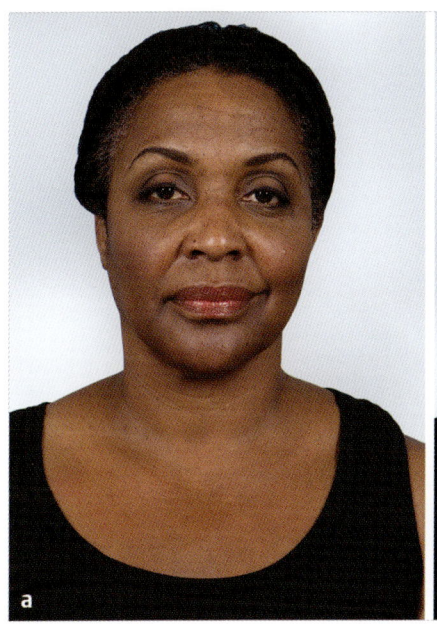 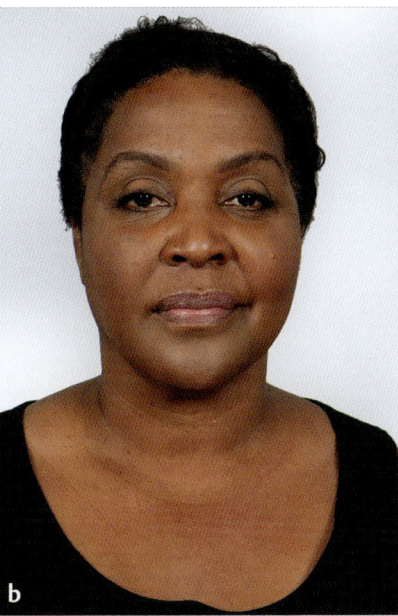

Fig. 16.14 Injectable poly-L-lactic acid (Sculptra, Galderma Inc.) case study. A 53-year-old patient treated with four vials Sculptra over 25 months. (a) Before treatment. (b) After treatment. (Courtesy Galderma, Inc.)

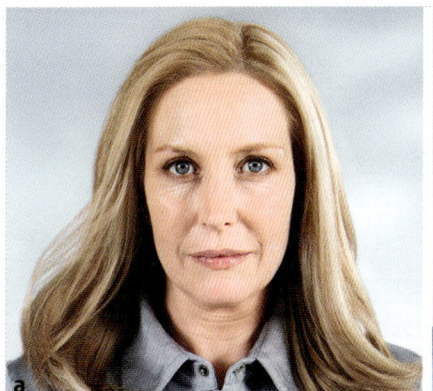 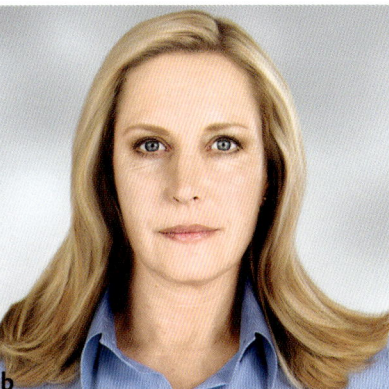

Fig. 16.15 Injectable poly-L-lactic acid (Sculptra, Galderma Inc.) case study. A 49-year-old patient treated with four vials of Sculptra over 25 months. (a) Before treatment. (b) After treatment. (Courtesy Galderma, Inc.)

16.7 Restylane

(see Chapter 2)

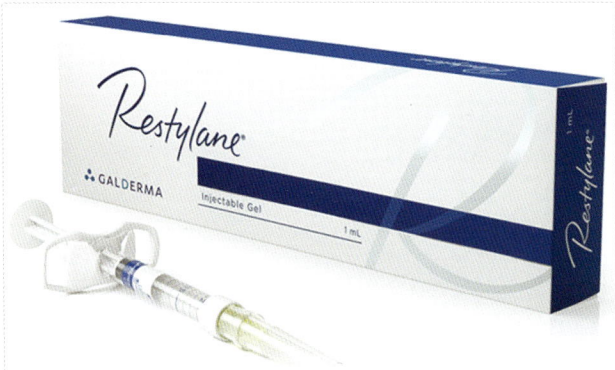

Fig. 16.16 Restylane (Galderma, Inc.). (Courtesy Galderma, Inc.)

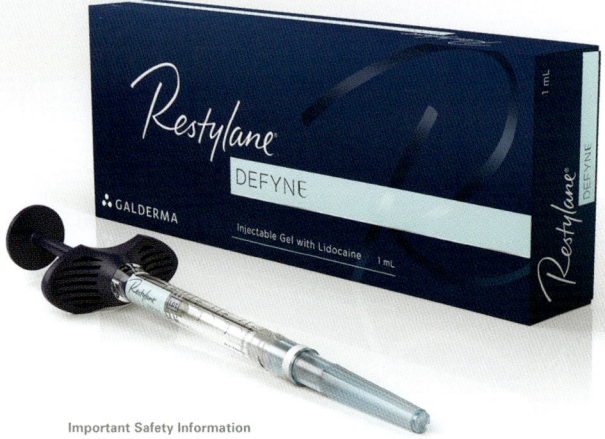

Fig. 16.17 Restylane Defyne (Galderma, Inc.). (Courtesy Galderma, Inc.)

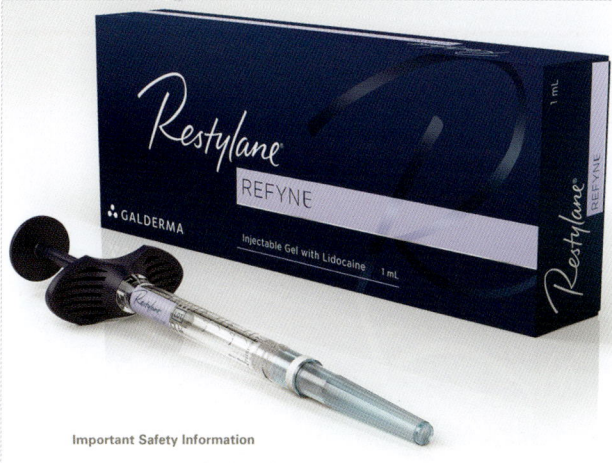

Fig. 16.18 Restylane Refyne (Galderma, Inc.). (Courtesy Galderma, Inc.)

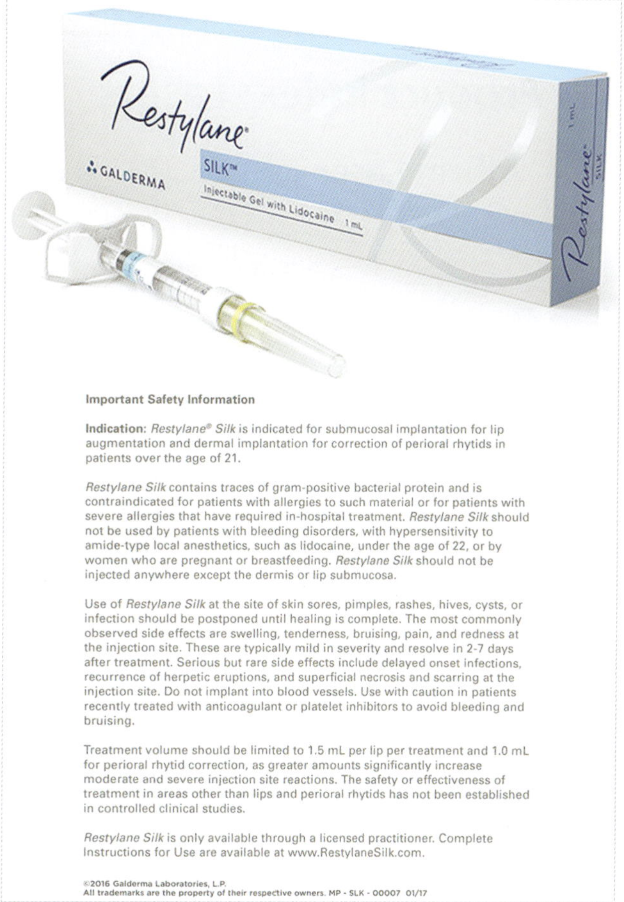

Fig. 16.20 Restylane Silk (Galderma, Inc.). (Courtesy Galderma, Inc.)

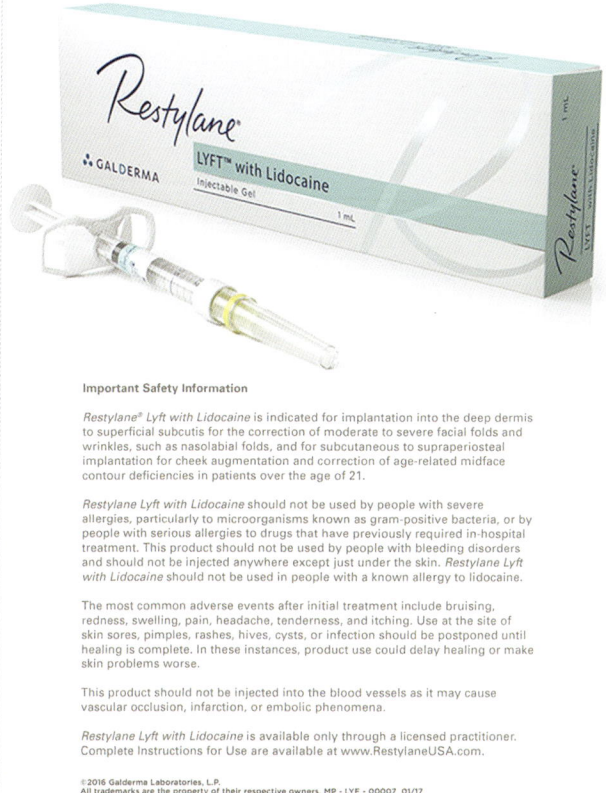

Fig. 16.19 Restylane Lyft (Galderma, Inc.). (Courtesy Galderma, Inc.)

17 Product Index: Lasers

17.1 Affirm Laser

(see Chapter 2)

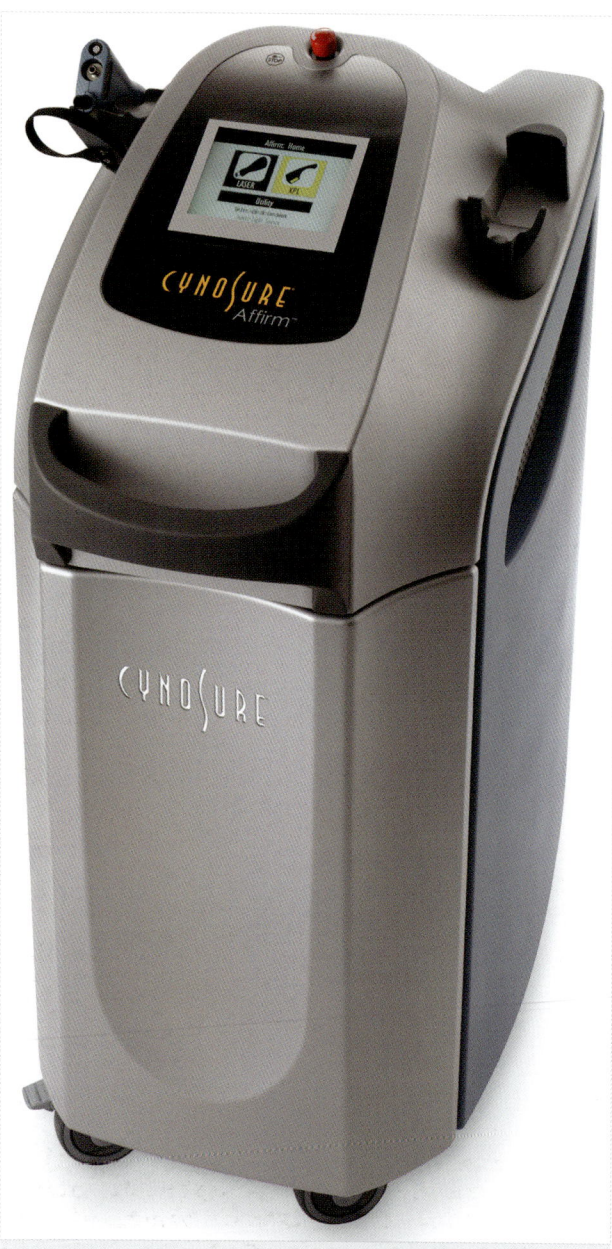

Fig. 17.1 Affirm laser (Cynosure, Inc.). (Courtesy Cynosure, Inc.)

17.2 BroadBand Laser (BBL)

(see Chapter 10)

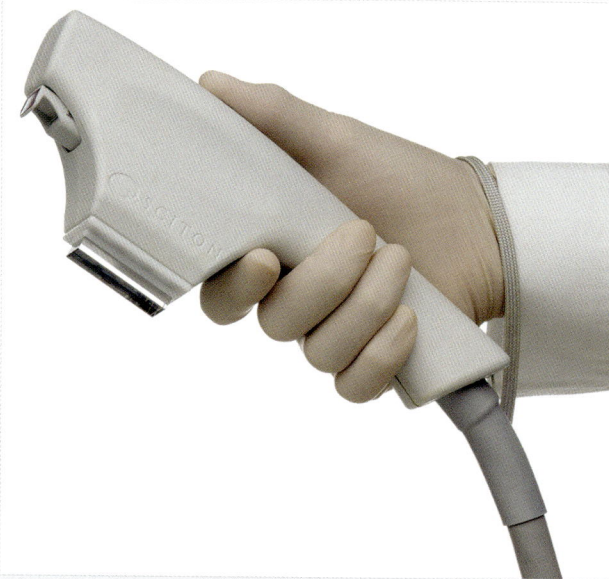

Fig. 17.2 BroadBand Laser (Sciton, Inc.). (Courtesy Sciton, Inc.)

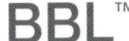
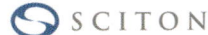

BEFORE / AFTER | Six months post 10 tx | courtesy of Chris W. Robb, MD, PhD

Parameters: 560 nm filter, 18 J/cm², 11 ms, 17 °C cooling

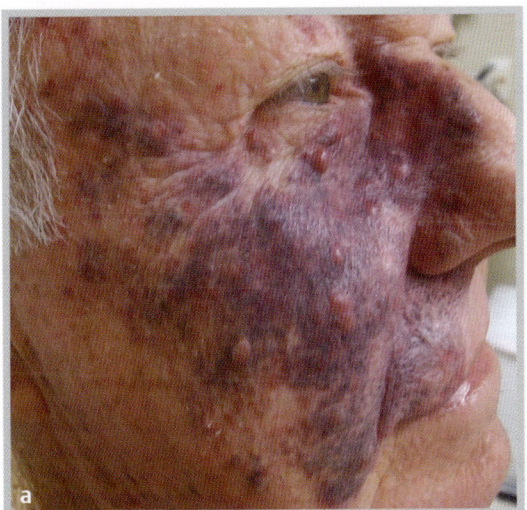
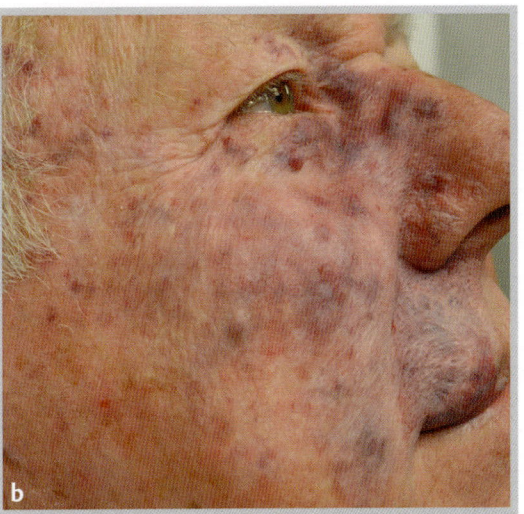

Fig. 17.3 (a) Before and (b) 6 months after 10 treatments with a BroadBand Laser from Sciton, Inc. 580 nm filter, 19 J/cm2, 11 ms, 17 °C cooling. (Courtesy Sciton, Inc.)

17.3 Cellulaze

(see Chapter 10)

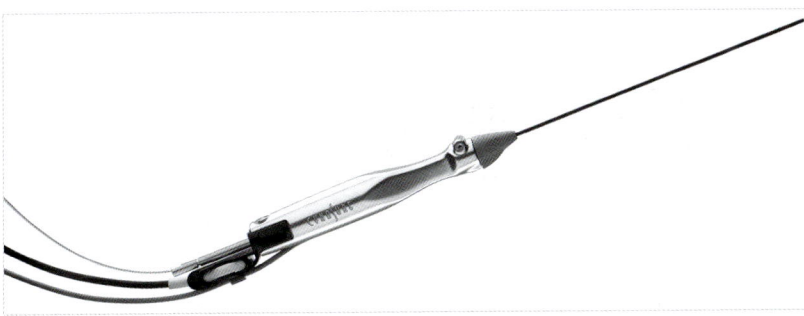

Fig. 17.4 Cellulaze handpiece (Cynosure, Inc.). (Courtesy Cynosure, Inc.)

17.4 ClearScan YAG

(see Chapter 2, Chapter 6)

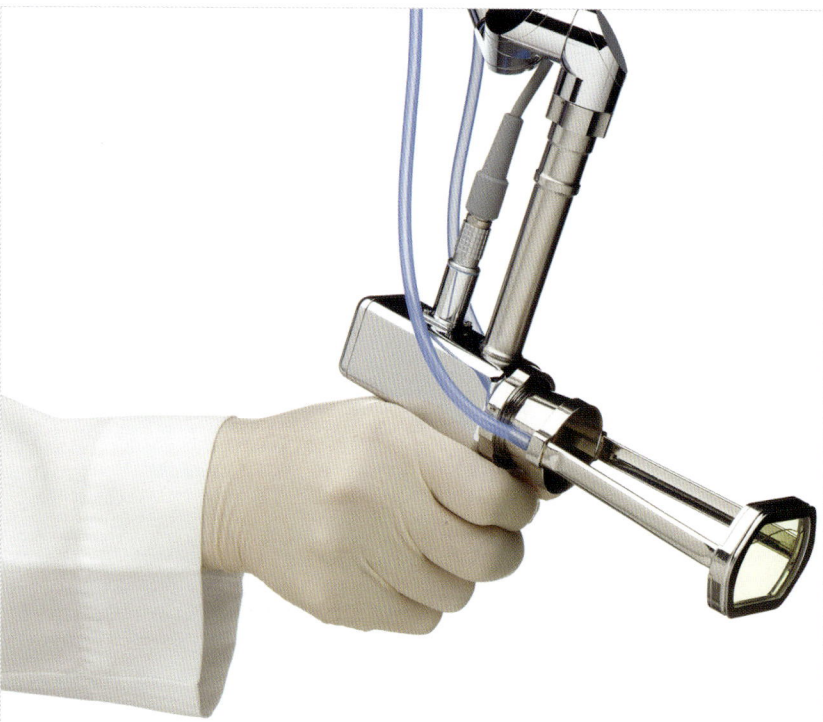

Fig. 17.5 ClearScan YAG (Sciton, Inc.). (Courtesy Sciton, Inc.)

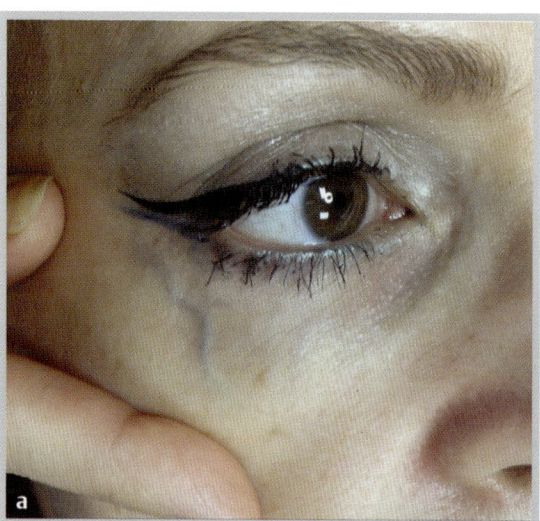
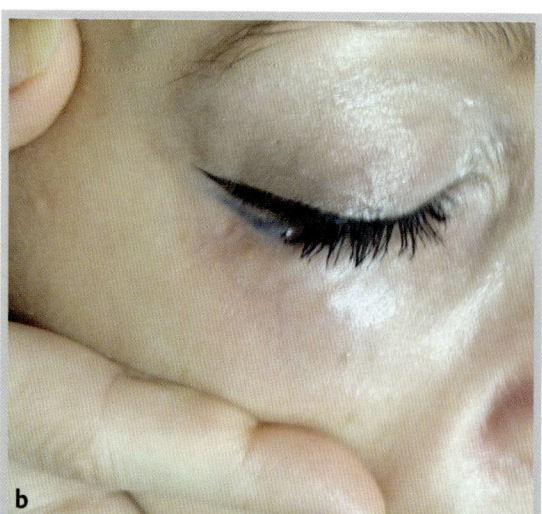

Fig. 17.6 (a) Before and (b) immediately after one treatment with the ClearScan YAG laser from Sciton, Inc. 115 J/cm2, 15 ms, 2.5 Hz, 5 °C cooling. (Courtesy Sciton, Inc.)

17.5 Contour TRL

(see Chapter 2)

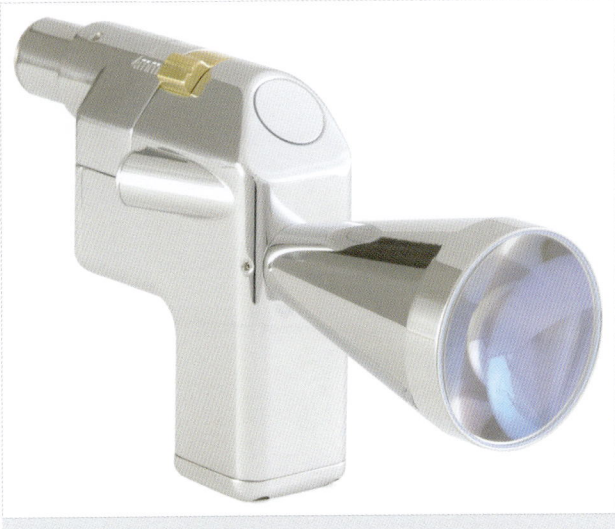

Fig. 17.7 Contour TRL (Sciton, Inc.). (Courtesy Sciton, Inc.)

BEFORE / AFTER | One month post 1 tx | courtesy of Sherrif Ibrahim, University of Rochester Medical Center

Contour TRL™
Parameters: 4 mm single spot, 100 µm ablation, multiple passes

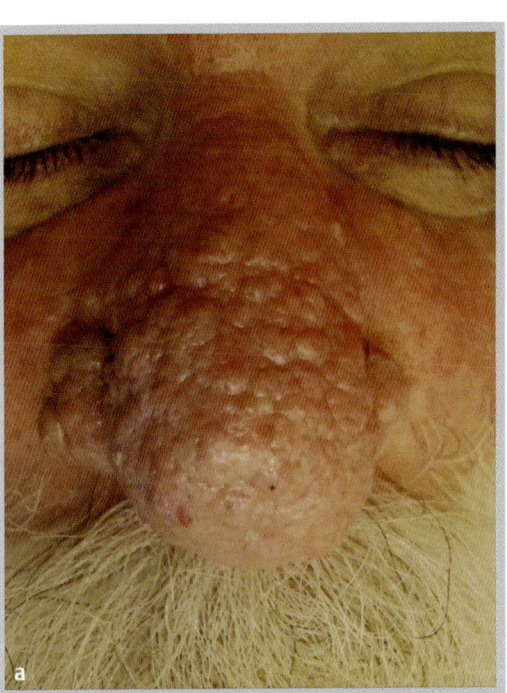
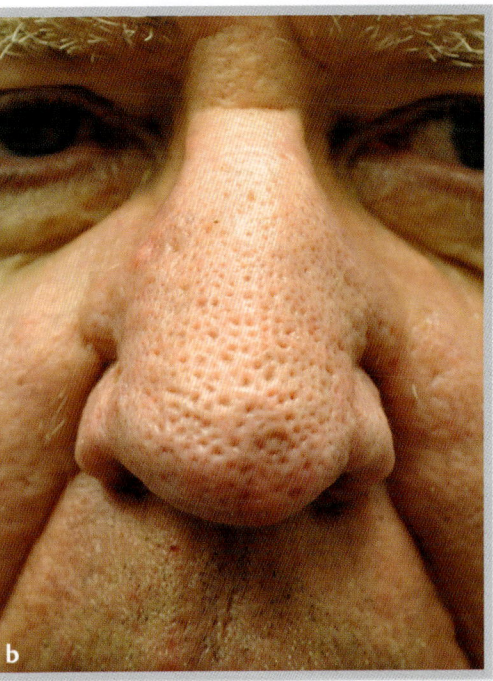

Fig. 17.8 (a) Before and (b) 1 month after treatment with the Contour TRL laser from Sciton, Inc. 4 mm single spot, 100 µm ablation, multiple passes. (Courtesy Sciton, Inc.)

Product Index: Lasers

17.6 CoolSculpting Cryolipolysis

(see Chapter 13)

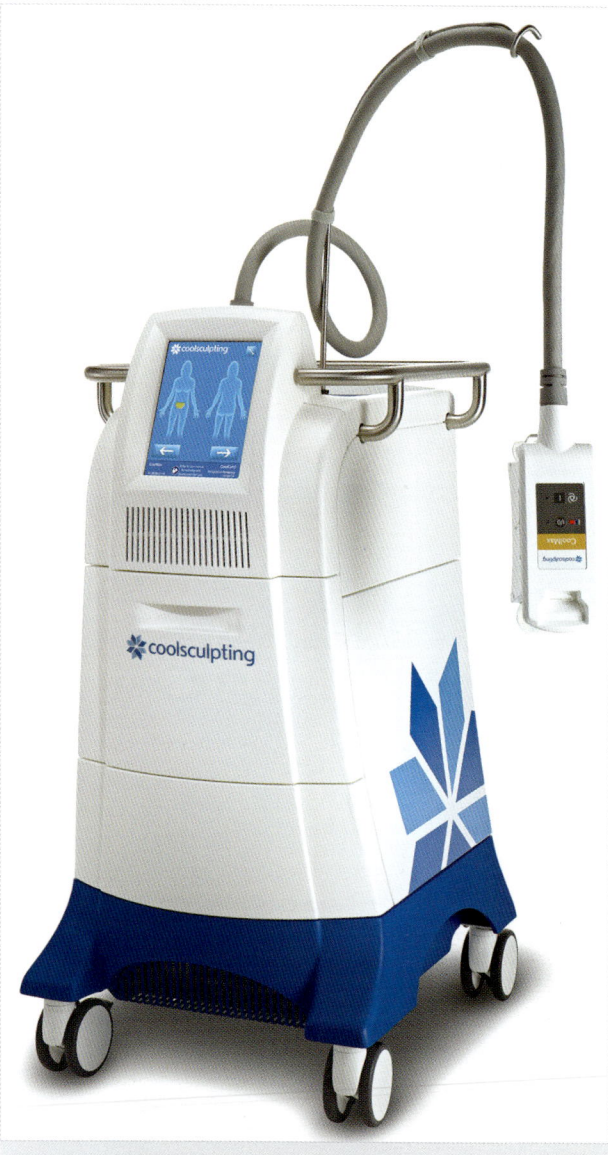

Fig. 17.9 CoolSculpting (ZELTIQ Aesthetics, Inc.) control unit. (Courtesy ZELTIQ Aesthetics, Inc.)

17.7 Halo Hybrid Fractional Laser

(see Chapter 2)

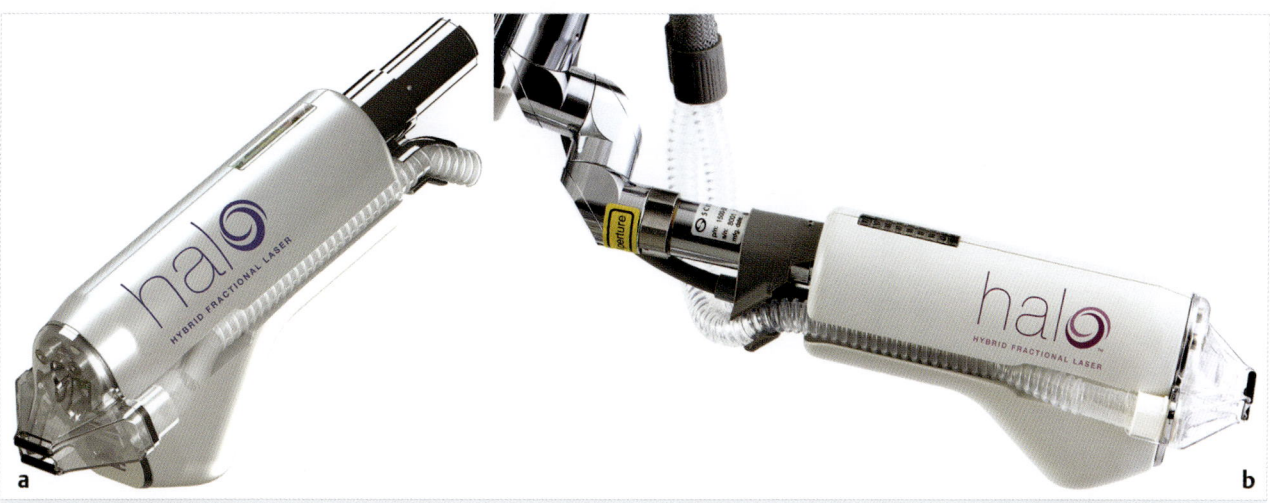

Fig. 17.10 (a,b) Halo Hybrid Fractional Laser (Sciton, Inc.). (Courtesy Sciton, Inc.)

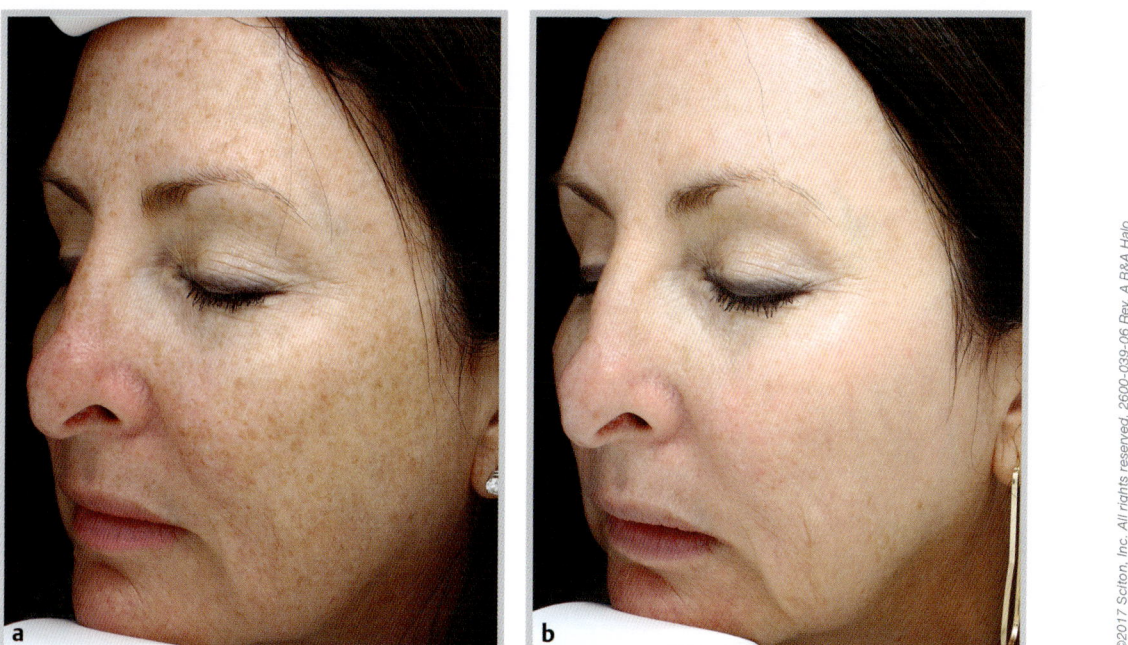

Fig. 17.11 (a) Before and (b) 1 month after treatment with the Halo Hybrid Fractional Laser from Sciton, Inc. 1470 nm 300 µm ablation, 20%. (Courtesy Sciton, Inc.)

Product Index: Lasers

17.8 Icon Fractional Laser

(see Chapter 2, Chapter 6)

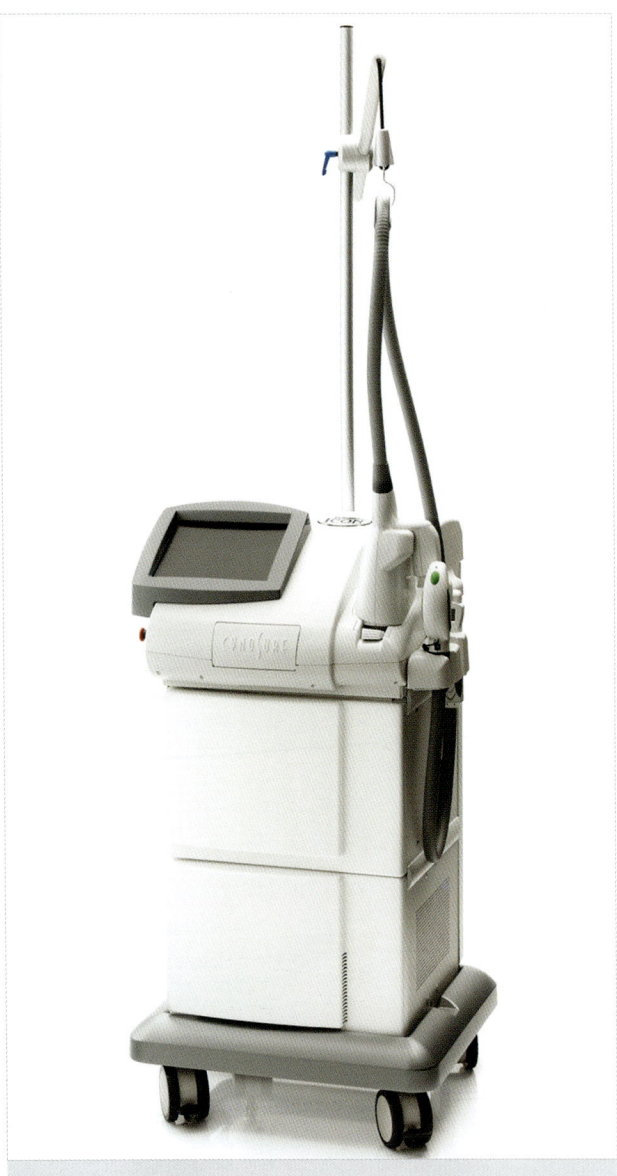

Fig. 17.12 Icon fractional laser (Cynosure, Inc.). (Courtesy Cynosure, Inc.)

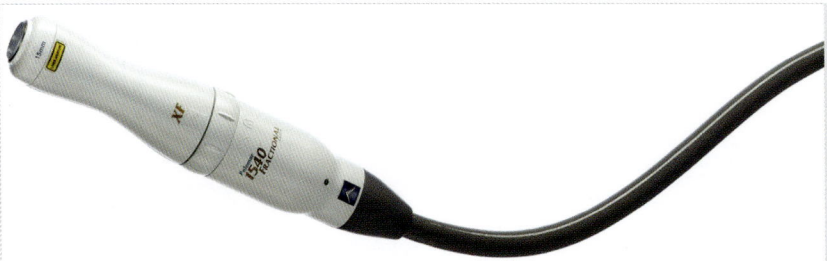

Fig. 17.13 1540 fractional laser handpiece (Cynosure, Inc.). (Courtesy Cynosure, Inc.)

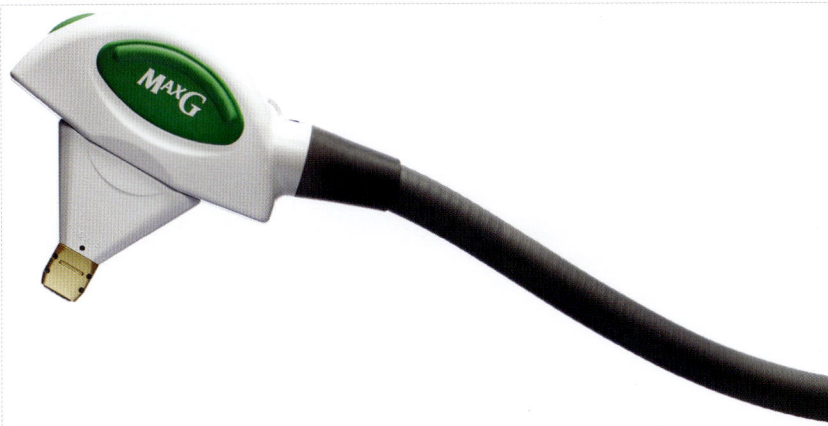

Fig. 17.14 MaxG fractional laser handpiece (Cynosure, Inc.). (Courtesy Cynosure, Inc.)

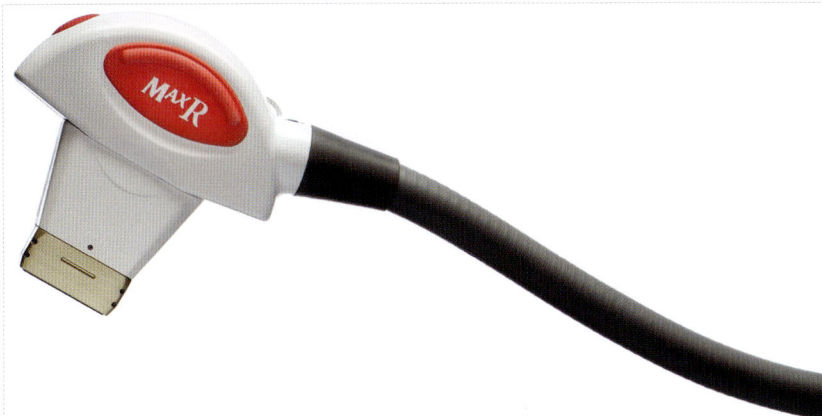

Fig. 17.15 MaxR fractional laser handpiece (Cynosure, Inc.). (Courtesy Cynosure, Inc.)

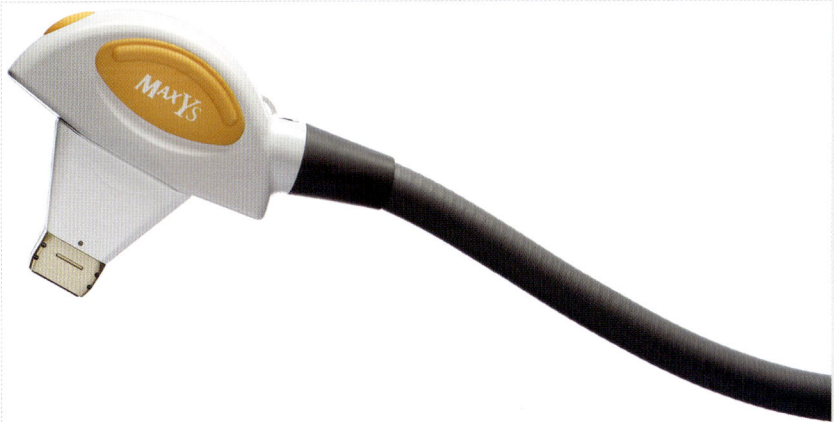

Fig. 17.16 MaxYs fractional laser handpiece (Cynosure, Inc.). (Courtesy Cynosure, Inc.)

17.9 Lutronic eCO$_2$ Laser

(see Chapter 2)

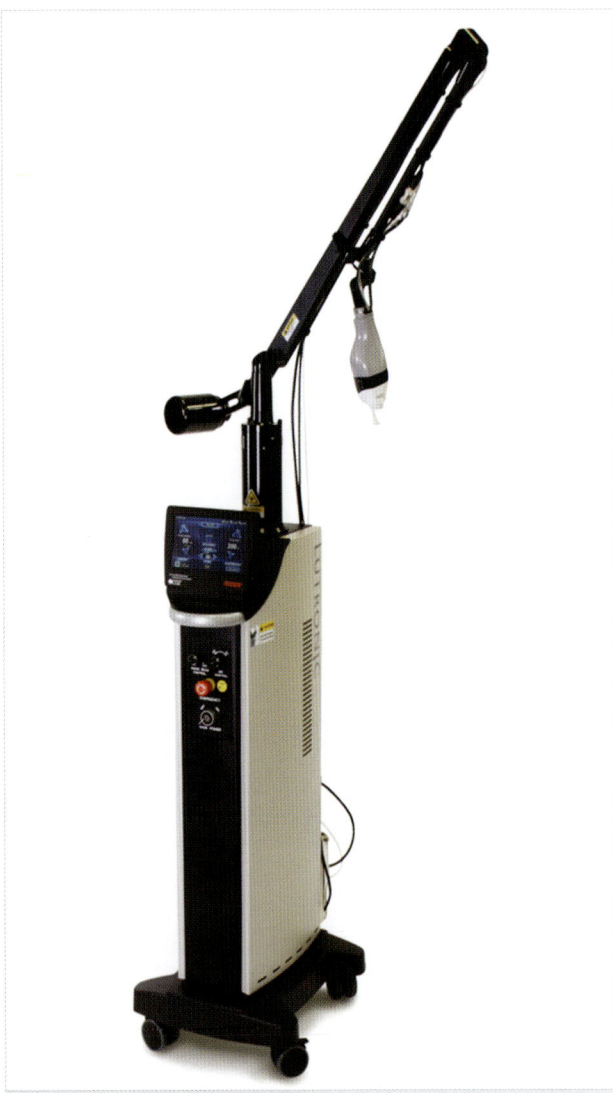

Fig. 17.17 Lutronic eCO$_2$ high speed fractional laser (Lutronic). (Courtesy Lutronic)

eCO2™ Rhytids & Dyschromia

Baseline   28 Post Tx

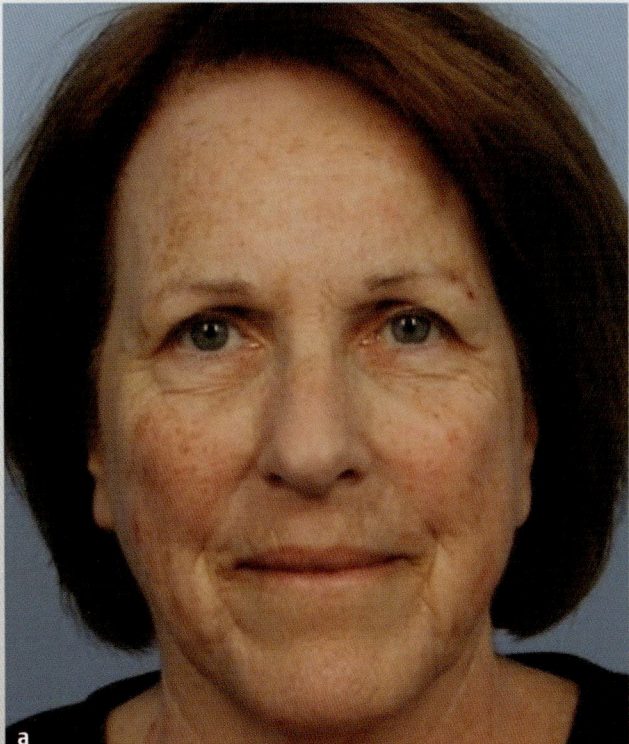
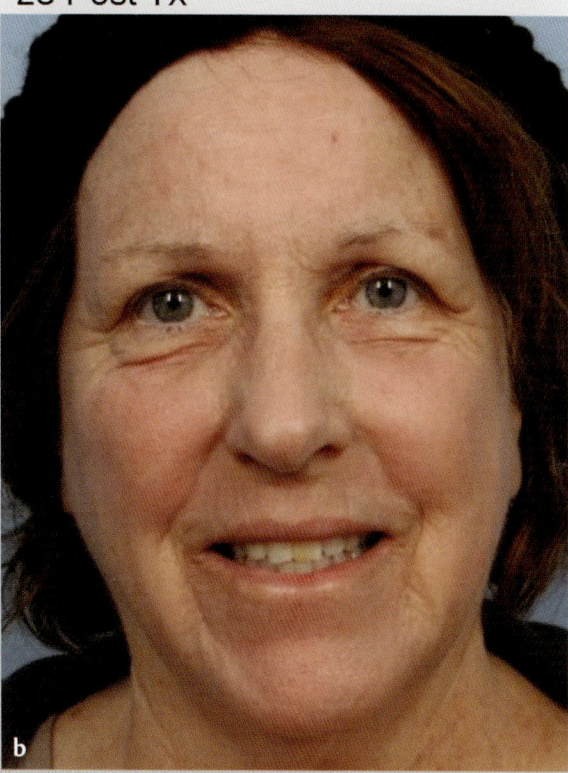

Courtesy of Melanie Palm, MD. (Solano Beach, CA)

Lateral Cheeks: 120 Tip – 80-90 mJ, density 100-150 spots per cm2
Rest of face: 120 Tip - 110 mJ, density 100-150 spots per cm2

Fig. 17.18 (a) Before rhytides and dyschromia and (b) after 28 laser treatments with the Lutronic eCO$_2$ high-speed fractional laser. Lateral cheek: 120 Tip 80–90 mJ, density 100–150 spots per cm^2; Rest of facial surface: 120 Tip 110 mJ, density 100–150 spots per cm^2. (Courtesy Melanie Palm, MD and Lutronic)

17.10 Microfocused Ultrasound

(see Chapter 2, Chapter 4, Chapter 5, Chapter 6, Chapter 11, Chapter 12)

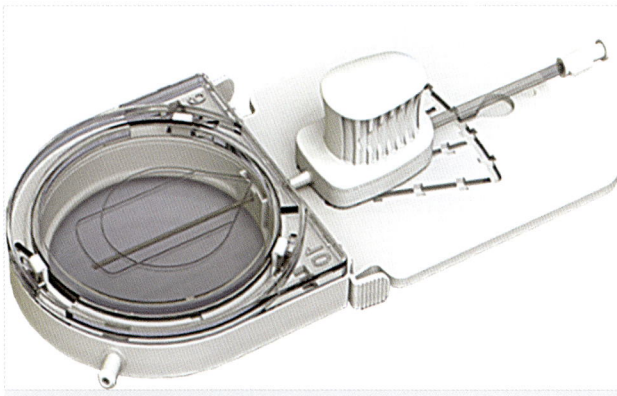

Fig. 17.19 Cellfina system anesthetic filtration device. (Cellfina is a registered trademark of Ulthera, Inc.)

Product Index: Lasers

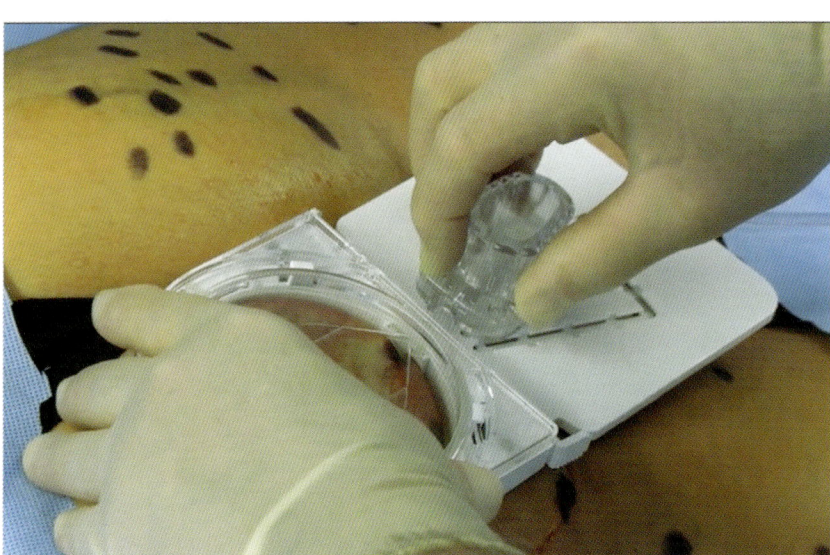

Fig. 17.20 Cellfina (Ulthera, Inc.) device in use. (Cellfina is a registered trademark of Ulthera, Inc.)

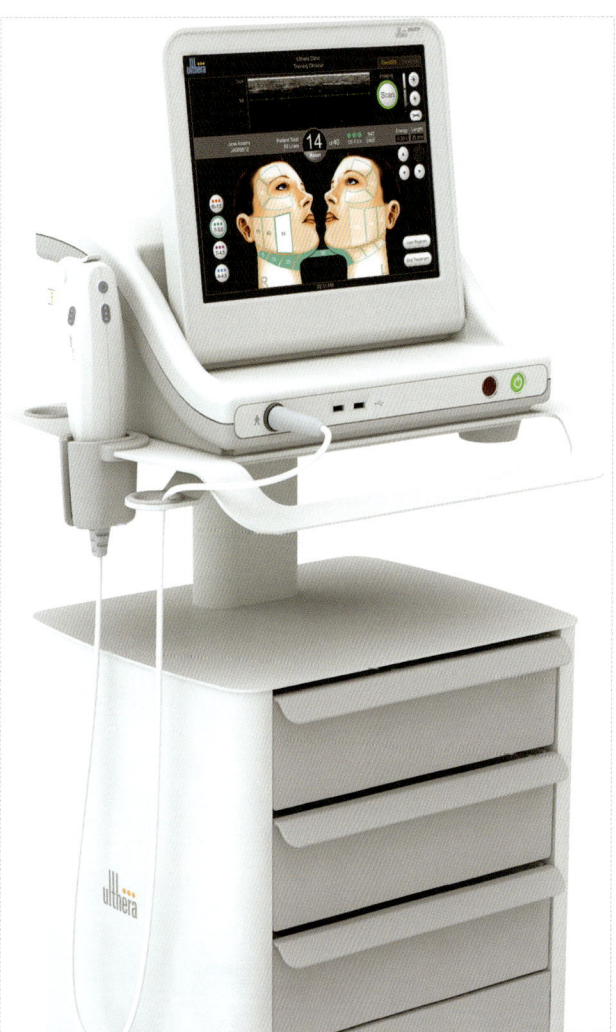

Fig. 17.21 Ultherapy (Ulthera, Inc.) system. (Ultherapy is a registered trademark of Ulthera, Inc.)

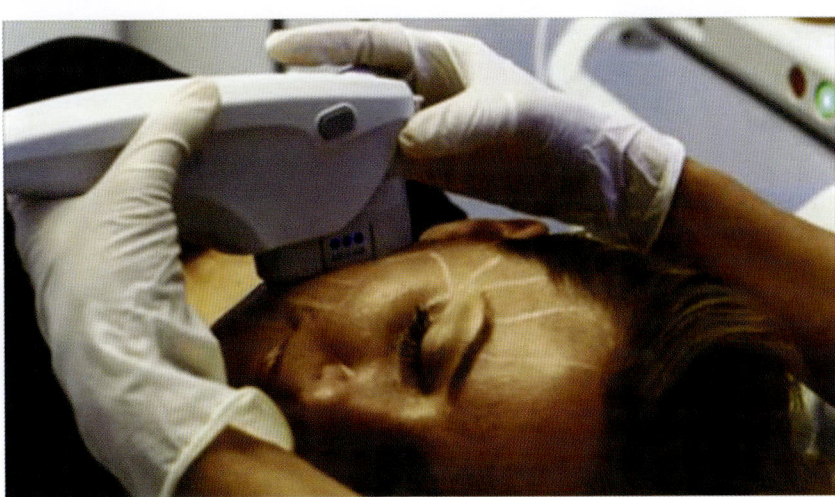

Fig. 17.22 Ulthera (Ulthera, Inc.) device in use. (Ultherapy is a registered trademark of Ulthera, Inc.)

17.11 Pellevé Fractional Laser

(See Chapter 2)

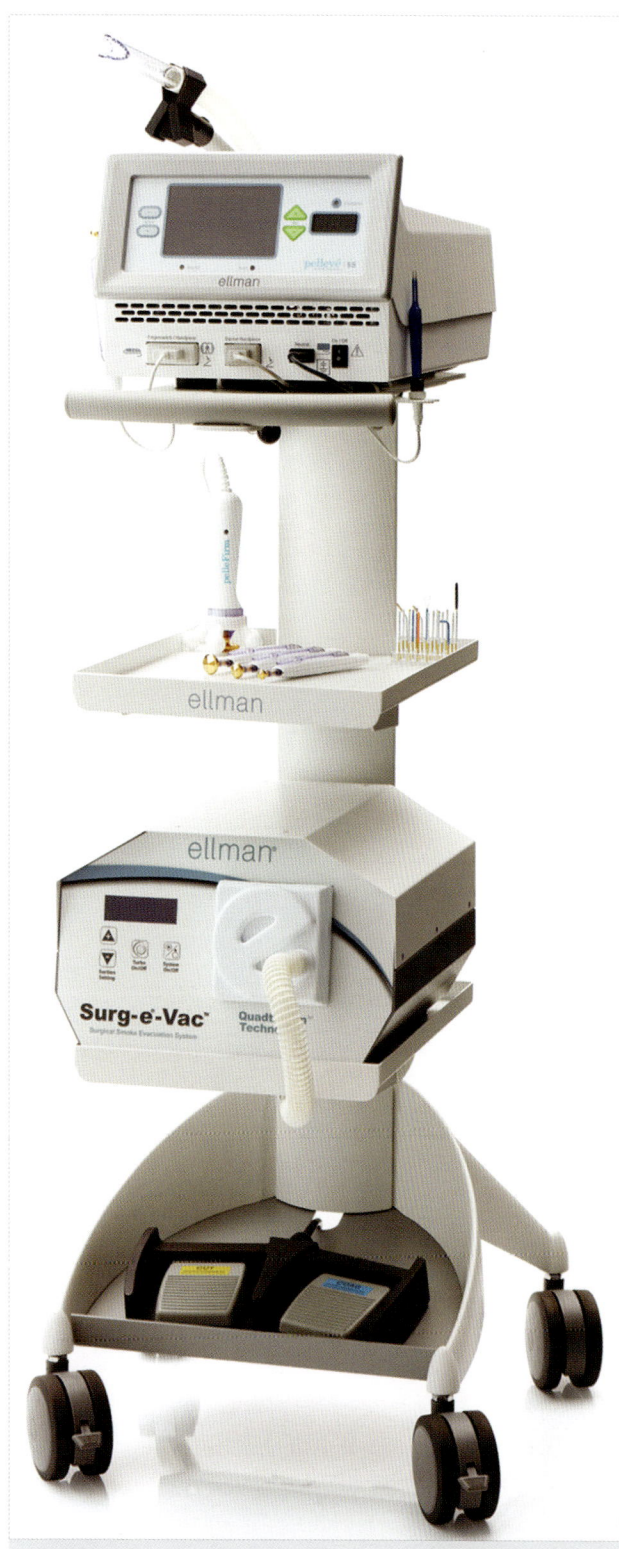

Fig. 17.23 Pellevé fractional laser (Cynosure, Inc.). (Courtesy Cynosure, Inc.)

17.12 ProFractional-XC

(see Chapter 2, Chapter 6)

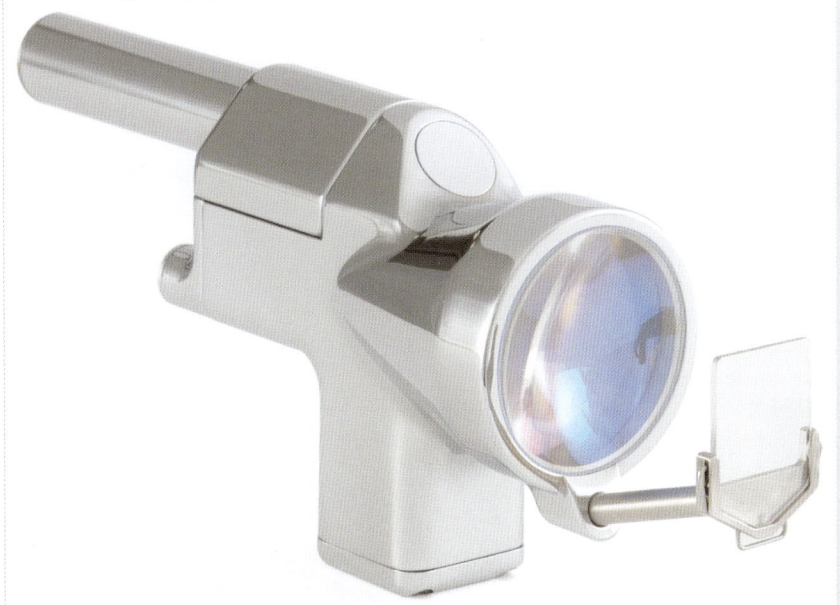

Fig. 17.24 ProFractional-XC (Sciton, Inc.). (Courtesy Sciton, Inc.)

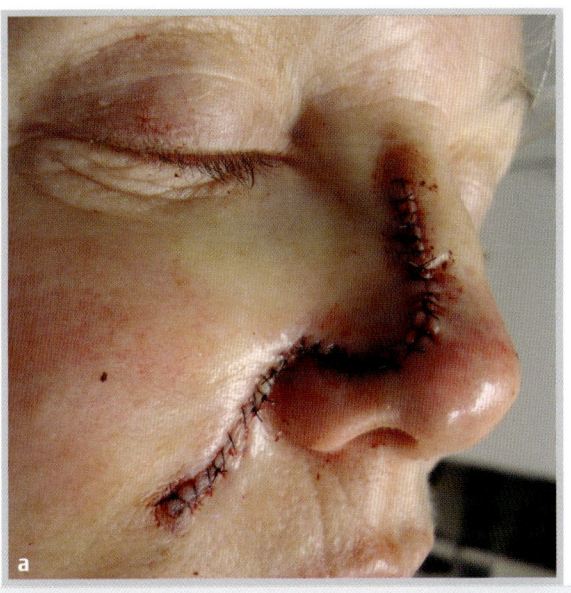
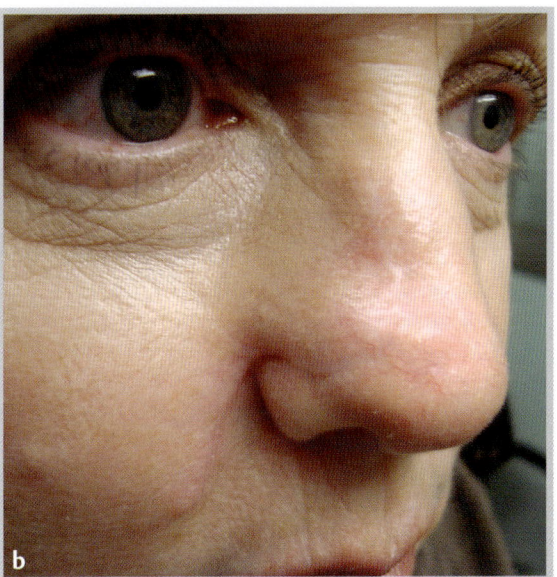

Fig. 17.25 (a) Before and (b) 3 months after 2 treatments with the ProFractional-XC from Sciton, Inc. 250–300 µm ablation, 11% density, coag 2. (Courtesy Sciton, Inc.)

17.13 SculpSure

(see Chapter 10)

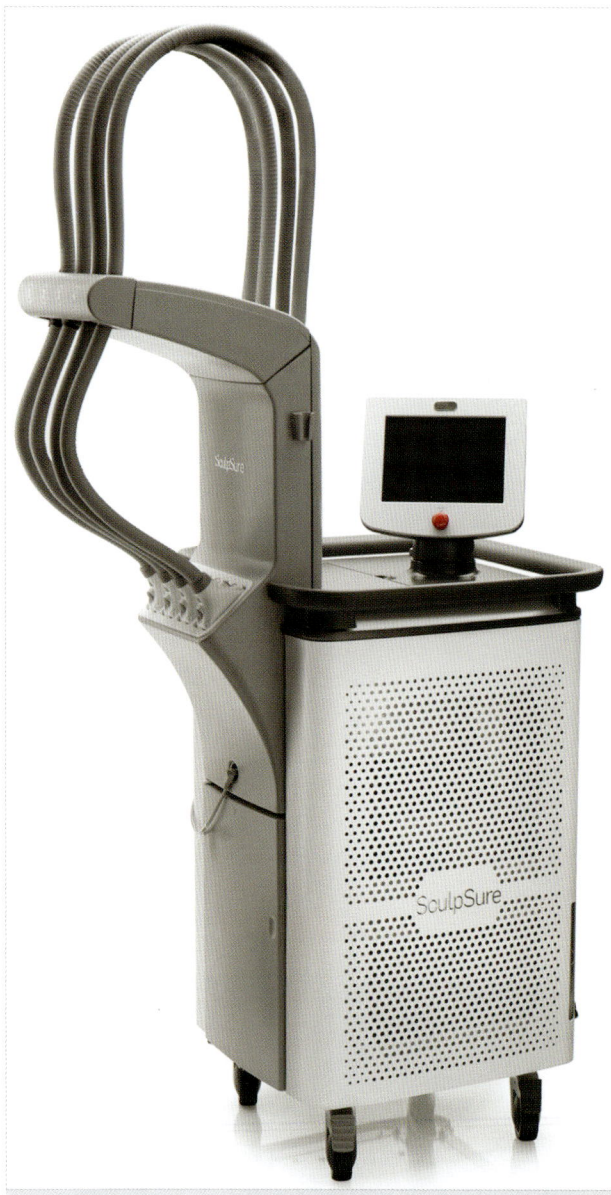

Fig. 17.26 SculpSure laser device (Cynosure, Inc.). (Courtesy Cynosure, Inc.)

17.14 SkinPen

(see Chapter 5)

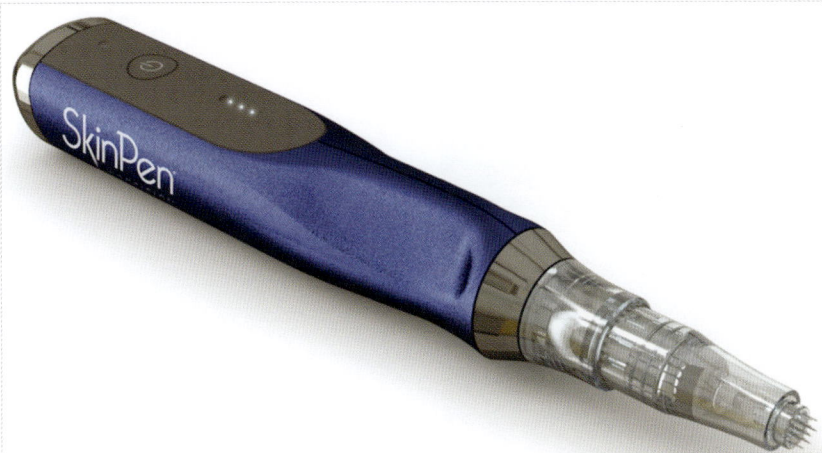

Fig. 17.27 SkinPen (Bellus Medical). (Courtesy Bellus Medical)

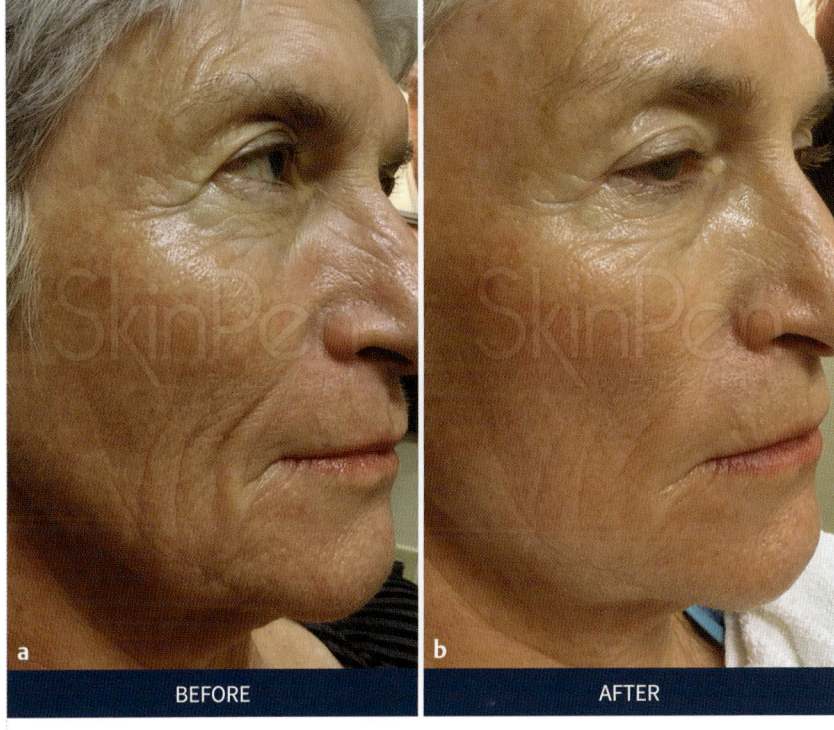

Fig. 17.28 This 66-year-old woman is shown **(a)** before and **(b)** after 2 treatments with the SkinPen by Bellus Medical. (Courtesy Bellus Medical)

Product Index: Lasers

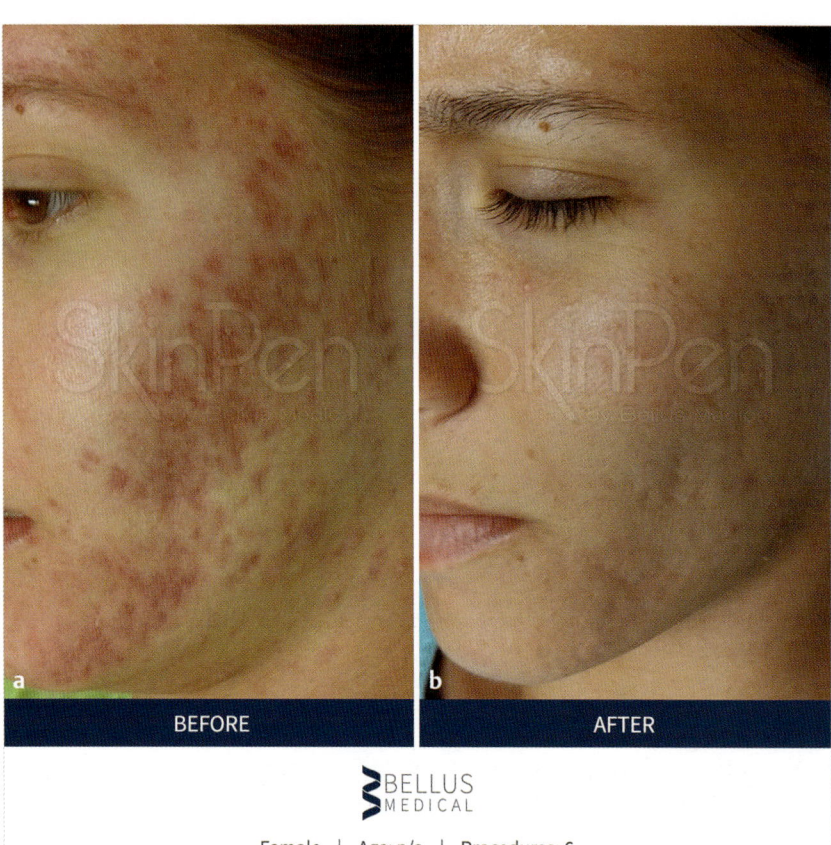

Fig. 17.29 This woman is shown **(a)** before and **(b)** after 6 treatments with the SkinPen from Bellus Medical. (Courtesy Bellus Medical)

17.15 Smartlipo

(see Chapter 9)

17.16 DOT SmartXide CO$_2$ Laser

(see Chapter 2)

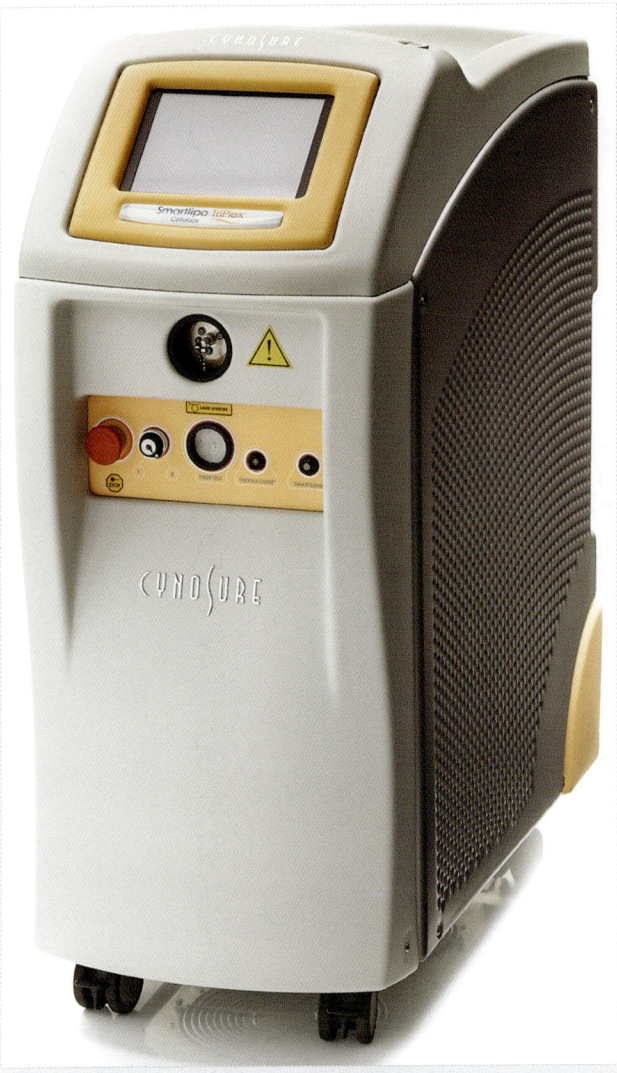

Fig. 17.30 Smartlipo laser (Cynosure, Inc.). (Courtesy Cynosure, Inc.)

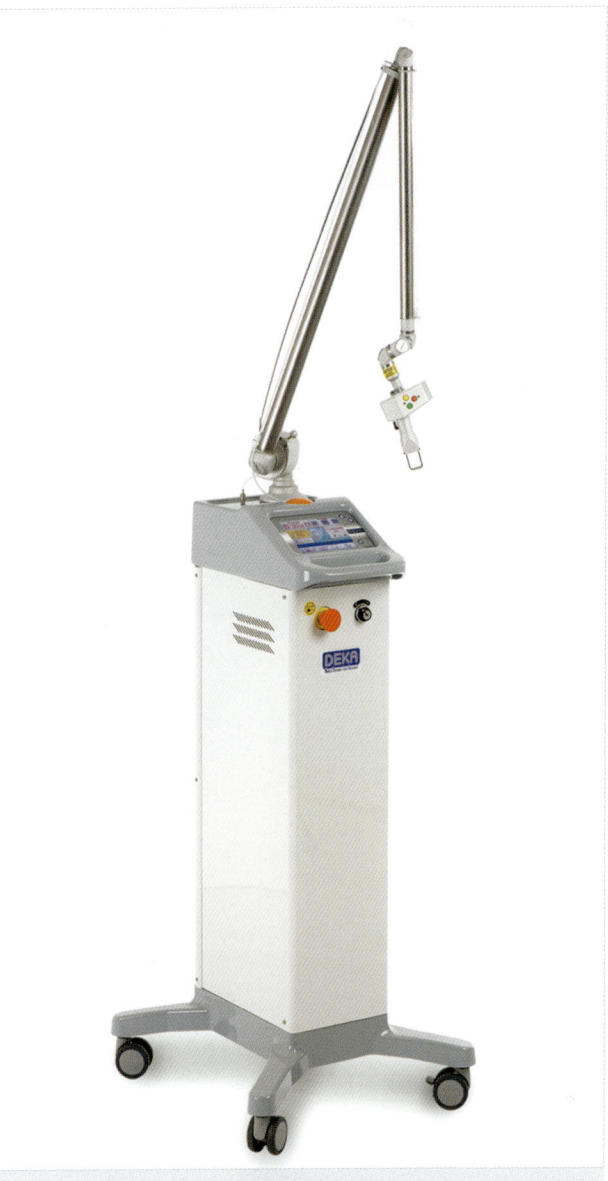

Fig. 17.31 DOT Therapy SmartXide CO$_2$ laser (DEKA M.E.L.A. s.r.l.). (Exclusive property of DEKA M.E.L.A. s.r.l.)

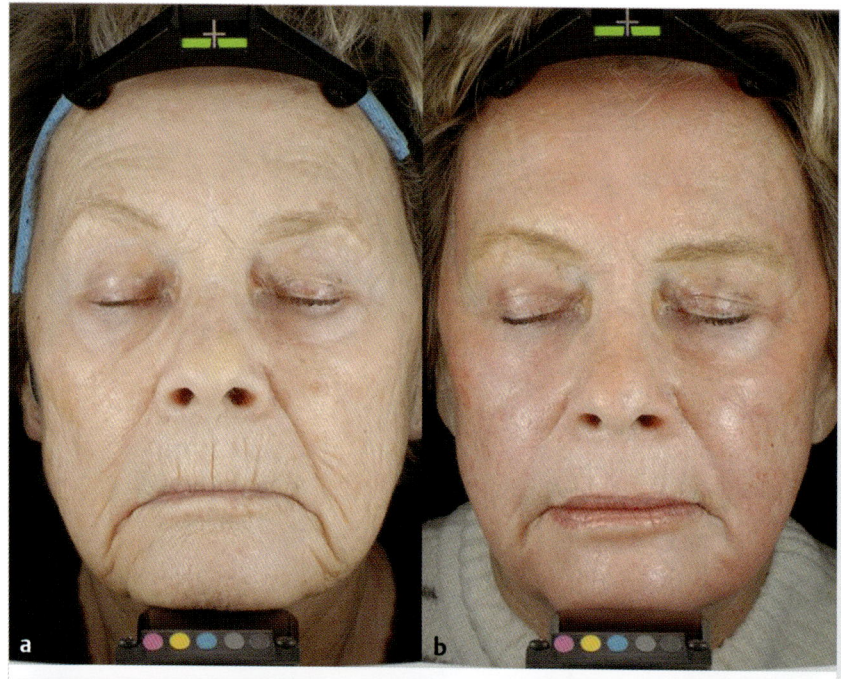
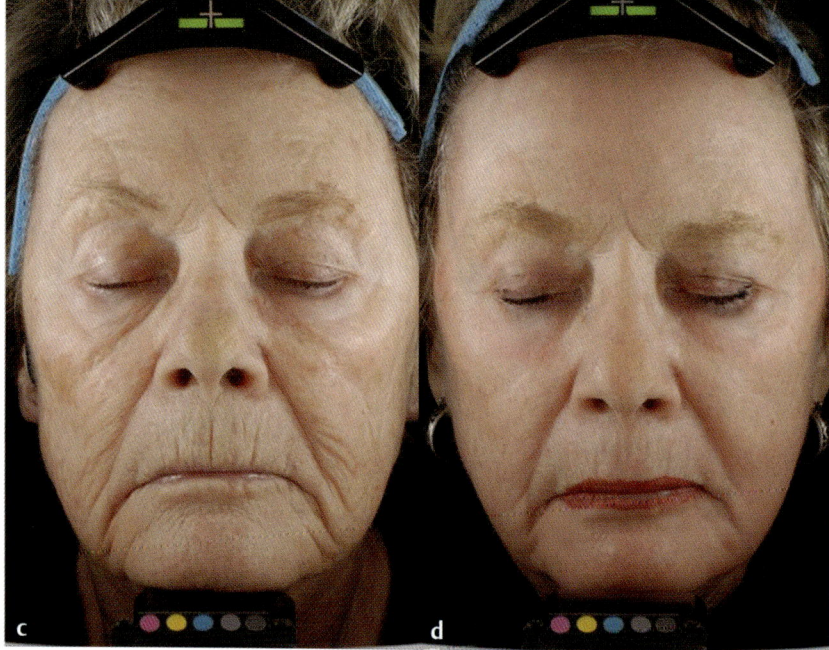

Fig. 17.32 (a,c) Before and **(b,d)** after DOT SmartXide CO_2 laser treatment. (The property of and procedures performed by Robert H. Gotkin, MD, FACS and Deborah S. Sarnoff, MD, FAAD, FACP. Courtesy DEKA M.E.L.A. s.r.l.)

17.17 ThermiRF Device

(see Chapter 9, Chapter 10, Chapter 11)

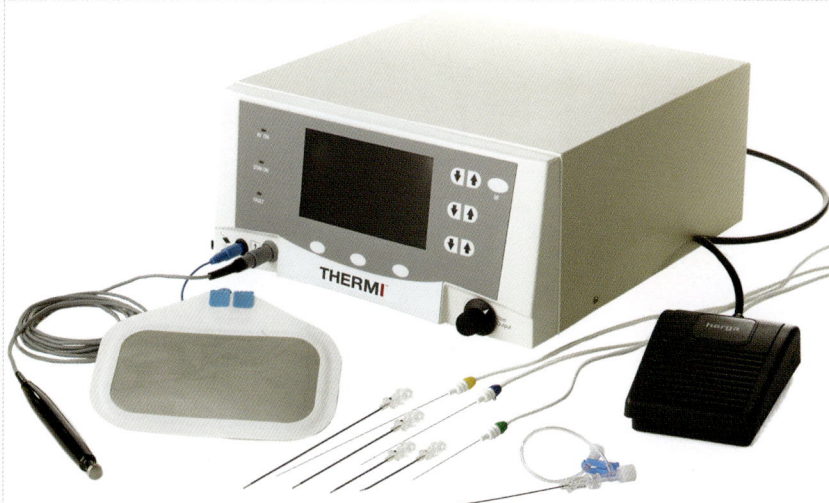

Fig. 17.33 ThermiRF Device (THERMI). (Courtesy ThermiGen, LLC, an Almirall Company)

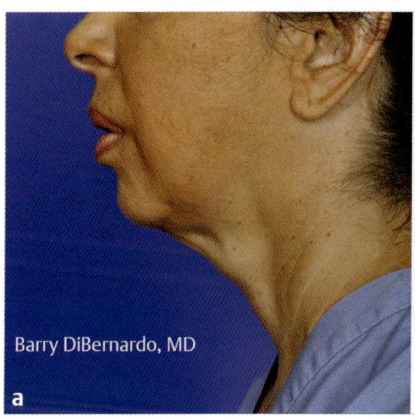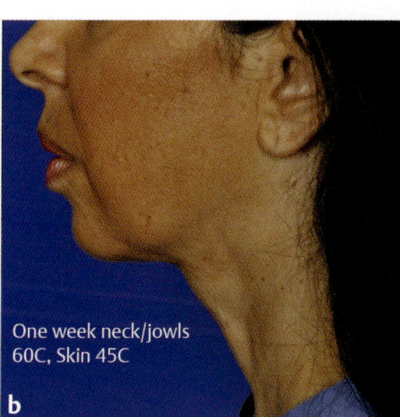

Fig. 17.34 (a) Before and (b) 1 week after ThermiTight application. (Courtesy THERMI, an Almirall Company)

Product Index: Lasers

17.18 Venus RF Devices

(see Chapter 4)

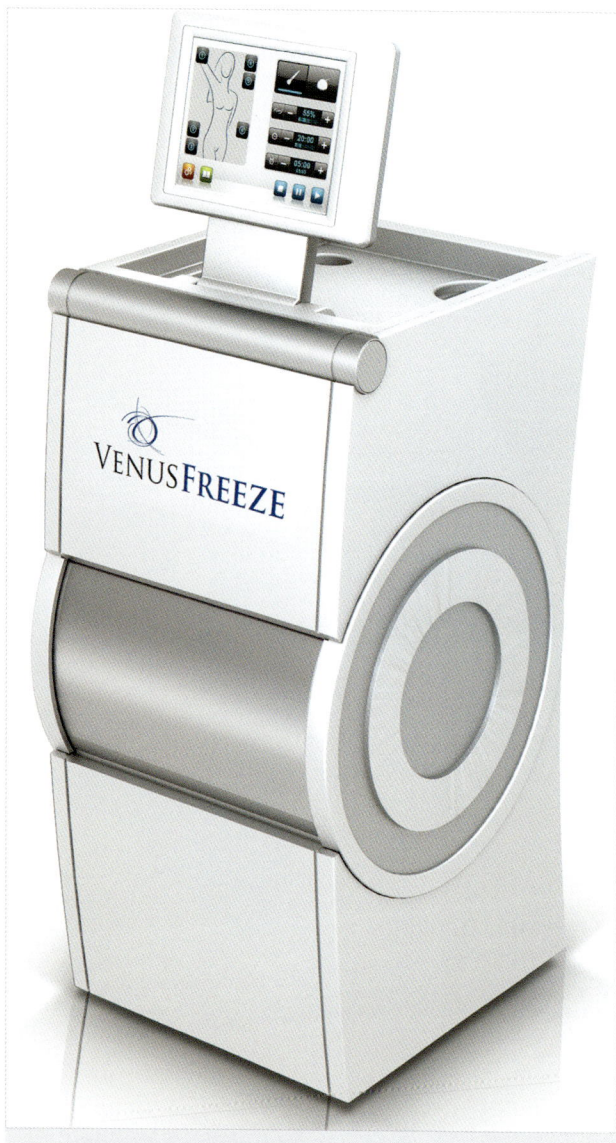

Fig. 17.35 Venus Freeze RF (Venus Concept) device. Licensed by Health Canada. (Courtesy Venus Concept)

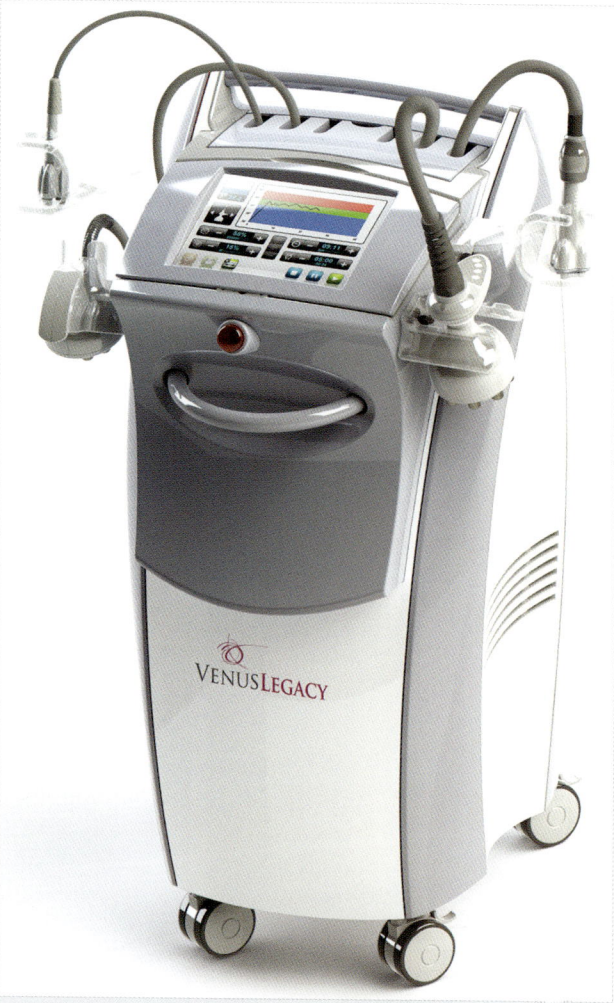

Fig. 17.36 Venus Legacy (Venus Concept) device. Licensed by the FDA. (Courtesy Venus Concept)

17.19 VISIA Complexion Analysis

(See Chapter 8)

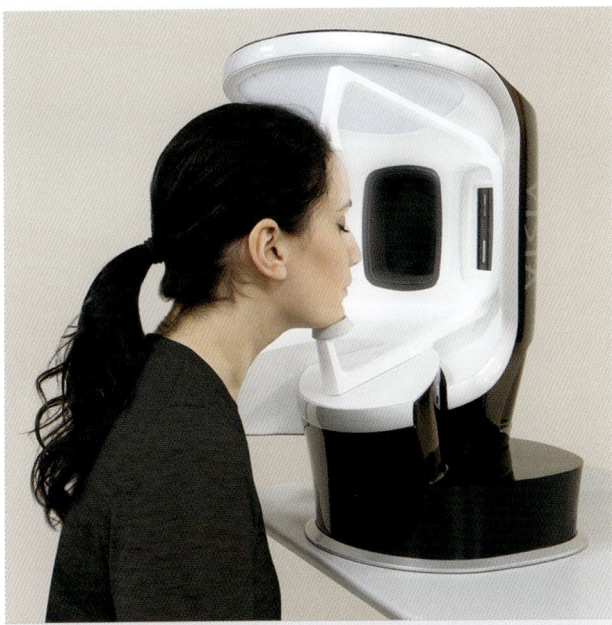

Fig. 17.37 VISIA Complexion Analysis System (Canfield Scientific). (Courtesy Canfield Scientific)

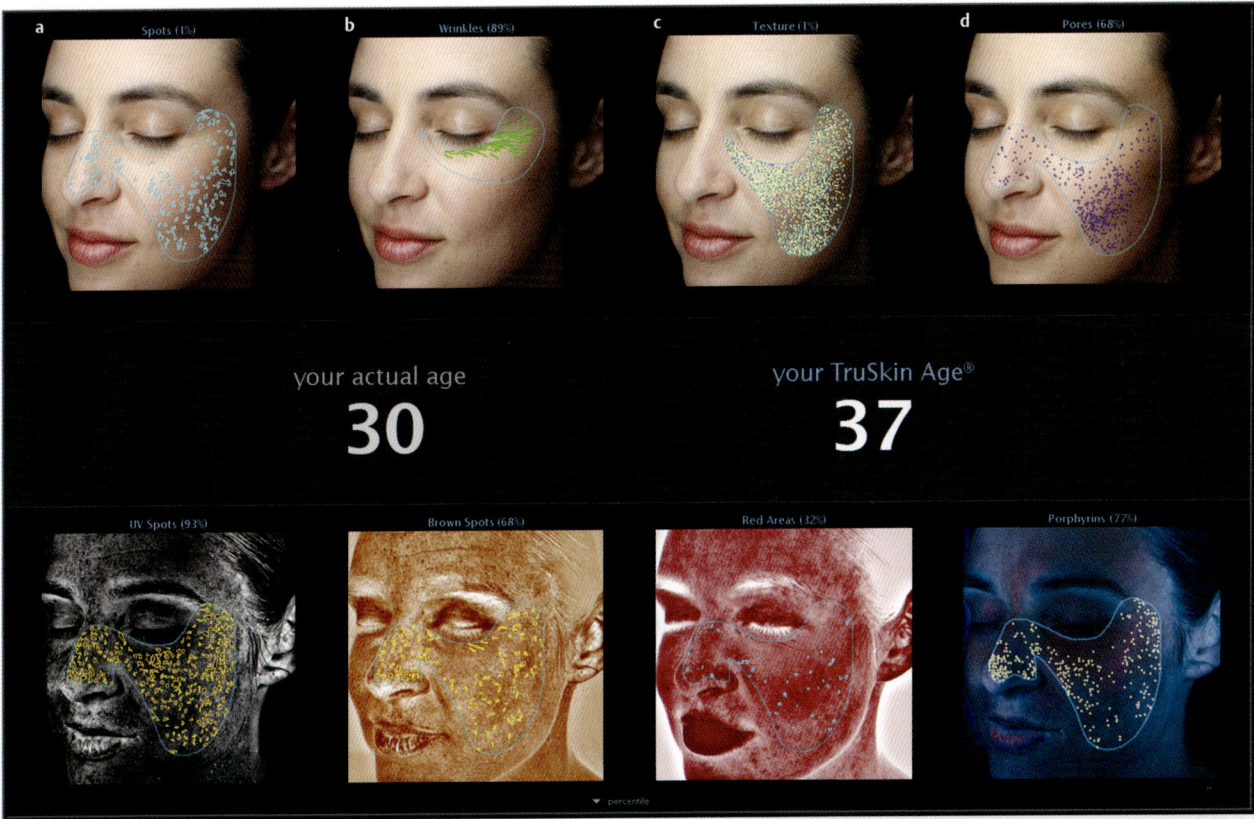

Fig. 17.38 Skin analysis using the VISIA Complexion Analysis System by Canfield Scientific. **(a, top)** Spots; **(a, bottom)** UV spots; **(b, top)** Wrinkles; **(b, bottom)** Brown spots; **(c, top)** Texture; **(c, bottom)** Red areas; **(d, top)** Pores; **(d, bottom)** Porphyrins. (Courtesy Canfield Scientific)

Index

Note: Page numbers set **bold** or *italic* indicate headings or figures, respectively.

3

3D imaging 162, *163–164*

5

5-Fluorouracil for keloidal and hypertrophic scars 49, *50*

7

7/47 effect 31

A

AbabotulinumtoxinA *169*
- *See also* See also Dysport

Abdomen
- cryolipolysis for *107*, 128, 134, 136, 138, 143, *143*
- liposuction for *107*
- radiofrequency for *107*
- stackable treatment for **38**, *41*

Ablative laser(s) **10**, *78*, **78**, 112, 152
- fractionated 11, *12–13*, *78*, **78**, 113, **114**, **116**, 152
- indications for use 152
- nonfractionated *10*, **10**, 152
- postprocedure care with 92
- use in conjunction with surgical procedures 81

Absorbable sutures 98, 160, 163

Acetaminophen
- for microfocused ultrasound 156
- for postprocedure pain 39

Acne
- eruptions laser skin resurfacing and 155
- intense pulsed light for *115*, **115**
- PIH in 47, *48*

Acne scarring
- fat injections for 116, *119*
- in skin of color 47
- -- ice-pick 47, *48*
- -- nonsurgical procedures for 47, *49*
- laser skin resurfacing for 34, 49, 116, *117*, *119*
- microneedling for *49*, 69, 72

Acquisition of novel technology **32**
- basic considerations in **33**
- business plan and 33
- market saturation versus 33
- questions before investment 32
- space considerations for 33
- trial period for 33

ActiveFX mode of CO2 laser 12, 16, 18, 61

Acyclovir 63

Adipocytolysis 108, 128
- *See also* See also Kybella (deoxycholic acid)

Adipose tissue 127
- *See also* See also specific fat reduction techniques
- cryolipolysis for **128**, **132**
- debulking of 134, 136, *137*, 138
- deoxycholic acid (Kybella) and 6, 9, **9**, 108, **128**, **151**, 159
- liposuction for 105, *106*, 107
- thickness of 136

Adjuncts nonsurgical
- after facial rejuvenation surgery **101**
- during facial rejuvenation surgery **95**

Adverse events **150**
- *See also* See also Complications

Advertising **126**
- direct-to-consumer 127
- strategies for 126, *127*

Aesthetic surgery, *see* See also specific procedures
- artistic tools of 2
- barriers to 30
- beauty as central concept of 1
- cardiac surgery parallels to 31
- common objectives of specialists in 163
- future of 5
- noninvasive core principles of 159
- plastic surgery versus 5
- self-identity in 5
- sequential changes over time 162, *163–166*

Affirm laser *176*, **176**

Akcal A. 70

Alam M. 9

Alarplasty internal in skin of color 53

Alexandrite laser
- for hair removal 49
- for pigmented lesions 64
- penetration depth of *62*

Alopecia microneedling for 69, 72

Amniotic membrane 161

Anesthesia 114

Angiogenesis microneedling and 69

Antibiotics
- and contact dermatitis 155
- and hyperpigmentation 75
- for acne 155
- for delayed healing syndrome 156
- for filler-related infections 153
- in hirsutism treatment 49
- postprocedure 67
- preprocedure 25, 63, 75, 155

Anticoagulants use before procedures 63, 75

Antihyperglycemic agents postprocedure avoidance of 39

Antiviral prophylaxis
- with laser skin resurfacing 14, 25, 39, 63, 67, 76, 155–156
- with light- and energy-based therapies 76
- with microneedling 72
- with stackable treatments 39, 67

Anxiolytics for procedures 114

Apoptosis of fat cells 132, 136

Argon laser penetration depth of *62*

Arms
- cryolipolysis for 134, 138, 143, *146*
- re-pigmentation for *91*, *92*

ArteFill 7

Asian skin hyperpigmentation in 44, *45*

Atrophic acne scars microneedling for 69

Autologous fat 7, 36

Autologous fillers 36–37

Axilla cryolipolysis for 128, 134, 143

Azelaic acid
- for acne 156
- for melasma 46, *47*
- for PIH 155

B

Bachelor E. P. 143

Back cryolipolysis for 128

Bacterial infections 25, 39, 67, 150, 153, 156
- *See also* See also specific types

Baker phenol peel 46

Banana rolls cryolipolysis for *146–147*

Barbed suture 98, 160, *161*

BBL (BroadBand laser) 109, *109*, **176–177**

Beauty
- concepts of **1**
- continuum of nonsurgical technology and 33
- proportion and harmony in 2, *4*
- role in today's culture 4
- skin clarity and 3
- skin of color and 42
- symmetry in 2, *3*

Beck Alex John 2

Bellafill 7, *52*

Belotero 7, *7*, 8, *167*, **167**
- for glabellar complex crow's-feet and forehead lines 14
- for perioral rejuvenation 17–18
- for skin of color *52*

Bernstein E. F. 143

Biases practitioner's 126

Biocompatibility 159, 163

Bipolar radiofrequency 88, *88*, 120

Blending, *see* See also specific techniques
- nonsurgical-surgical **95**
- stackable treatment 12, 31

Bleomycin for keloidal and hypertrophic scars 49, *50*

Blepharoplasty
- fat grafting for 98
- laser skin resurfacing for **16**, *97*, **97**, 116, *117*–118, 130
- lower lid techniques in 97
- microfocused ultrasound for **16**
- neuromodulators for **14**, **98**
- nonsurgical **14**
- nonsurgical adjuncts during surgery for 95, **97**
- skin of color and *53*, **53**, *54*
- soft tissue fillers for **14**, **98**
- stackable treatment for **38**, **38**, *65*
- treatment plans and results 14
- trends in 97

Body/body areas
- aesthetic challenges of 104, 109
- assessing skin laxity in **107**
- basic approach of energy for **105**
- basic approach of pharmacology in **105**
- commentary on **109**
- cryolipolysis for **107**
- dyspigmentation for **109**, **109**
- gravity and 104
- inside-out techniques for 107–108
- laser treatment for 108, *108*, 109, *109*
- liposuction for 105, *106*, 107, *107*
- microfocused ultrasound for 108–109
- outside-in techniques for 107–108
- radiofrequency for 107, *107–108*, 109
- skin contour irregularities in **108**
- skin laxity in etiology and issues of **104**
- skin lifting on
- -- economic issues in **105**, 109
- -- nonsurgical-surgical blend for **104**
- -- selecting surgical and nonsurgical options for **105**
- soft tissue fillers for 105, 107, 109
- stackable treatment for general sequence for **37**

Boey G. E. 142

BoNT, *see* See Botulinum neuromodulator

Both Sides Of (Beck's photography project) 2

Botox (botulinum toxin type A) 2, 7, *168*, **168**
- *See also* See also Botulinum neuromodulator
- for frontalis muscle 14, **51**
- for glabellar complex 14
- for lateral orbital rhytids 14, *168*
- for neck rejuvenation 22
- for perioral rejuvenation 17
- for skin of color **51**

Botulinum neuromodulator (BoNT) 2, 6, **151**
- allergic reactions to 155
- antibody formation with 155
- as adjunct after surgery **101**
- as adjunct during surgery **97–98**, **100**
- as workhorse of injectable agents 6
- complications of 23, **154**
- contraindications to 7, 151
- contraindications to relative 151, **151**
- duration (longevity) of 32
- for blepharoplasty **14**, **98**
- for browlifting 14, **97**
- for frontalis muscle **14**
- for glabellar complex 14
- for lateral orbital rhytids 14, *15*
- for neck rejuvenation 22, **100**
- for perioral rejuvenation 17
- for skin of color *51*, **51**
- increasing use and patient demand 60
- indications for **151**
- patient selection for **7**
- pretreatment planning for 32
- serotypes of 7

Index

- stackable treatments with 12, 62, 64
Bovine collagen 7
Brassiere rolls cryolipolysis for 134, 138, 143, *143*, 145
BroadBand laser (BBL) 109, *109*, 176–177
Brow lift, *see* See Browplasty
Browplasty
- fat grafting for 96
- laser skin resurfacing for 16, *96*, **96**
- microfocused ultrasound for 9, 16, *17*, **96**
- microneedling for 97
- neuromodulators for 14, 97
- nonsurgical 14
- nonsurgical adjuncts during surgery for 95, **95**, *96*
- radiofrequency for 97
- skin of color and 53, **53**, *54*
- soft tissue fillers for 14, **96**
- treatment plans and results 14
Business plan 33
Buttocks cryolipolysis for *146–147*

C

Calcium gluconate as activator in PRP 70
Calcium hydroxylapatite (Radiesse) 7, 8
- for midface 20
- for perioral rejuvenation 17
- for skin of color 52
- in stackable treatment 63
-- longevity effects in 62
-- with monopolar radiofrequency 61
-- with ultrasound 61
Candida albicans 67
Canfield Imaging Systems 162
- Vectra 3D system 143, 162, *163–164*
- VISIA Complexion Analysis System 83, *84–85*, 89, *197*, **197**
Cardiac surgery parallels to aesthetic surgery 31
Casabona G. 61
Cellfina system anesthetic filtration device *185–186*
Cellulaze 108, 177, **177**
Cellulite 37, 104, 108, *108*, 147
Cheeks
- fat grafting for 98
- microneedling with PRP for 70
- suture lifts for **98**
Chemical browlift 14
Chemical peels
- as adjunct after surgery **101**
- as adjunct during surgery **99**
- deep 46, *48*
- for acne scarring 49
- for melasma 45–46, *47*
- for perioral rejuvenation **99**
- for postinflammatory hyperpigmentation 116
- medium 46, *48*
- priming with skin lightening agent before 47
- superficial 46, *48*
Chest
- depigmentation for 109
- male cryolipolysis for 134, 143
- photorejuvenation for 83, *86*
- re-pigmentation for 91, *92*
Chin

- cryolipolysis for 134
- microfocused ultrasound for 20, *22*, 100
Chromophores
- intense pulsed light and 81, 112, 153
- laser treatment and 112, 129
- light- and energy-based therapies and 75–76, 112, 114
- stackable treatments and 64
Classification of skin types 44, **44**
Clear + Brilliant fractionated diode laser 11
ClearScan YAG 178, **178**
Clostridium botulinum toxin 2, 6
- *See also* See also Botulinum neuromodulator
CO2 lasers 10, 78, *78*, 112, *114*, 152
- ActiveFX mode of 12, 16, 18, 61
- clinical results of 78, *79–80*
- complications with 116
- continuous wave (CW) mode 10
- cross-hatching with 114, *115*
- DeepFX mode of 12, 16, 18, 61
- DOT SmartXide 193, *194*
- for keloidal and hypertrophic scars 50
- for perioral rejuvenation 18
- for periorbital region 16, *16*
- for skin of color 50, *50*, 54, 79, *80*
- fractionated 12, *12–13*, **114**
- in stackable treatment
-- effect on filler longevity 62
-- with neuromodulators 62
-- with soft tissue fillers 61
- Lutronic eCO2 184, **184**, *185*
- nonfractionated 10
- penetration depth of 62
- postprocedure care with **116**
- use in conjunction with surgical procedure 81, *81*
Coherence of lasers 129
Collagen
- body treatments and 105
- deoxycholic acid and 128
- in skin of color 43–44
- in stackable treatment with monopolar radiofrequency 61
- principle of thermal disruption and 111
Collagen induction therapy 69
- *See also* See also Microneedling
Collimation of lasers 129
Combined treatments, *see* See Stackable treatment
Communication patient–practitioner 126
Compliance patient **93**
Complications 23
- *See also* See also specific procedures
- commentary on **157**
- cryolipolysis **145**
- deoxycholic acid (Kybella) 25, **155**, 159
- intense pulsed light 116, *119*, **157**
- key points on **150**
- laser skin resurfacing 25, **116**, **155**
- light- and energy-based therapies *93*, **116**
- microfocused ultrasound 25, 39, 121, **156**
- neuromodulator 23, 25, **154**
- nonsurgical-surgical blend **102**

- patient selection and 150, **150**
- preventing and managing **150**, **153**
- radiofrequency 39, **120**
- skin of color 42, 45, *45*
- soft tissue filler 24, 39, **153**
- stackable treatment **39**, **66**
Comprehensive contouring 134, 136, *137*, 139
Constantian M. B. 4–5
Contact dermatitis 25, 43, 155
Contour irregularities **108**, 134, *135*
Contour TRL 179, **179**
Contouring procedures (body) 105
- *See also* See also specific procedures
- abdominal stackable treatment for **38**, *41*
- comprehensive 134, 136, *137*, 139
CoolAdvantage 138, *139*, 140, 147
CoolCore 138, *139*, 142, 146
CoolCore Advantage 138
CoolCurve+ 138, *139*
CoolCurve+Advantage 138
CoolFit 138, *139*, 142, 145
CoolFit Advantage 138
CoolMax 138, *139*
CoolMini 136, 138, *139*, 140, *141–142*, 147
CoolSculpting 37–38, *40–41*, **128**, 132, **180**
- advantages to 128
- applicators for 136, *139*
-- cupped-plated 138, 147
-- flat-plated 136, 138
-- new development of 147
-- nonvacuum (nonsuction) 136, 138, *139*
-- placement of 140, *141*
-- vacuum 136, *139*, 140, *141*
- background of 132, 136
- business perspective on 134, 136
- clinician pager and monitoring in 140
- commentary on **148**
- common treatment areas 138
- complications of **145**
- contraindications to 136
- cost of 128
- cryodermadstringo in 136, *137*, 145
- debulking with 134, 136, *137*, 138
- disadvantages of 128
- duration of treatment 140
- efficacy of 143
- error message in 140
- FDA-approved uses of 134, 136
- for comprehensive contouring 134, 136, *137*, 139
- for contour irregularities after liposuction 134, *135*
- future of **147**, 159
- key points on **132**
- long-term effects of 132, *133*
- machine (system) for 136, **138**, **180**
- massage and 38, 132, 138, 142
- mechanism of action 132, 136
- multiple procedures performed with 134, *135*, 136, 140
- off-label uses of 128, 134, 143
- patient assessment and marking for 139
- patient experience/comfort in 140, *142*
- patient positioning for 140, *142*
- patient selection for **136**

- pillows for 140, *142*
- posttreatment care in **142**
- Pretreatment Skin Wipe for 140
- results of 143, **143**, *144–147*
- skin laxity and 136, 159
- technique for **136**
- thermal protection in 132, *133*, 140
- thickness of adipose tissue and 136
- Treatment to Transformation Protocol 145
CoolSmooth Pro 138, *139*, 142, 144
Corrugator supercilii muscles 14
Corticosteroids
- for hirsutism 49
- for keloidal and hypertrophic scars 49, *50*
- for melasma 46
Creative license 93
Crepiness of body skin 104, 108
Cross-hatching 8, *9*, 20, 114, *115*
Crow's-feet (lateral orbital rhytids)
- laser skin resurfacing for 16
- neuromodulators for 14, *15*, 168
- soft tissue fillers for 14
- stackable treatment for **38**, *38*, *40*
Cryodermadstringo 136, *137*, 145
Cryolipolysis **128**, 132, **180**
- advantages to 128
- applicators for 136, *139*
-- cupped-plated 138, 147
-- flat-plated 136, 138
-- new development of 147
-- nonvacuum (nonsuction) 136, 138, *139*
-- placement of 140, *141*
-- vacuum 136, *139*, 140, *141*
- background of 132, 136
- business perspective on 134, 136
- clinician pager and monitoring in 140
- commentary on **148**
- common treatment areas 138
- complications of **145**
- contraindications to 136
- cost of 128
- counterfeit non-FDA-approved systems of 145, *148*
- cryodermadstringo in 136, *137*, 145
- debulking with 134, 136, *137*, 138
- disadvantages of 128
- duration of treatment 140
- efficacy of 143
- error message in 140
- FDA-approved (CoolSculpting) 134, 136
- for comprehensive contouring 134, 136, *137*, 139
- for contour irregularities after liposuction 134, *135*
- future of **147**, 159
- in stackable treatment 36–37
- integration into practice 134
- key points on **132**
- long-term effects of 132, *133*
- machine (system) for 136, **138**, **180**
- massage and 38, 132, 138, 142
- mechanism of action 132, 136
- multiple procedures performed with 134, *135*, 136, 140
- off-label uses of 128, 134, 143
- on porcine tissue 132, *134*
- patient assessment and marking for 139

Index

- patient experience/comfort in 140, *142*
- patient positioning for 140, *142*
- patient selection for **136**
- pillows for 140, *142*
- posttreatment care in **142**
- Pretreatment Skin Wipe for 140
- results of *143*, **143**, *144–147*
- skin laxity and 136, 159
- technique for **136**
- thermal protection in 132, *133*, 140
- thickness of adipose tissue and 136
- Treatment to Transformation Protocol 145
Cryotherapy for keloidal and hypertrophic scars 49, *50*
Cupid's bow aging and 17
Cupped-plated applicators for cryolipolysis 138, 147
Cytolytic therapy 6
- *See also* See also Kybella (deoxycholic acid)

D

Daher Marcelo 26
Dalá Salvador 1, *1*, 5
Dayan S. H. 31
Debulking of adipose tissue 134, 136, *137*, 138
Decision-making
- on devices 130
- practitioner's 126
Deep chemical peels 46, *48*
DeepFX mode of CO2 laser 12, 16, 18, 61
Delayed healing syndrome 156
Deoxycholic acid (Kybella) 6, **9**, 108, **128**, **151**, *170*, **170**
- case studies of *171–172*
- complications of **25**, **155**, 159
- contraindications to 9
- contraindications to relative **152**
- efficacy of 159, *160*
- for neck rejuvenation **22**, *23–24*, *171–172*
- future considerations for 159
- indications for **152**
- injection technique for 22
- patient selection for **9**
- postprocedure care with 22
Depressor anguli oris (DAO) muscle 17, 24, 65
Depressor labii muscle 24
Depth of penetration by noninvasive devices 62, *62*
Dermabrasion
- for melasma 47
- for skin of color 42, 54, 57
Dermapen 161
Dermaroller for skin of color 51
Dermatosis papulosa nigra (DPN) 44, *45*
Dermis in skin of color 43–44
Diakonova Elena Dmitrievna (Gala) 1, *1*
Diode lasers 11
- ablative 11
- for hair removal 49
- nonablative 11, *11*
- penetration depth of 62
Direct-to-consumer advertising (DTCA) 127
Divine Proportions 2, *4*

DOT SmartXide CO2 laser **193**, *194*
DREAM procedure 161
DualSculpting 134, *135*
Dyschromia 42–44, *44*, 76
Dyspigmentation in body areas *109*, **109**
Dysport 7, **169**
- for frontalis muscle 14
- for glabellar complex 14
- for lateral orbital rhytids 14
- for neck rejuvenation 22
- for perioral rejuvenation 17
- for skin of color 51

E

Ectropion 25, 156
Eflornithine hydrochloride for hirsutism 49
EGF, *see* See Epidermal growth factor
Elastin
- body treatments and 105
- in skin of color 43
Embolization of soft tissue fillers 24, 153
Endothelial cells microneedling with PRP and 69
EndyMed PRO 51
Epidermal growth factor (EGF) 69
Equestrian cold panniculitis 132, 136
Erbium glass lasers 11, *11*, 61
Erbium laser penetration depth of *62*
Erbium:yttrium-aluminum-garnet (Er:YAG) lasers 10, 78, *78*, 112, *114*, 152
- complications with 116
- for melasma 47
- for midface 99
- fractionated 12, *12*
- in stackable treatment 61
- indications for 113
- nonfractionated 10
- postprocedure care with **116**
- technical steps for micropeel **114**
Erythema
- postinflammatory acne and 47
- prolonged 25, 72, 116
Ethnic skin, *see* See Skin of color
Exogenous ochronosis 46, *46*
Eyebrow ptosis neuromodulators and 23, 154
Eyelid ptosis neuromodulators and 23, 25, 154

F

Facelift nonsurgical **20**
- *See also* See also Facial rejuvenation
Facial aging
- etiology of 60, 74
- genetic component of 74
- lifestyle effects on 74
- perceived aesthetic appearance 74
- sequential imaging of 162, *163*
- younger skin versus older skin 74
Facial motor nerve microfocused ultrasound and 25
Facial rejuvenation, *see* See also specific techniques
- amniotic membrane for 161
- demand and use for 6
- in skin of color **54**, *56*
- – keloidal and hypertrophic scarring in 54

- – SMAS plication for 54, *56*
- laser skin resurfacing for 6, **10**, 78, *79*, 116, *117–118*
- lipolytic therapies for 6, **9**
- microfocused ultrasound for 6, **9**
- neuromodulators for 6, **6**
- nonsurgical **6**
- nonsurgical adjuncts after surgery for **101**
- nonsurgical adjuncts during surgery for **95**
- nonsurgical-surgical blend for **95**
- patient selection for 6
- sequential changes over time 162, *163–165*
- soft tissue fillers for 6, 7, **7**
- stackable treatment for **12**, **37**
- suture lift for **98**, 160, *161–162*, 163
- technologies for review of **6**
Famciclovir 63
Fanning 8, *9*, 20
Fat grafting **7**
- as adjunct after surgery 102
- as adjunct during surgery 96, **98**
- for acne scarring 116, *119*
- for blepharoplasty **98**, *98*
- for browlifting 96
- for hands 83, *87*
- for midface **98**, *98*
- for stackable treatment 36, 113
Fat reduction **127**
- *See also* See also specific techniques
- cryolipolysis for **128**, **132**, **180**
- debulking for 134, 136, *137*, 138
- deoxycholic acid (Kybella) for 6, 9, **9**, 108, **128**, **151**, 159, **170**
- liposuction for 105, *106*, 107, 127
- Smartlipo for **193**, *193*
FDA, *see* See Food and Drug Administration
Fibroblasts
- deoxycholic acid and 128
- in skin of color 43
- microneedling with PRP and 69
Financial (business) issues
- acquisition of novel technology **32**
- advertising **126**
- business model for aesthetic devices 130
- business plan 33
- cost of CoolSculpting 128
- cost of microfocused ultrasound 128
- cost of skin lifting on body **105**, 109
- cryolipolysis 134, 136
- role of industry **127**
Fitzpatrick Skin Type (FST) 44, **44**, 76, **77**
Flanks cryolipolysis for 128, *133*, 134, 136, 138, *143*, *144*
Flat-plated applicators for cryolipolysis **136**, 138
Focused ultrasound, *see* See Microfocused ultrasound
Follicular unit extraction (FUE) 129, *129*
Follicular unit transplantation (FUT) 129, *129*
Food and Drug Administration (FDA) 67, 127, 130
- on combining modalities 60, 67
- on cryolipolysis 128, 134, 136
- on deoxycholic acid (Kybella) 6, 9, 128, 151, 155

- on Dysport 7
- on Er:YAG laser 10
- on microfocused ultrasound 9, 96, 100, 121, 128
- on ReLume laser 90
- on Silhouette InstaLift 160
- on skin of color 51–52
- on skin tightening 100
- on soft tissue fillers 6, 8
Forearm re-pigmentation for 91, *92*
Forehead lines
- laser skin resurfacing for 16
- microneedling with PRP for 70
- neuromodulators for 14
- radiofrequency for 89, *89*
- soft tissue fillers for **14**
- stacked treatment for **38**, *38*
Fractional radiofrequency 120
Fractionated laser technology 10–11, 113
Fractionated laser(s)
- ablative 11, *12–13*, 78, *78*, 113, **114**, **116**, 152
- CO2 12, *12–13*, **114**, **116**
- nonablative 11, *11*, 78, *78*
- postprocedure care with **116**
Fraxel re:pair system 13
Freezing, *see* See Cryolipolysis
Frontalis muscle **14**
- neuromodulator complications of 14, *15*, 23
Fungal infections 150, *151*, 156
FUT, *see* See Follicular unit transplantation
Future considerations
- biocompatibility in 159
- key points on **159**
- modalities in **159**

G

Gala (Elena Dmitrievna Diakonova) 1, *1*
Gatherwright J. R. 163
Glabellar complex **14**
- laser skin resurfacing for 16
- neuromodulators for **14**
- soft tissue fillers for **14**
- stackable treatment for **38**, *38*, 40
Glycolic acid
- for acne 156
- for PIH 155
Glycolic acid peels
- for acne scarring 49
- for melasma 47
Golden Ratio 2, *4*
Granulomatous reactions to soft tissue fillers 154
Gravity and skin laxity in body 104
Growth factors in platelet-rich plasma 69, 73

H

Hair transplantation microfollicular **129**
- follicular unit extraction for 129, *129*
- follicular unit transplantation for 129, *129*
Halo hybrid fractional laser **18**, *19*, **181**, *181*
Hands
- photorejuvenation for 83, *87*

201

Index

- soft tissue filler for 83, *87*
Harmony and beauty 2, *4*
Hemoglobin as chromophore 75, 112, *114*, 129
Herpes simplex virus (HSV)
- injectable fillers and 150, *151*
- laser skin resurfacing and 25, 67, 155–156
- microneedling and 72
- prophylaxis against 39, 67, 72, 76, 155–156
- stackable treatment and 39
High-intensity focused ultrasound (HIFU) 111
Hip rolls cryolipolysis for 138
Hirsutism
- in skin of color *48*, **49**
- laser hair removal for *49*, *50*
HSV, *see* See Herpes simplex virus
Human papilloma virus (HPV) 150
Hyaluronic acid 2, 7, *7*
- See also See also specific products
- as adjunct after surgery 103
- Belotero *167*, **167**
- complications of 24, 154
- cross-linking of 8
- for nasojugal groove/tear trough 15
- for perioral rejuvenation 17
- for skin of color 30, 42, *52*, 56
- gel hardness of 8
- gel swelling of 8
- hydrophilic nature of 8
- imaging of sequential effects 162
- in stackable treatment 63
- -- longevity effects in 62
- -- with lasers 61–62, 113
- -- with monopolar radiofrequency 61
- -- with ultrasound 61
- JuvÃ©derm *169*, **169**
- properties and clinical performance of 8
- temperature tolerance of 62
- with microneedling 70
Hyaluronidase 7, 25, 154
Hybrid approach 32
Hybrid fractional laser (Halo) **18**, *19*, *181*, **181**
Hybrid practices 127, 130
Hydroquinone
- for acne scarring 49
- for hirsutism 49
- for melasma 46, *47*
- with laser skin resurfacing 54, 79, 155
- with light- and energy-based therapies 76
Hylaform for skin of color *52*
Hyperpigmentation, *see* See also specific types
- assessment for LAEBT 76
- in skin of color 44, *44*
- re-pigmentation and risk of 90
- underlying hypervascularity with 76, *79*
Hypertrophic scarring
- facelift and 54
- histology of 49
- in skin of color *45*, **49**
- keloid scars versus 49
- laser skin resurfacing and 25, 156
- light- and energy-based therapies and 76
- microneedling with PRP and 72

- nonsurgical treatment options for *49*, *50*
Hypervascularity
- and aging 74
- and hyperpigmentation 76, *79*
- and LAEBT 75–76
- and photorejuvenation 82, *82*, *87*
Hypopigmentation
- causes of 89, *90*
- laser skin resurfacing and 155
- postprocedure in skin of color 45
- re-pigmentation for 72, **89**
- treating role in practice 92

I

Ice-pick acne scars in skin of color *47*, *48*
Icon fractional laser *182*, **182**, *183*
IGF, *see* See Insulin-like growth factor
Imaging studies 162
- sequential changes over time 162, *163–166*
- Vectra 3D system 143, 162, *163–164*
- VISIA Complexion Analysis System 83, *84–85*, 89, *197*, **197**
Imiquimod for keloidal and hypertrophic scars 49
Industry role of 127
Infection, *see* See also specific types
- bacterial 25, 39, 67, 150, 153, 156
- fungal 150, *151*, 156
- laser skin resurfacing and 14, 25, 39, 63, 67, 76, 155–156
- patient education on 67
- soft tissue fillers and 150, *151*
Infection prevention 66
- antibiotic prophylaxis for 25, 63, 67, 75, 155
- antiviral prophylaxis for
- -- with laser skin resurfacing 14, 25, 39, 63, 67, 76, 155–156
- -- with light- and energy-based therapies 76
- -- with microneedling 72
- -- with stackable treatments 39, 67
- postprocedure 67
Informed consent for light- and energy-based therapies 76, 93
Infrared (IR) device in stackable treatment
- with neuromodulators 62
- with soft tissue fillers 62
Injectable bioactive agents 6
- See also See also Neuromodulators, See also Soft tissue fillers
Injection techniques for soft tissue fillers 8, *9*
Inside-out body lifting 107–108
Inside-out neck tightening 100, **100**
Instalift (Silhouette Instalift) 98, 160, *161–162*
Insulin-like growth factor (IGF) 69
Intense pulsed light (IPL) 11, **112–113**, *114*, **153**
- advantages of 153
- as adjunct to surgical procedures 83, *85*
- chromophores for 81, 112, 153
- clinical results of *83*, **83**, *84–88*
- complications of 116, *119*, *157*
- contraindications to **153**

- definition of area and blending for 82
- for acne *115*, **115**
- for body areas 109, *109*
- for chest 83, *86*, *109*
- for hands 83, *87*
- for neck region 83, *86*
- for periorbital region 87, *88*
- for photorejuvenation 81, 116, *118*
- for postinflammatory hyperpigmentation 116
- for rosacea 87, *87*
- for skin of color 82, 93, 157
- hypervascularity and 82, *82*, 87
- in stackable treatment
- -- with neuromodulators 62
- -- with soft tissue fillers 61
- -- with ultrasound and soft tissue fillers 61
- indications for 113, **153**
- laser versus 113
- pain management in 157
- patient selection for *113*, 157
- postprocedure care with 92
International normalized ratio (INR) 63
Internet
- advertising/marketing via 126
- globalization of facial aesthetic surgery via 126
Invasive therapy declining interest in 31
Ionizing radiation 74
IPL, *see* See Intense pulsed light
IR, *see* See Infrared (IR) device
Irritant contact dermatitis 25, 43, 155
Irritants and skin of color 43–44
Isotretinoin use before procedures 63, 75

J

Jacono A. A. 162
Jordan D. R. 66
Jowling soft tissue fillers for 20, *34*
JuvÃ©derm *169*, **169**
- for nasojugal groove/tear trough 15
- for skin of color *52*
JuvÃ©derm Volbella 8, 26, *170*
JuvÃ©derm Volift 8
JuvÃ©derm Voluma 7, *7*, 8
- as adjunct after surgery 103
- duration (longevity) of 36
- for midface 20, *21*
- for skin of color *52*
- for stackable treatment 38
JuvÃ©derm Voluma XC *170*
JuvÃ©derm XC 7, *7*, 8

K

Keloidal scars 43, 45
- difficulty in treating 49
- examining skin for 45
- facelift and 54, *56*
- histology of 49
- hypertrophic scars versus 49
- laser skin resurfacing and 76, 156
- light- and energy-based therapies and 76
- microneedling with PRP and 72
- nonsurgical treatment options for *49*, *50*

Kenkel J. M. 9, 121
Keratinocytes microneedling with PRP and 69
Knees cryolipolysis for 134, 138, 143
Kojic acid 46, 76
KTP laser, *see* See Potassium titanyl phosphate (KTP) laser
Kybella (deoxycholic acid) 6, **9**, 108, **128**, **151**, *170*, **170**
- case studies of *171–172*
- complications of **25**, **155**, 159
- contraindications to 9
- contraindications to relative **152**
- efficacy of 159, *160*
- for neck rejuvenation **22**, *23–24*, *171–172*
- future considerations for 159
- indications for **152**
- injection technique for 22
- patient selection for **9**
- postprocedure care with 22

L

LAEBT, *see* See Light- and energy-based therapies
Lambros Val 162
Laser hair removal 129
- in skin of color *49*, *50*
Laser skin resurfacing 6, **10**, 130, **152**
- ablative **10**, *78*, **78**, 152
- ancillary use of 75
- antibiotic prophylaxis for 25, 63, 67, 155
- antiviral prophylaxis with 14, 25, 39, 63, 67, 76, 155–156
- as adjunct after surgery **101**
- as adjunct during surgery **96–97**, **99–100**, 129
- body location and 76
- case examples of **116**
- chromophores for 75, *75*, 76
- classes of lasers for 10
- clinical results of **78**, *79–80*, 116
- combined with surgical procedure *81*, **81**
- combining modalities of **77**
- commentary on 124
- complications of **25**, **116**, **155**
- contraindications to 14, 63, 75
- contraindications to relative **152**
- delayed healing syndrome in 156
- expected short-term side effects of **156**
- for acne scarring **34**, *49*, **116**, *117*, *119*
- for blepharoplasty **16**, *97*, **97**, 116, *117*, 130
- for browlifting **16**, *96*, **96**
- for cellulite 108
- for keloidal and hypertrophic scars *49*, *50*
- for melasma 45, *47*, **47**
- for midface **99**
- for neck rejuvenation 100, **100**, *101*, 116, *118*
- for perioral rejuvenation *18*, **18**, *19*, *78*, *80*, *99*, **99**
- for periorbital region *16*, **16**
- for skin of color 50, **54**, *57*, *79*, *80*, 152
- in pregnant patients 75
- in stackable treatment 36

Index

-- complications of 66
-- effect on filler longevity 62
-- percentage of correction 37
-- same-day considerations for 63
-- with neuromodulators 62
-- with radiofrequency treatment 77
-- with soft tissue fillers 60–62, 113
-- with soft tissue fillers and ultrasound 61
- indications for 152, **152**
- informed consent and information for 76
- medications complicating 75, 76
- minimizing focus and recovery time in 78
- nonablative **152**
- nonsurgical incorporating **78**
- pain management for 114
- patient age and 76
- patient selection for **13**, 75, **113**
- penetration depth in 62, *62*
- postprocedure care with **16**, 39, 77, 102, **116**, 155
- pretreatment protocol for **77**
- recovery times in estimated 115, **115**
- relative absorption of light energy in 75, *112*
- safety of **75**
- scarring with 25, 76, 156
- skin analysis for **76**, 77
- stackable treatments with 12
- supplements adversely impacting 75, 76
- technical steps and treatment plan for **114**
- understanding technology of **77**
Laser(s) 10, **112**, **129**
- *See also* See also specific devices and procedures
- ablative **10**, *78*, 112
- ablative fractionated 11, *12–13*, 78, *78*, 113, **114**, **116**, 152
- ablative nonfractionated 10, *10*
- business model for 130
- chromophores for 112, *112*
- coherence of 129
- collimation of 129
- commonly used 112
- ideal pulse width versus vessel diameter *111*
- intense pulsed light versus 113
- maintenance of 93
- monochromaticity of 129
- nonablative *78*, 112, **116**, **152**
- nonablative fractionated 11, *11*, 78, *78*
- nonablative nonfractionated 11, *11*
- parameters for operating 111, **111**
- principle of thermal disruption and 111
- product index **176**
- properties of 129
- selection of device 112, *112*, 113, *114*
Lateral orbital rhytids
- laser skin resurfacing for 16
- neuromodulators for **14**, *15*, *168*
- soft tissue fillers for **14**
- stackable treatment for *38*, **38**, *40*
Levator labii superioris 17
Light- and energy-based therapies (LAEBT) **74**, 112

- *See also* See also Laser skin resurfacing, See also Photorejuvenation, See also Radiofrequency (RF)
- ablative *78*, **78**, 92
- ancillary use of 75
- antiviral prophylaxis for 76
- body location and 76
- case examples of **116**
- chromophores for 75, *75*, 76, 112, *112*, *114*
- clinical results of **78**, *79–80*, **116**
- combined with surgical procedure **81**, *81*
- combining modalities of **77**
- commentary on **93**, 124
- complications and shortcomings for **93**, **116**
- contraindications to 75
- creative license in **93**
- for photorejuvenation **81**, 92
- for re-pigmentation **89**
- for skin of color 79, *80*
- in pregnant patients 75
- informed consent and information for 76, 93
- keloid/hypertrophic scarring in 76
- maintenance of devices **93**
- medications complicating 75, 76
- minimizing focus and recovery time in 78
- nonablative **78**
- nonsurgical incorporating **78**
- operator experience with **93**
- patient age and 76
- patient compliance in **93**
- patient expectations for **93**
- patient selection for **75**, **113**
- postprocedure care with **77**, 92, **116**
- pretreatment protocol for **77**
- recovery times in estimated 115, **115**
- relative absorption of light energy in 75, *112*
- safety of **75**
- selection of device 112, *112*, 113, *114*
- skin analysis for **76**, 77
- supplements adversely impacting 75, 76
- technical steps and treatment plan for **114**
- understanding technology of **77**
Linear threading 8, *9*
- for nasojugal groove/tear trough 16
- for perioral rejuvenation 17
Lipolytic therapies 6, **9**
- *See also* See also Kybella
Liposuction 105, *106*, 107, 127
- abdominal *107*
- contour irregularities after 134, *135*
- radiofrequency-assisted *106*
- salvage 109
- Smartlipo **193**, *193*
Lips (perioral rejuvenation)
- chemical peels for **99**
- fat grafting for **99**
- laser skin resurfacing for *18*, **18**, *19*, 78, *80*, 99, **99**
- microneedling with PRP for 70
- neuromodulators for **17**
- nonsurgical adjuncts during surgery for **99**

- nonsurgical procedures for **17**
- radiofrequency for 89, *89*
- soft tissue fillers for **17**, *18–19*, 34, **99**
- stackable treatment for **38**, *39*, **65**
- treatment plans and results **17**
Longevity on nonsurgical approaches 32, 36
Lowe N. J. 162
Lowe P. 162
Lower face
- laser skin resurfacing for **18**
- microfocused ultrasound for 20
- microneedling with PRP for 70
- musculature of 17, *18*
- neuromodulators for **17**
- perioral rejuvenation in **17**
- radiofrequency for 89, *89*
- soft tissue fillers for **17**
- stackable treatment for **66**
- treatment plans and results **17**
Lumbar rolls cryolipolysis for 138
Lutronic eCO2 laser 184, **184**, 185

M

Macrophages microneedling with PRP and 69
Magnetic field generation 31
Maintenance device **93**
Malar augmentation **19**
- anatomic landmarks for 20, *20*
- soft tissue fillers for **19–20**, *21*
- treatment plans and results **19**
Malar fat pad 19
Malar prominence 19
Marginal mandibular nerve Kybella injections and 22
Marionette lines 17, *18*
- neuromodulators for 17
- soft tissue fillers for **34**
- stackable treatment for **38**, *39*
Market saturation 33
Marketing (advertising) **126**
- direct-to-consumer 127
- ideal blend in 127
- pull 126–127, *127*
- push 126, *127*
- strategies for 126, *127*
Massage
- and cryolipolysis 38, 132, 138, 142
- and soft tissue fillers 16, 66–67, 153–154
Mast cells in skin of color 43
MaxG fractional laser handpiece 183
MaxR fractional laser handpiece 183
MaxY fractional laser handpiece 183
Medical device companies 127
Medications and LAEBT 75, 76
Medium chemical peels 46, *48*
Meier J. D. 162
Melanin
- absorption of light energy 75, *112*
- as chromophore 75, 112, *112*, *114*, 129
- in skin of color 43–44, 51
- lack in hypopigmentation 89, *90*
Melanocytes in skin of color 43
Melanosomes in skin of color 43–44
Melasma 44, **45**, *46*
- risk of PIH with 45
- treatment options for 45, *47*

- triple combination topical therapy for 46, *47*
Mentalis muscle 17, 24, *65*
Mephisto appearance 14, *15*
Mequinol for melasma 46
Methicillin-resistant Staphylococcus aureus 63
MFUS, *see* See Microfocused ultrasound
Michalany N. 61
Michelangelo 2
Microchannels in microneedling 69, 72
Microdermabrasion
- for melasma **47**
- for skin of color 42
Microfocused ultrasound (MFUS) 6, **9**, **120**, **128**, **152**, **185**, *186–187*
- advantages of 128
- as adjunct after surgery **101**
- as adjunct during surgery **96**, **99–100**, 102
- BMI and 121
- business model for 130
- case example of **121**
- Cellfina anesthetic filtration device for *185–186*
- complications of **25**, 39, **121**, 156
- contraindications to **152**
- contraindications to relative 152
- cost of 128
- disadvantages of 128
- duration (longevity) of 32
- Few's experience with 31
- for body 108
- for browlifting 9, **16**, *17*, **96**
- for face **20**
- for lower face and chin 20
- for midface 20
- for neck rejuvenation 9, **20**, 26, 100, **100**, *118*, 121, *122–123*, 128, *128*
- for periorbital region **16**
- for skin of color 50, *51*
- in stackable treatment 36–37, 63–64
-- complications of 66
-- with IPL and soft tissue fillers 61
-- with soft tissue fillers 61–62, 67
- indications for **152**
- mechanism of action 152
- pain management in 121, 156
- patient selection for **9**, **121**, 152
- penetration depth of 62, *62*
- postprocedure care with **17**, 39, **121**
- results of **121**
- technical steps and treatment plan for **121**
- warnings on combining with other modalities 60
Microfollicular hair transplantation **129**
- follicular unit extraction for 129, *129*
- follicular unit transplantation for 129, *129*
Microneedling
- as adjunct after surgery **101**
- background on 69
- for acne scarring *49*, 69, 72
- for browlifting 97
- for melasma 47, *47*
- for neck rejuvenation 100, **100**
- for repigmenting skin 72
- for skin tightening in skin of color 50, *51*

Index

- future considerations in 161
- with platelet-rich plasma 69, 161
-- antiviral prophylaxis in 72
-- case examples of 71
-- commentary on 72
-- complications and shortcomings of 72
-- efficacy of 70
-- horizontal and vertical passes in 70
-- needle depth in 70, 72
-- patient preparation for 70
-- patient selection for 70
-- postprocedure care in 70, 72
-- results of 71, 71
-- technical steps and treatment plan for 70
-- treatment process for 70
-- versus microneedling with vitamin C 70

Micropeel Er:YAG laser for 114
Microthermal (microscopic) treatment zones (MTZs) 10, 113
Midface
- anatomic landmarks of 20, 20
- fat grafting for 98, 98
- laser skin resurfacing for 99
- microfocused ultrasound for 20
- microneedling with PRP for 70
- nonsurgical adjuncts during surgery for 95, 98
- nonsurgical augmentation of 19
- skin of color and procedures in 54
- soft tissue fillers for 15, 19, 20, 21, 98
- stackable treatment for 23, 38
- surgical options for 98
- suture lifts for 98
- treatment plans and results 19–20

Migration of soft tissue fillers 66
Minimally invasive devices 60
- See also See also specific devices
- decision-making on 130
- role of industry 127

Minimally invasive procedures 6
- See also See also specific procedures

Mirror images (symmetry) 2, 3
Molluscum contagiosum 150
Monochromaticity of lasers 129
Monopolar radiofrequency 88, 88, 120
- combined with soft tissue fillers 60

MRSA (methicillin-resistant Staphylococcus aureus) 63
MTZs, see See Microthermal (microscopic) treatment zones
Multipolar radiofrequency 120
Munavalli G. S. 143
Mycobacterium atypical 67
Myobloc 7

N

Nasojugal groove
- soft tissue fillers for 15, 16
- Tyndall effect in 16, 24

Nasolabial folds 17
- laser skin resurfacing for 18
- skin of color and procedures for 54
- soft tissue fillers for 17, 18, 34
- stackable treatment for 23, 38

Nd:YAG laser, see See Neodymium: yttrium-aluminum-garnet (Nd:YAG) laser
Neck aging stigmata of 20

Neck contouring, see See Neck rejuvenation
Neck lift, see See Neck rejuvenation
Neck rejuvenation 20
- inside-out 100, 100
- IPL (photorejuvenation) for 83, 86
- Kybella for 22, 23–24, 171–172
- laser skin resurfacing for 100, 100, 101, 116, 118
- microfocused ultrasound for 9, 20, 26, 100, 100, 116, 118, 121, 122–123, 128, 128
- neuromodulators for 22, 26, 100
- nonsurgical adjuncts during surgery for 99
- nonsurgical laxity reduction and lifting for 100
- off-label technologies for 100
- outside-in 100, 100
- platysmal bands in 22, 24, 26, 27, 100, 121
- radiofrequency for 100
- radiofrequency microneedling for 100, 100
- scarring risk in 100
- treatment plans and results 20

Necrosis soft tissue fillers and 23–24, 66
Neodymium:yttrium-aluminum-garnet (Nd:YAG) laser 11, 11, 114
- for acne scarring 49
- for hair removal 49
- for neck rejuvenation 100
- for vascular lesions 114
- in stackable treatment with soft tissue fillers 61
- indications for 113
- penetration depth of 62

NeoGraft 129
Nerve blocks 114
Neuromodulators 2, 6, 6, 151
- acquisition of novel technology 32
- advantages of 31
- as adjunct after surgery 101
- as adjunct during surgery 97–98, 100, 103
- complications of 23, 25, 154
- contraindications to 7
- duration (longevity) of 32
- for blepharoplasty 14, 98
- for browlifting 14, 97
- for frontalis muscle 14
- for glabellar complex 14
- for lateral orbital rhytids 14, 15
- for neck rejuvenation 22, 26, 100
- for perioral rejuvenation 17
- for periorbital region 14
- for skin of color 42, 51, 51
- increasing use and patient demand 60
- patient selection for 7
- postprocedure care with 39
- pretreatment planning for 32
- stackable treatments with 12, 62, 64
-- with lasers 62

Neutrophils microneedling with PRP and 69
Nodules soft tissue fillers and 66, 154
Nonablative laser skin resurfacing 10
Nonablative laser(s) 78, 112
- fractionated 11, 11, 78, 78
- indications for use 152
- nonfractionated 11, 11

- postprocedure care with 116
Nonablative radiofrequency 88
Nonfractionated lasers
- ablative 10, 10, 152
- nonablative 11, 11
Noninvasive devices 60
- See also See also specific devices
- decision-making on 130
- depth of penetration 62, 62
- role of industry 127
Noninvasive therapy 30
- See also See also Nonsurgical technology
Nonresponders
- options for 40
- rate of 40
- stackable treatment and reducing rate of 36, 40
Nonsurgical salvage procedures 111
- liposuction in 109
Nonsurgical technology, see See also specific procedures techniques
- 7/47 effect in 31
- acquisition of 32
-- basic considerations in 33
-- business plan and 33
-- market saturation versus 33
-- questions before investment 32
-- space considerations for 33
-- trial period for 33
- advantages of 31
- background of 30
- cervicofacial rejuvenation 6
- commentary on 130
- continuum of beauty and 33
- decision-making on 126, 130
- duration (longevity) of effects 32, 36
- efficacy and safety of 130
- FDA approval of 130
- Few's evolving experience with 30
- future considerations 159
- imaging studies and 162
- incorporation into practice 30, 126
- increasing use and patient demand 60, 95, 95, 111
- patient desires and 126, 130
- physician advertising of 126
- practical considerations on 31
- practitioner's decision-making on 126
- pretreatment planning for 32
- pros and cons versus surgery 31
- psychological and practical results of 31
- pushing limits in severe cases 130
- quiet revolution of 30
- sequential changes from over time 162, 163–165
- surgical perfection versus 30
Nonsurgical-surgical blend 121
- adjuncts after facial rejuvenation surgery 101
- adjuncts during facial rejuvenation surgery 95
- commentary on 102
- complications and shortcomings of 102
- enhancement procedures 111
- for blepharoplasty 95, 97
- for browlifting 95, 95, 96
- for facial rejuvenation 95
- for midface 95, 98
- for neck 99

- for perioral area 99
- for skin lifting on body 104
- goal for 95
- ideal candidates for 124
- LAEBT and surgery 81, 81
- photorejuvenation and surgery 83, 85
- postoperative care in 102
- salvage procedures 111
-- See also See also Nonsurgical salvage procedures
Nonvacuum applicators for cryolipolysis 136, 138, 139
Novel technology acquisition of 32

O

Ochronosis exogenous 46, 46
OnabotulinumtoxinA 168
- See also See also Botox
Oral commissure soft tissue fillers for 17
Orbicularis oculi muscle 14, 19
Orbicularis oris muscle 17
Original handpiece of Clear + Brilliant laser 11
Osteoblasts microneedling with PRP and 69
Outside-in body lifting 107–108
Outside-in neck tightening 100, 100

P

Package inserts/warnings on combining treatments 60, 67
Pain management 37, 114
- for intense pulsed light 157
- for microfocused ultrasound 121, 156
Panchaprateep R. 143
Park K. Y. 62
Patient compliance 93
Patient desires 126, 130
Patient expectations for light- and energy-based therapies 93
Patient selection 30
- and complications 150, 150
- for cryolipolysis 136
- for facial rejuvenation 6
- for intense pulsed light 113, 157
- for Kybella 9
- for laser skin resurfacing 13, 75, 113
- for light- and energy-based therapies 75, 113
- for microfocused ultrasound 9, 121, 152
- for microneedling with PRP 70
- for neuromodulators 7
- for radiofrequency 120
- for soft tissue fillers 8
- for stackable treatment 36, 63
Patient-practitioner communication 126
PCI (percutaneous collage induction) 69
- See also See also Microneedling
PDGF, see See Platelet-derived growth factor
PDL laser penetration depth of 62
Peau d'orange 17
Pellevé fractional laser 188, 188

204

Index

Penetration depth on noninvasive devices 62, *62*
Percutaneous collagen induction (PCI) 69
- *See also* See also Microneedling

Perioral rejuvenation
- chemical peels for **99**
- fat grafting for **99**
- laser skin resurfacing for *18*, **18**, *19*, *78*, *80*, *99*, **99**
- microneedling with PRP for 70
- neuromodulators for **17**
- nonsurgical **17**
- nonsurgical adjuncts during surgery for **99**
- radiofrequency for 89, *89*
- soft tissue fillers for **17**, *18–19*, *34*, **99**
- stackable treatment for **38**, *39*, *65*
- treatment plans and results **17**

Periorbital complications neuromodulator 23

Periorbital region, *see* See also specific anatomy and procedures, See also specific procedures
- laser skin resurfacing for *16*, **16**
- microfocused ultrasound for **16**
- microneedling with PRP for 70
- nonsurgical procedures for **14**
- photorejuvenation for 87
- skin of color and procedures in *53*, **53**, *54*
- soft tissue fillers for **14**
- stackable treatment for **38**, **38**, *40*
- treatment plans and results **14**

Peritrochanteric areas cryolipolysis for 138

Perlane *7*, *20*, *52*
- *See also* See also Restylane Lyft

PermeÃ¡ handpiece of Clear + Brilliant laser 11

Phi 2
Phidias 2
Phosphatidyl choline 9, 108

Photorejuvenation **81**, *116*, *118*
- as adjunct to surgical procedures 83, *85*
- clinical results of *83*, **83**, *84–88*
- definition of area and blending for 82
- for chest 83, *86*
- for hands 83, *87*
- for neck region 83, *86*
- for periorbital region 87
- for rosacea 87, *87*
- hypervascularity and *82*, *82*, 87
- in skin of color *82*, *93*
- neck treatment in 83
- postprocedure care in 92

PIE, *see* See Postinflammatory erythema
PIH, *see* See Postinflammatory hyperpigmentation

Pillows for cryolipolysis 140, *142*
Pimecrolimus for melasma 47
Platelet-derived growth factor (PDGF) 69, 73
Platelet-poor plasma 70
Platelet-rich plasma (PRP)
- animal studies of 69
- applications across fields 69
- definition of 69
- equivocal or deleterious effects of 69

- growth factors in 69, 73
- in vitro studies of 69
- microneedling with **69**, 161
- -- antiviral prophylaxis in 72
- -- case examples of **71**
- -- commentary on 72
- -- complications and shortcomings of 72
- -- efficacy of 70
- -- horizontal and vertical passes in 70
- -- needle depth in 70, 72
- -- patient preparation for **70**
- -- patient selection for **70**
- -- postprocedure care in 72
- -- results of *71*, **71**
- -- technical steps and treatment plan for **70**
- -- treatment process for **70**
- -- versus microneedling with vitamin C 70
- -- preparation of 69, **70**

Platysmal band myotomy 26, *27*
Platysmal band(s)
- microfocused ultrasound and 26, 121
- neuromodulators and 22, *24*, 26, 100

Polaris RF device 13, 89, *89–90*
Poly lactic co-glycolic acid (PLGA) sutures 160
Poly-L-lactic acid 8
- *See also* See also Sculptra
Polymethylmethacrylate, *see* See Bellafill
Polypodium leucotomos 155
Pomade acne 47
Porcine tissue cryolipolysis on 132, *134*

Postinflammatory erythema (PIE) acne and 47
Postinflammatory hyperpigmentation (PIH) 44
- acne and 47, *48*
- deep chemical peels and 46
- examining skin for 45
- hirsutism and *48*, 49
- intense pulsed light and 116, *119*
- laser skin resurfacing and 14, 25, 47, 54, 116, 152, 155
- melasma and risk of 45
- soft tissue fillers and 56
- treatment of 116

Postprocedure care
- with cryolipolysis **142**
- with Kybella 22
- with laser skin resurfacing **16**, 39, 77, 102, **116**, 155
- with light- and energy-based therapies **92**, **116**
- with microfocused ultrasound **17**, 39, **121**
- with microneedling with PRP 70, **72**
- with neuromodulator treatment 39
- with nonsurgical-surgical blend **102**
- with re-pigmentation 90
- with soft tissue fillers **16**, 39
- with stackable treatment **39**, **66**, 67
- written handout on 66

Potassium titanyl phosphate (KTP) laser 112–113, *114*
- indications for 113
- penetration depth of *62*

Pozner J. N. 103

Pregnancy light- and energy-based therapies in 75
Pressure therapy for keloidal scars 49
Pretreatment planning **32**
Pretreatment Skin Wipe for cryolipolysis 140
Product index
- fillers 167
- lasers 176
ProFractional-XC *189*, **189**
Proportion and beauty 2, *4*
PRP, *see* See Platelet-rich plasma
PRPen 161
Pseudofolliculitis barbae in skin of color *48*, 49
Pseudomonas aeruginosa 156
Ptosis
- assessment for stackable treatment 37
- eyebrow neuromodulators and 23, 154
- eyelid neuromodulators and 23, *25*, 154
Pull marketing 126–127, *127*
Push marketing 126, *127*
Pushing limits in severe cases 130

R

Radiesse (calcium hydroxylapatite) 7, 8
- for midface 20
- for perioral rejuvenation 17
- for skin of color 52
- in stackable treatment 63
- -- longevity effects in 62
- -- with monopolar radiofrequency 61
- -- with ultrasound 61
Radiofrequency (RF) 31, **116**
- as adjunct after surgery **101**
- background of 88
- bipolar 88, *88*, 120
- blind to skin color types 88
- clinical results of *89*, **89**, *90*
- complications of 39, **120**
- contraindications to 120
- facial recovery from 88
- for acne scarring 49
- for body 107, *107–108*
- for browlifting 97
- for forehead lines 89, *89*
- for keloidal and hypertrophic scars 50
- for neck rejuvenation 100, **100**
- for perioral rejuvenation 89, *89*
- for photorejuvenation 81
- for skin resurfacing 10, 13, *13*
- for skin tightening in skin of color 50, *51*
- fractional 120
- future considerations in 161
- goal of 88
- improvements in 89
- in stackable treatment 37, 63–64, 77
- -- with soft tissue filler 60
- maintenance of devices 93
- mechanism of action 88, *88*, 116
- monopolar 88, *88*, 120
- -- combined with soft tissue fillers 60
- multipolar 120
- nonablative **88**
- patient selection for **120**
- penetration depth of *62*
- Polaris device for 13, 89, *89–90*

- protective barriers with 88
- series of treatments with 88
- technical steps and treatment plan for **120**
- ThermiRF device for 161, *195*, **195**
- ThermiTight for **120**, *195*
- types of 120
- Venus devices for 37–38, *40–41*, *196*, **196**
Radiofrequency-assisted liposuction (RFAL) 106
Re-pigmentation 89
- clinical results of *91*, **91**, *92*
- for chest 91, *92*
- for forearm 91, *92*
- for retroauricular region 91, *91*
- microneedling for 72
- postprocedure care in 90
- risk of hyperpigmentation in 90
- role in practice 92
Regional nerve blocks 114
ReLume laser for re-pigmentation 90, *91–92*
Restylane 7, *7*, 8, *174*, **174**
- for nasojugal groove/tear trough 15, *16*
- for perioral rejuvenation 17, *18–19*, *34*
- for skin of color 30, *52*
Restylane Defyne 174
Restylane Lyft (Perlane) 7, *7*, 8, *52*, 175
- as adjunct after surgery 103
- for midface and malar augmentation 20
- for skin of color 52
Restylane Refyne 175
Restylane Silk 7, *7*, 8, *175*
- for glabellar complex crow's-feet and forehead lines 14
- for perioral rejuvenation 17–18
Retin-A postprocedure avoidance of 39
Retinoic acid
- for acne 156
- with laser skin resurfacing 54, 155
Retinol postprocedure avoidance of 39
Retroauricular region re-pigmentation in 91, *91*
RFAL, *see* See Radiofrequency-assisted liposuction
Rhinoplasty nonsurgical **22**
- skin of color and *53*, *55*
- soft tissue fillers for 22
- treatment plans and results **22**
Rhytid(s)
- body contouring irregularities 108
- lateral orbital
- -- laser skin resurfacing for 16
- -- neuromodulators for **14**, *15*, *168*
- -- soft tissue fillers for 14
- -- stackable treatment for **38**, *38*, *40*
- midface
- -- anatomy and 19
- -- soft tissue fillers for 19
- -- vertical perioral 17
- -- laser skin resurfacing for **18**
- -- neuromodulators for **17**
- -- soft tissue fillers for **17**
Rhytidectomy in skin of color 54
RimabotulinumtoxinB (Myobloc) 7
Rosacea photorejuvenation for 87, *87*
Ruby laser
- for hair removal 49

205

Index

- penetration depth of 62
Rucinol for melasma 47

S

Saltz R. 143
Salvage nonsurgical **111**
- liposuction for 109
Same-day stackable treatments 63
Sasaki G. H. 142–143
Scars, see See Hypertrophic scarring, See Keloidal scars
Scott Allen 6
SculpSure 108, 190, **190**
Sculptra 7, 8, 173, **173**
- case studies of 173
- for skin of color 52
- in stackable treatment 63
-- with monopolar radiofrequency 61
-- with ultrasound and lasers 61
- warnings on combining with other modalities 60
Seborrheic keratoses 45
Self-identity aesthetic surgery and 5
Sequencing of stackable treatment 36, **36**
- general for body 37
- general for face 37
Sequential changes imaging of 162, 163–166
Serial puncture 8, 9
- for nasojugal groove/tear trough 16
- for perioral rejuvenation 17
Sexual dimorphism 3
Silhouette Instalift 98, 160, 161–162
Silhouette Soft 160
Silicone gel sheeting for keloidal and hypertrophic scars 49, 50
Silicone liquid with monopolar radiofrequency 61
Skin aging
- etiology of 60, 74
- genetic component of 74
- lifestyle effects on 74
- perceived aesthetic appearance 74
- sequential imaging of 162, 163
- younger skin versus older skin 74
Skin assessment
- for light- and energy-based therapies 76
- for stackable treatment 37
Skin care **121**
Skin clarity and beauty 3
Skin excision procedures 107
Skin flaps microneedling with PRP and 70
Skin hygiene 74
Skin laxity 104, **104**
- See also See also specific procedures
- assessment of **107**
- cryolipolysis and 136, 159
- gravity and 104
- surgery for 113
Skin lifting on body
- aesthetic challenges in 104, 109
- assessing skin laxity for **107**
- basic approach of energy for **105**
- basic approach of pharmacology in **105**
- commentary on 109
- economic issues in **105**, 109
- inside-out techniques for 107–108
- laser treatment for 108, 108, 109

- microfocused ultrasound for 108–109
- nonsurgical-surgical blend for **104**
- outside-in techniques for 107–108
- radiofrequency for 107, **108**, 109
- skin lifting on **105**
- soft tissue fillers for 105, 109
Skin lightening agents
- for melasma 45, 47
- priming for chemical peel with 47
- with laser skin resurfacing 54, 79, 155
- with light- and energy-based therapies 76
Skin of color **42**
- acne in 47
- acne scarring in 47
-- ice-pick 47, 48
-- nonsurgical procedures for 47, 49
- adverse events/complications for 42, 45, **45**
- aesthetic consultation on **44**
- commentary on 52
- concept of beauty and 42
- dermis of 43–44
- dyschromia in 42–44, **44**
- facial rejuvenation in **54**, 56
-- keloidal and hypertrophic scarring in 54
-- SMAS plication for 54, 56
- hirsutism in 48, **49**
- hypertrophic scarring in 45, **49**, 54
- IPL (photorejuvenation) in 82, 93, 157
- irritant susceptibility/resistance in 43–44
- keloidal scars in 43, 45, **49**, 54
-- difficulty in treating 49
-- facelift and 56
-- nonsurgical treatment options for 49, 50
- key points on **42**
- laser hair removal in 49, 50
- laser skin resurfacing in 50, **54**, 57, 79, 152
- melanin in 43–44, 51
- melanocytes and melanosomes of 43–44
- melasma in 44, **45**, 46
-- risk of PIH with 45
-- treatment options for 45, 47
-- triple combination topical therapy for 46, 47
- microfocused ultrasound for 50, 51
- neuromodulators for 42, 51, **51**
- nonsurgical procedures for **45**, 54
- patient history on 45
- periorbital rejuvenation in 53, **53**, 54
- retaining ethnic identity in 52
- rhinoplasty (nonsurgical) in 53, 55
- skin tightening in **50**, 51
- soft tissue fillers for 30, 42, **51**, 52, **56**
- statistics on aesthetic surgery for persons with 42, **42**
- stratum corneum of 43–44
- structure and function of **43**
- sun protection/damage in 43, 51
- transepidermal water loss in 43
Skin tightening **127**
- See also See also Microfocused ultrasound, See also Radiofrequency (RF)

- cryodermadstringo and 136, 137, 145
- for neck **100**
- in skin of color **50**, 51
- in stackable treatment 64
- nonablative radiofrequency for 88
- principle of thermal disruption in 111
Skin types **42**, 76
- classification of 44, **44**
- Fitzpatrick 44, **44**, 76, 77
SkinPen 191, **191**, 192
Smartlipo 193, **193**
SmartXide CO2 laser 193, **194**
Smooth muscle cells microneedling with PRP and 69
Snap test for ectropion risk 156
Soft tissue deflation 113
Soft tissue fillers 6, **7**, **150**
- acquisition of novel technology 32
- advantages of 31
- as adjunct after surgery **102**, 103
- as adjunct during surgery **96**, **98**
- autologous 36–37
- biocompatibility of 159
- comparison of 7
- complications of 24, 39, **153**
-- early 153, **154**
-- late 154, **154**
- contraindications to 63
- contraindications to relative **151**
- currently available 7
- duration (longevity) of 36
- erroneous placement of 153
- FDA approval of 6
- Few's experience with 30
- for blepharoplasty **14**, **98**
- for body 105, 107
- for browlifting **14**, **96**
- for forehead lines **14**
- for glabellar complex **14**
- for hands 83, 87
- for lateral orbital rhytids **14**
- for midface and malar augmentation **15**, 19, **20**, **21**, **98**
-- anatomic landmarks for 20
- for nasojugal groove/tear trough **15**, 16
- for nonsurgical facelift **20**
- for periorbital region **14**
- for perioral rejuvenation **17**, 18–19, 34
- for periorbital region **14**
- for rhinoplasty **22**
- for skin of color 30, 42, **51**, **52**, **56**
- granulomatous reactions to 154
- ideal characteristics of 7
- in stackable treatment 36
-- complications of 66
-- longevity effects in 62
-- morphology effects in 64
-- percentage of correction 37
-- same-day considerations in 63
-- selection of substance 63
-- with IPL and ultrasound 61
-- with lasers 60–62, 113
-- with monopolar radiofrequency 60
-- with ultrasound 61–62, 67
- increasing use and patient demand 60
- indications for **151**
- infection and infection prevention with 150, 151
- injection techniques for 8, 9

- massage and 16, 66–67, 153–154
- migration of 66
- off-label uses of 150
- overcorrection with 153–154
- patient selection for **8**
- postprocedure care with **16**, 39
- product index **167**
- rapid-injection rapid-flow rates for 66
- stackable treatments with 12
- synthetic 7, **8**, 36–37
- temperature tolerance of 62
- Tyndall effect with 16, 24, 154
Solar lentignes 44, 45, 99, 101
Sommeling C. E. 70
Sophora-alpha for melasma 47
Spock-like appearance 14, **15**
St. John's wort postprocedure avoidance of 39, 75
Stab-and-stick method of hair transplantation 129, 129
Stackable treatment 12, 31
- blending considerations in **36**
- case examples of **38**, **64**, 65–66
- commentary on **67**
- commercial concern in 67
- complications and shortcomings of **39**, 66
- comprehensive care in 36
- concerns over filler and laser treatments 63
- filler selection for 63
- frequently used 37
- individualization of 37
- key points on **36**
- light- and energy-based therapies **77**, 113
- literature review of **60**
- package inserts/warning on 60, 67
- patient expectations for 36
- patient selection in **36**, 63
- percentages of correction in 37
- postprocedure care in **39**, **66**, 67
- practitioner hesitancies in 60
- preoperative considerations in 63
- ptosis assessment for 37
- reducing nonresponder rate with 36, 40
- regulatory issues in 67
- results of **38**, **64**
- same-day considerations in 63
- sequencing in 36, **36**
-- general for body 37
-- general for face 37
- skin assessment for 37
- skin tightening in 64
- technical steps in **37**, 63
- tips for **63**
- treatment plan for 37
- volume assessment for 37
Staphylococcal infection 63, 150, 156
Staphylococcus aureus 63
Stem cells microneedling with PRP and 69
Stevens W. Grant 134, 143
Stoica B. 66
Stratum corneum in skin of color 43–44
Streptococcal infections 150, 156
Striae 104, 108
Submental liposis 6, 9
- See also See also Kybella (deoxycholic acid)

206

Index

Suborbicularis orbital fat (SOOF) 19
Sun protection
 – for melasma 45
 – for skin of color 43, 51
 – in skin care 121
 – postprocedure 39
Superficial chemical peels 46, *48*
Superficial muscular aponeurotic system (SMAS) plication for skin of color 54, *56*
Supplements and LAEBT 75, *76*
Surgery
 – nonsurgical adjuncts after **101**
 – nonsurgical adjuncts during **95**
 – nonsurgical enhancement with **111**
 – nonsurgical salvage after 109, **111**
 – nonsurgical treatments blended with **95**
 –– *See also* See also Nonsurgical-surgical blend
Surgical perfection versus nonsurgical techniques 30
Suture lifts **98**, 160, *161–162*, 163
Swelling stackable treatments and 63–64, 66
Swift Arthur 2, *4*
Symmetry 2, *3*
Synthetic fillers *7*, **8**, 36–37

T

Tattoo ink as chromophore 129
Tattoo removal 129
TCPs, *see* See Thermal coagulation points
Tear trough soft tissue fillers for **15**
TEWL (transepidermal water loss) 43
TGF-α, *see* See Transforming growth factor-alpha
TGF-β, *see* See Transforming growth factor-beta
Thermal coagulation points (TCPs) 9, 120
Thermal disruption principle of 111
Thermal injury prevention in cryolipolysis 132, *133*, 140

ThermiRF device 161, *195*, **195**
ThermiTight **120**, *195*
Thighs cryolipolysis for 128, 134, 138, 143, *144–145*
Thread (suture) lifting **98**, 160, *161–162*, 163
Thulium laser *11*, 62
Tissue regeneration microneedling and 69
Titan infrared nonablative heating device *51*
Tobacco cessation postprocedure 39
Toxins (neurotoxins), *see* See Neuromodulators
Tram track scars 72
Tranexamic acid for melasma 47
Transepidermal water loss (TEWL) 43
Transforming growth factor-alpha (TGF-α) 69
Transforming growth factor-beta (TGF-β) 69
Tretinoin
 – for acne scarring *49*
 – for melasma 46, *47*
 – postprocedure avoidance of 39
Trial period of new technology 33
Triamcinolone acetonide for keloidal and hypertrophic scars *49*, *50*
Trichloroacetic acid for acne scarring *49*
Triple-combination topical therapy for melasma 46, *47*
Tyndall effect 16, 24, 154
Tyrosinase in skin of color 43

U

Ulthera, *see* See Microfocused ultrasound
UltraPulse Encore laser *12*
Ultrasonic energy therapy 128
 – *See also* See also Microfocused ultrasound
Ultrasound **120**
 – high-intensity focused 111

 – microfocused, *see* See Microfocused ultrasound
Upper face
 – laser skin resurfacing for **16**, *96*, **96**
 – microfocused ultrasound for **16**, 20, **96**
 – microneedling with PRP for 70
 – neuromodulators for **14**, **97**
 – nonsurgical adjuncts during surgery for **95**, **97**
 – nonsurgical procedures for **14**
 – radiofrequency for 89, *89*
 – skin of color and procedures in *53*, **53**, *54*
 – soft tissue fillers for **14**, **96**
 – stackable treatment for *38*, **38**
 – treatment plans and results **14**
UV-induced hyperpigmentation 44

V

Vacuum applicators for cryolipolysis 136, *139*, 140, *141*
Valacyclovir 63
Vascular absorption of light energy 75, 112, *112*
Vascular endothelial growth factor (VEGF) 69
Vascular lesions
 – Nd:YAG laser for **114**
 – pretreatment in stackable treatment 64
Vascular occlusion soft tissue fillers and 24, 153
Vectra 3D system 143, 162, *163–164*
VEGF, *see* See Vascular endothelial growth factor
Venus Freeze 37–38, *40–41*, 196
Venus Legacy 196
Venus RF devices 37–38, *40–41*, 196, **196**
Vermilion show
 – aging and 17
 – soft tissue fillers for 17
Vertical perioral rhytids 17

 – laser skin resurfacing for **18**
 – neuromodulators for **17**
 – soft tissue fillers for **17**
Vinegar soaks 66–67
VISIA Complexion Analysis System 83, *84–85*, 89, *197*, **197**
Vitamin C microneedling with 70
Vitamin E postprocedure avoidance of 39
Volift 8
Volume assessment for stackable treatment 37
Volume restoration 98
 – *See also* See also Fat grafting, See also Soft tissue fillers

W

Warfarin use before procedures 63, 75
Warnings on combining treatments 60, 67
Wasilenchuk J. L. 142
Water
 – absorption of light energy 75, *112*
 – as chromophore (laser target) 75, 78, 112, *112*, 114, 129

X

Xeomin 7
 – for frontalis muscle 14
 – for glabellar complex 14
 – for lateral orbital rhytids 14
 – for neck rejuvenation 22
 – for perioral rejuvenation 17
 – for skin of color *51*

Z

Zelickson B. D. 143, 145
Zimmer percussion 142
Zyderm 7
Zygomaticus major muscle 17, 19